Handbook of Hepatology

Handbook of Hepatology

Editor: Dinah Beck

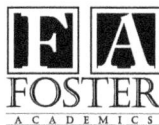

FA FOSTER ACADEMICS

www.fosteracademics.com

www.fosteracademics.com

FA FOSTER
ACADEMICS

Cataloging-in-Publication Data

Handbook of hepatology / edited by Dinah Beck.
    p. cm.
Includes bibliographical references and index.
ISBN 978-1-63242-681-9
1. Hepatology. 2. Gastroenterology. I. Beck, Dinah.
RC845 .H36 2019
616.362--dc23

Foster Academics,
118-35 Queens Blvd., Suite 400,
Forest Hills, NY 11375, USA

ISBN 978-1-63242-681-9 (Hardback)

Contents

Preface

Hepatology is a branch of medicine, which is aimed at the treatment and management of the disorders of the gallbladder, liver, biliary tree and pancreas for overall health. This domain is mostly involved in the study of the diseases and complications related to alcohol consumption and viral hepatitis. Some of the other diseases and medical conditions studied under this domain include storage disease of liver, gastrointestinal bleeding due to liver damage, jaundice, ascites, etc. Hepatitis B and C are the leading cause of liver cancers. In the modern world where alcohol consumption is gradually on the rise, the cases of incidence of cirrhosis and other conditions are also increasing. This makes research in hepatology very important. The various studies that are constantly contributing towards clinical advances and evolution of hepatology are examined in detail in this book. Also included herein is a detailed explanation of the various practices and procedures of hepatology. This book is a vital tool for all researching or studying hepatology as it gives incredible insights into emerging trends and concepts.

This book is a comprehensive compilation of works of different researchers from varied parts of the world. It includes valuable experiences of the researchers with the sole objective of providing the readers (learners) with a proper knowledge of the concerned field. This book will be beneficial in evoking inspiration and enhancing the knowledge of the interested readers.

In the end, I would like to extend my heartiest thanks to the authors who worked with great determination on their chapters. I also appreciate the publisher's support in the course of the book. I would also like to deeply acknowledge my family who stood by me as a source of inspiration during the project.

Editor

Early Experience of Helical Tomotherapy for Hepatobiliary Radiotherapy

Carole Massabeau,[1,2] Virginie Marchand,[1] Sofia Zefkili,[1] Vincent Servois,[3] François Campana,[1] and Philippe Giraud[1,4]

[1] Department of Radiation Oncology and Medical Physics, Institut Curie, 75005 Paris, France
[2] Department of Radiation Oncology, Institut Claudius Regaud, 31052 Toulouse, France
[3] Department of Radiology, Institut Curie, 75005 Paris, France
[4] Department of Radiation Oncology, European Georges Pompidou Hospital, 75015 Paris,
Paris Descartes University, 75005 Paris, France

Correspondence should be addressed to Carole Massabeau, cmassabeau@hotmail.com

Academic Editors: A. Irisawa, C. Karaca, and B. Mauro

Helical tomotherapy (HT), an image-guided, intensity-modulated, radiation therapy technique, allows for precise targeting while sparing normal tissues. We retrospectively assessed the feasibility and tolerance of the hepatobiliary HT in 9 patients. A total dose of 54 to 60 Gy was prescribed (1.8 or 2 Gy per fraction) with concurrent capecitabine for 7 patients. There were 1 hepatocarcinoma, 3 cholangiocarcinoma, 4 liver metastatic patients, and 1 pancreatic adenocarcinoma. All but one patient received previous therapies (chemotherapy, liver radiofrequency, and/or surgery). The median doses delivered to the normal liver and to the right kidney were 15.7 Gy and 4.4 Gy, respectively, below the recommended limits for all patients. Most of the treatment-related adverse events were transient and mild in severity. With a median followup of 12 months, no significant late toxicity was noted. Our results suggested that HT could be safely incorporated into the multidisciplinary treatment of hepatobiliary or pancreatic malignant disease.

1. Introduction

Majority of patients who develop either liver malignancy (metastasis or hepatobiliary primaries) have unresectable disease [1, 2]. Moreover, after first resection of liver lesions, recurrences are observed in two thirds of patients despite the use of systemic chemotherapy. In recent years, several new methods of nonsurgical ablation of liver malignancies have been tested, such as radiofrequency ablation, but also cryotherapy, laser hyperthermia, intra-arterial therapies, or ethanol injection, with variable success [3]. Until recently, radiotherapy of hepatic malignancies was playing a limited role due to the well-known limited radiotolerance of the liver [4, 5]. Recently, there is an increasing interest for modern radiotherapy as an attractive alternative, because it is noninvasive and not limited by anatomical issues associated with other therapies as the size, multiplicity and location of liver lesions [6]. New radiation techniques

including intensity modulated radiation therapy (IMRT), image-guided radiation therapy (IGRT), and stereotactic radiosurgery make it possible to deliver optimally high doses to the target volume with minimal effect on adjacent radiosensitive tissues.

Literature concerned with modelling liver tolerance indicate that high doses of radiation therapy can be delivered without significant toxicity, as long as a certain amount of normal liver is spared [7, 8]. The liver parenchyma is composed of numerous functional subunits that tolerate substantial focal injury prior to any clinical sequelae. Partial liver irradiation to high doses is, consequently, possible if adequate normal liver parenchyma can be spared [9]. The risk of RT-induced liver disease (RILD) is increasing with the preexisting liver disease and with dosimetric parameters among which the most important were identified to be the mean liver dose and the volume of liver receiving more than 30 Gy [10]. With the development of new technologies and

TABLE 1: Patient and disease characteristics.

Patient	Sex	Age	Performance Status (ECOG)	Primary tumour site	Previous therapies	Location/number/size of liver lesions
1	M	51	0	Rectum Ad.	Partial liver resection CT Pelvic RT RF	Hepatic dome 3 lesions (34; 10; 9 mm)
2	M	42	0	Cholangio	Biliary stent CT	Diffuse periductal infiltration Not measurable
3	F	73	2	Colon Ad.	CT Colon surgery	Posterior to the right portal branch 1 lesion (20 mm)
4	F	60	0	Pancreatic Ad.	CT Biliary Stent Partial liver resection	Pancreatic mass 1 lesion (40 mm)
5	F	72	0	Cholangio.	Extensive hepatobiliary surgery	Hilar region (no macroscopic disease)
6	M	64	1	Colon Ad.	Colon surgery CT	Perihilar metastasis 1 lesion (70 mm)
7	M	63	0	HepatoC.	Left hepatectomy Partial liver resections CT	Adjacent to the hepatic vein trunk (1 lesion-36 mm)
8	F	80	0	Colon Ad.	CT Partial liver resection RF	Hepatic dome 1 lesion (10 mm)
9	F	48	1	Cholangio	No[a]	Hilar infiltration (20 mm)

Abbreviations: HT: helical tomotherapy; M: male; F: female; Ad: adenocarcinoma; Cholangio: cholangiocarcinoma; HepatoC: hepatocarcinoma; CT: chemotherapy; RT: radiation therapy; RF: radiofrequency ablation [a]The patient 9 underwent an abdominal irradiation for Hodgkin lymphoma thirty years ago.

techniques, we are able to focus the radiation more precisely on the lesion to provide a higher dose to the tumor [11, 12]. Helical tomotherapy (HT), an image-guided, intensity-modulated radiotherapy system, can allow for simultaneous and precise targeting of multiple lesions, while sparing normal tissues [13]. The objective of the current study was to review our initial experience using HT for irradiation of hepatobiliary malignant disease.

2. Cases Presentation

2.1. Patients and Treatment. Between May 2008 and July 2010, 9 patients who underwent a course of HT (Hi-Art system, TomoTherapy, Madison, wis, USA) in the Radiation Department of the Institut Curie for malignant hepatic lesions entered in our study. The baseline characteristics of the nine enrolled patients as well as the treatment details are listed in Table 1. A total of 7 patients received chemotherapy prior to irradiation, 5 underwent previous hepatic surgery, and 2 underwent previous radiofrequency ablation. Patient 7 was a 63-year-old man whose hepatitis

B-related hepatocarcinoma (Child-Pugh class A disease) was initially treated with a left lobectomy. When a multifocal recurrence occurred, both chemotherapy and two segmental liver resections were performed, leading to one year of clinical remission before another local recurrence, presented as a single 3.6 cm lesion. Since the location of this lesion (directly adjacent to the median hepatic vein) precluded surgical management and RF ablation, patient 7 was referred for the HT. Two of the 3 cholangiocarcinoma patients were treated in a curative intent in a neoadjuvant setting according to the Mayo Clinic protocol. This is a protocol combining neoadjuvant concurrent chemoradiotherapy with capecitabine and cadaver donor liver transplantation for patients with operatively confirmed stage I and II hilar cholangiocarcinoma. Concurrent capecitabine which could be used as an irradiation sensitizer, was started on the first day of irradiation, half in the morning and half in the evening, for the duration of the radiation therapy [14]. All patients provided written informed consent before HT started. HT was performed to deliver the prescribed dose in 27 or 30 daily fractions, 5 days a week. Before each treatment,

TABLE 2: Dosimetric constraints for each organ at risk: recommended dose-volume limits from Quantec [15] and French guidelines [16].

Normal liver	Median dose <28 Gy (in 2-Gy fractions)
	V30 < 50%[a]
Right kidney	Maximum dose of 20 Gy to the total kidney
	Mean dose < 18 Gy[a]
Right lung	V20 < 20%[a]
Spinal cord	Maximum dose of 45 Gy

[a]Vx: Percentage of the organ at risk receiving more than x dose.

a megavoltage CT scan in the HT Hi-Art system was made to adjust table position and to verify the position of the tumor and vital organs.

2.2. Tomotherapy Planning. Patients were immobilized for initial simulation and for treatment with the two arms above the head in a body frame. Simulation was performed in a large bore computed tomography (CT) (Aquilion LB, Toshiba medical, Puteau, France SA) of 90 cm aperture. Images were acquired with 3-mm slice thickness from the mid-neck to the pelvis. Intravenous contrast was used to facilitate the appreciation of the tumour volume. Planning images are obtained by a four-dimensional CT (4D-CT) to assess respiratory motion. Regular breathing can lead to organ motions up to several centimeters which are taken into account by adding a specific margin around the target volume. The CT data was transferred to a linac-based planning system (Eclipse 3D version 8.1; Varian Medical Systems Inc., Palo Alto, USA) for delineating target volume and organs at risk (OAR). The gross tumour volume (GTV) was contoured manually corresponding to the tumour volume seen in the CT scan and in the co registered MRI images [17]. No specific size limit was placed on the tumor diameter. A margin of 1 cm to account for microscopic disease extension was added to the GTV to define the clinical target volume (CTV). An additional safety margin for liver movement caused by breathing and other nonspecific setup error was placed around the CTV to define the final planning target volume PTV (PTV) [18, 19]. For the OAR, the entire liver, the kidneys, the spinal cord, and the lungs were outlined. The normal liver was defined as the total liver minus the GTV. The CT images and accompanying contours were exported to the HT planning system (HiART Version 2, Tomotherapy Inc., Madison USA) for planning. According to the International Commission on Radiation Units and Measurements reports [20], the dosimetric planning objectives consisted of achieving full uniform dose coverage of the target, while keeping the dose to critical structures below their tolerance. The PTV must receive between 95% and 107% of the prescribed dose. For organs at risk (OAR), the dosimetric constraints have been set based on previously published toxicity data reviewed in the QUANTEC recommendations [21]. For partial liver irradiation, the median normal liver dose must be under 28 Gy (in 2-Gy fractions) for primary liver cancer and under 32 Gy (in 2-Gy fractions) for liver metastases. The French

guidelines recommended to give less than 26 Gy in the total liver and to restrict to 50% the volume of normal liver receiving 30 Gy or more [16]. The total kidney must receive less than 20 Gy and the mean kidney dose must stay below 18 Gy; the maximum dose to the spinal cord was 45 Gy, and the percentage of the right lung receiving 20 Gy or more, must be limited to 20% (Table 2).

2.3. Dosimetric Results. The dosimetric results are listed in Table 3. The doses to the target volumes always met their prescription constraint. The median liver V30 was 12% (6–37.2), well below the 50% recommended limit, while the median liver dose was 15.7 Gy (9.7–25.9) (recommended limit: 28 Gy). The median dose delivered to the right kidney was 4.4 Gy (1.5–9.7) and remained less than the recommended constraint of 18 Gy. The same observation can be made for the lungs, the left kidney, and the spinal cord) (data not shown). The distributions of isodoses for the patient 8 and 9 are shown in Figures 1 and 2.

2.4. Acute and Late Toxicities. Toxicities were assessed using the Radiation Therapy Oncology Group/National Cancer Institute Common Toxicity Criteria, version 3 morbidity scale [15], every week during the HT course to address side effects and monitor laboratory values. All but one patient completed the prescribed treatment. One of the two cholangiocarcinoma patient prematurely stopped HT for recurrent cholangitis on day 3rd of the radiation treatment, effectively treated with antibiotics, stent revision and surgery. As shown in Table 4, only minor toxicities developed during treatment. Most of the treatment-related adverse events were transient and mild in severity, with no case of direct treatment-related death. The hematologic and hepatic disorders occurred 1-2 weeks after the start of treatment and regressed spontaneously without interfering with the scheduled delivery of HT. We reported 1 thrombopenia grade 2 leading to 5 days of capecitabine interruption. The thrombopenia was most likely to be related to the capecitabine than the HT.

One patient experienced cytolysis grade 2, ten weeks after the HT course. A persistent thrombopenia grade 2 and cholestasis grade 1 (more than 4 months) occurred in one patient with progressive disease confirmed 4 months after the end of the radiation treatment. No radiation-induced liver disease was reported during the months following the HT.

2.5. Disease Outcome. After completing chemoradiotherapy, follow up was performed at 1–3 month intervals thereafter. The tumor response was assessed with follow-up CT scans. At study analysis, all but one patient, who died from progressive disease, were still alive. The median duration of followup after the HT course was 12 months (4–32). The cholangiocarcinoma patient treated in a neoadjuvant setting underwent successful cadaveric liver transplant 3 months after chemoradiotherapy with a complete histological response and remains disease-free 2 years later as the cholangiocarcinoma patient treated in an adjuvant setting. The pancreatic adenocarcinoma patient remains disease-free

TABLE 3: Treatment characteristics and dosimetric results.

Patients	Radiation dose per fraction (/F)	Concurrent capecitabine (mg·m²·day)	Median dose to the PTV[a]	PTV[a] volume (cc)	Normal liver Volume[b] (cc)	Normal liver V30[c] (%)	Median normal liver dose (Gy)	Median right kidney dose (Gy)
1	54 Gy 2 Gy/F	no	56.6	417.7	1244	8	25.5	1.7
2	54 Gy 2 Gy/F	1500	57.2	381	1726.2	37	25.9	5.3
3	60 Gy 2 Gy/F	1500	61	268	1424,3	12	12.1	1.5
4[d]	54 Gy 60 Gy 2 Gy/F	1500	55.5[e] 61.6[f]	671.9 143.5	1653.9	7,5	13.2	9.7
5	54 Gy 1.8 Gy/F	1600	54.1	174.6	892.9	17.5	15.7	4.4
6	54 Gy 1.8 Gy/F	no	54	262.6	857	30	22.1	2.1
7	60 Gy 2 Gy/F	no	61.1	121	1160.1	10	14.3	1.6
8	54 Gy 2 Gy/F	1500	54	93.9	1272.3	6	9.7	4.5
9[d]	54 Gy 60 Gy 2 Gy/F	1500	54[e] 59.8[f]	275.9 221.7	1484.1	37.2	25.6	4.5

[a]PTV: planning target volume; [b]Normal liver volume: liver volume minus PTV; [c]V30: percentage of the normal liver receiving 30 Gy or more; [d]For patient 4 and patient 9, two levels of dose were prescribed: 54 Gy to the PTV 1 (gross tumour volume (GTV) + 2 cm margin) and 60 Gy to the PTV2 (GTV + 1 cm margin); [e]Median dose to the PTV1; [f]Median dose to the PTV.

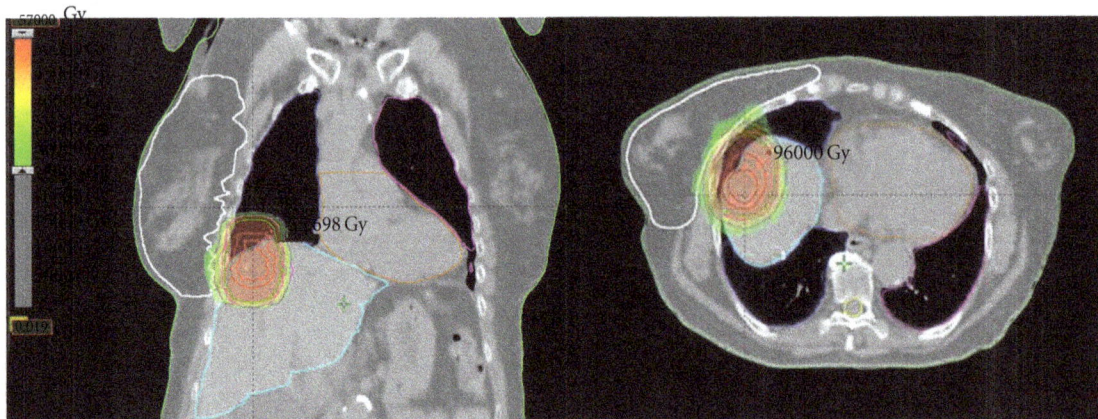

FIGURE 1: Distribution of isodoses with HT treatment planning in the patient 8 (hepatic dome metastasis) in axial and frontal representation. The different doses as well as the target volumes/organs at risk are represented with different colors. Red color represents the target volume dose (>54 Gy). Green color represents lower radiation doses of 30 Gy.

during 10 months then bone metastasis and local progression occurred. The hepatocellular carcinoma patient attained complete clinical remission after the helical Tomotherapy. Two years later, however, this patient experienced lung metastasis and local hepatic progression. Only one in-field progression (progression of disease inside the targeted tumor volume) occurred in the melanoma metastatic patient (patient 1), who died from his progressive disease, while the 2 colorectal metastatic patients developed exclusively out-of-field (patient 8) and distant progression without local relapse (patient 9).

3. Discussion

3.1. General and Technical Issue. Radiation oncology has seen the development of new technology which offers significant improvements in local control and reductions in toxicity. Increased doses >50 Gy with non-3D techniques improved tumor control marginally but were associated with a relatively high incidence of liver and gastrointestinal toxicity [10, 22]. Recently, the modulated intensity radiotherapy has allowed local radiation to the liver to be performed safely and have yielded promising results for dose escalation [23].

(a)

(b)

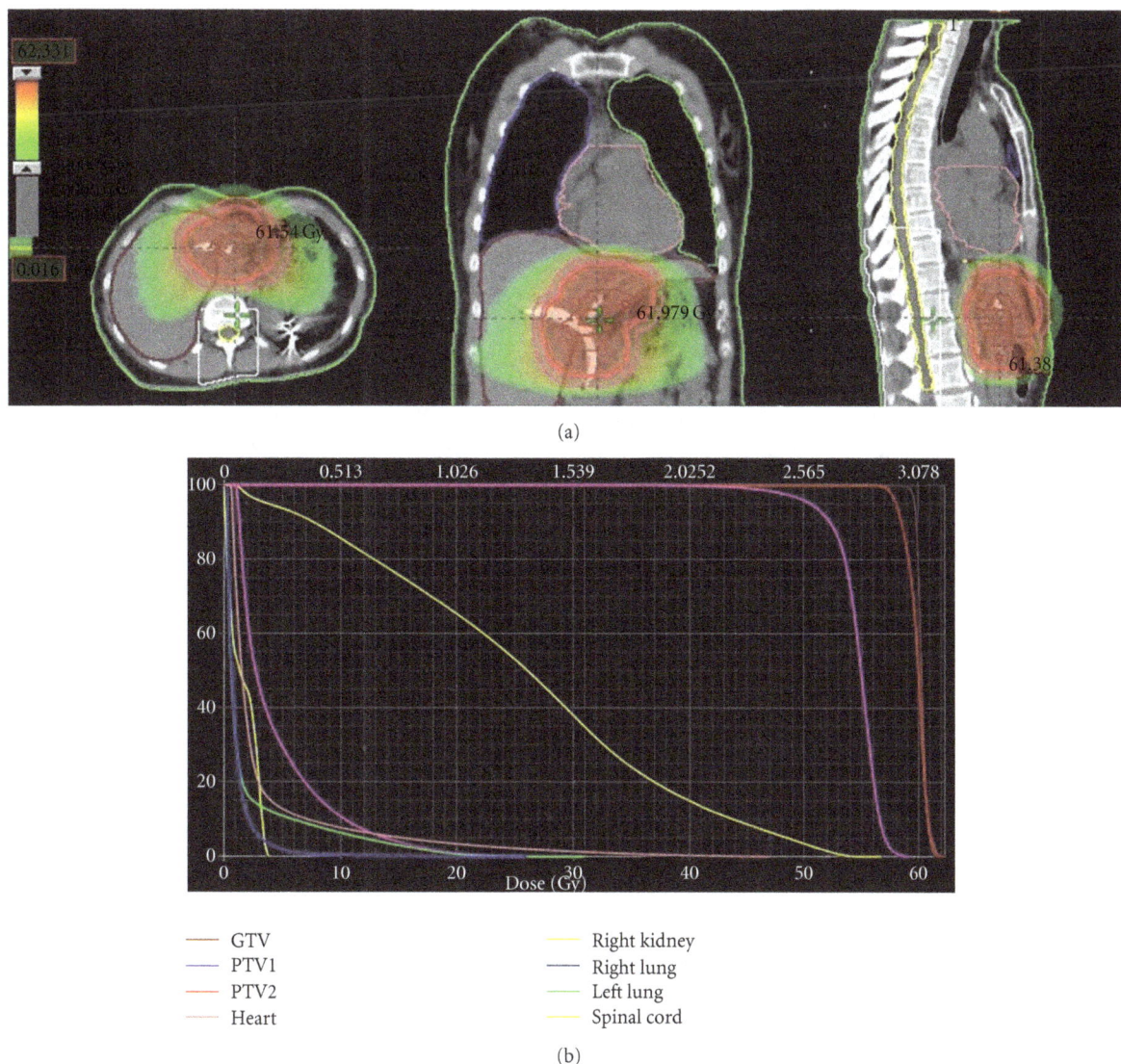

FIGURE 2: Distribution of isodoses with HT treatment planning in the patient 9 (cholangiocarcinoma) and the corresponding dose-volume histogram. The different doses as well as the target volumes/organs at risk are represented with different colors. Red color represents the target volume dose (>54 Gy). Green color represents lower radiation doses of 30 Gy.

TABLE 4: Acute clinical and biological adverse events: maximum toxicity grade per patient (Radiation Therapy Oncology Group/National Cancer Institute Common Toxicity Criteria, version 3) [15].

Patient	Nausea	Pain	Diarrhea	Fatigue	Thrombopenia	Cytolysis	Cholestasis
Patient 1	0	0	0	0	1	1	1
Patient 2	0	0	0	1	2	0	1
Patient 3	0	0	0	1	0	0	1
Patient 4	0	0	0	0	0	0	0
Patient 5	1	0	0	1	0	0	0
Patient 6	0	0	0	0	0	0	0
Patient 7	0	0	0	0	1	0	0
Patient 8	0	0	0	1	1	0	0
Patient 9[a]	1[a]	1[a]	0	1[a]	0	1[a]	4[a]

[a]Symptoms were not related to the HT but most likely to biliary stent obstruction with cholangitis, which is a major concern in cholangiocarcinoma patients.

We report here our early experience of the use of the modulated intensity with HT for irradiation of hepatobiliary malignant disease in 9 patients with several clinical settings. The HT was not limited by the tumour size, the tumour location, the multiplicity of lesions as well as a previous history of abdomen irradiation or a preexistant liver disease. Helical tomotherapy, a new type of RT, combines megavoltage computed tomography (CT) imaging with an intensity-modulated RT system. Such a combination allows for the delivery of precise RT to the tumor area while sparing normal tissues. In addition, this system can perform simultaneous RT of multiple lesions during the course of rotational fan beam RT delivery. This device is an ideal tool for delivering multifocal and high-dose radiation treatment and allows the irradiation at different dose levels in a single treatment session. With regard to radiation toxicity, in our study, treatment was feasible, safe, and very well tolerated with only mild and transient clinical or biological adverse effects. No patient developed the clinical syndrome of radiation-induced liver disease (RILD). This syndrome is known to be related to the volume of normal liver receiving more than 30 Gy [15]. By incorporating the analysis of the histogram dose volume in the treatment planning process, algorithms could allow us to better adjust the prescribed dose and regimens [24]. Data from our study indicate that the HT planning achieved to give a highly conformal treatment plan sparing as much normal liver as possible and respecting the recommended dose-volume limits, making it possible to deliver a radiation dose of 54 Gy or more, in a standard regimen (2 Gy per fraction).

3.2. HT for Liver Malignancies. Hepatocellular carcinoma (HCC) is one of the most common malignant diseases worldwide. Only 10% to 15% of patients are candidates for curative surgery because of the size of the tumour, disease multifocality, early vascular invasion, decompensated liver disease, or poor performance status [25]. Some alternative treatments, such as percutaneous ethanol injection, radiofrequency ablation, and transcatheter arterial chemoembolization, tend to be more effective in small tumours (from <2 cm to 4 cm in greatest dimension) but have some contraindications as they are invasive techniques. No standard treatment has been established in locally advanced HCC [26]. External beam irradiation therapy for HCC has been used infrequently because of the limited tolerance of the entire liver [6, 22, 27]. Case series data published by Dawson et al. [28] have shown median survivals of 11 to 15 months with the use of radiation in unresectable hepatobiliary cancer, which compares favorably with other modalities. Three-dimensional conformal and more recently IMRT has come to be recognized as a potentially option for advanced HCC, since it may enable the safe escalation of the dose to the tumor [28–31]. McIntosh et al. [32] reported initial experience with IMRT (50 Gy in 20 fractions) plus capecitabine for patients who had large HCC lesions, with acceptable toxicity and promising local control. Besides, another approach, the stereotactic body radiation therapy (SBRT) consisted of the delivery of a high tumor dose with an extreme precision in only few fractions

of very high dose (10 or 20 Gy per fraction). This represents a promising noninvasive treatment for unresectable small HCC previously successfully tested in liver metastasis [33–37].

Until recently, modern radiation therapies were studied for *liver metastatic* patients by the way of symptom palliation [25]. The liver metastases derived most often from colorectal cancer, whose prognosis has really changed in recent years, suggests the need for an effective local treatment. The resectability rate is reported to be only 25%. The recent spread of interstitial therapies and radiofrequency has further increased the possibilities of liver metastasis treatment [3, 38, 39]. The stereotactic body radiation therapy (SBRT) has been shown to be an effective, well-tolerated treatment but the tumor size might be a limiting factor. Baisden et al. [24] proposed a model based on the planning target volume (PTV) and liver volume to predict the maximum tolerable dose (MTD) delivered to a lesion by HT-based SBRT. Exactly how high the dose should be for each treatment, how many fractions in total are optimal, and how much time should pass between treatments are still to be resolved. For metastatic liver patients with an acceptable performance status, without active systemic disease, we argue that a standard regimen (2 Gy per fraction, during 6 weeks) of the well-tolerated HT could be as interesting alternative in particular for the large and/or multiple lesions.

Intrahepatic cholangiocarcinoma (ICC) is a rare hepatic malignancy that for the 30% patients with unresectable disease is uniformly fatal [40]. Systemic chemotherapy has been disappointing in regard to its efficacy, with most regimens resulting in a median survival of 6 to 12 months [41]. There has been great interest in other modalities of treatment, particularly intra-arterial therapies, and conformal radiotherapy, such as IMRT [42–44]. Baisden et al. reported the feasibility and acceptable tolerance of photodynamic therapy and concurrent chemoradiotherapy with HT (50 Gy in 25 fractions) in 10 unresectable hilar cholangiocarcinoma [45]. The most promising results have been achieved with combinations of these techniques, with the use of neoadjuvant chemoradiotherapy prior to orthotopic liver transplantation at the Mayo Clinic [46]. This approach has provided improved histological response as well as a better outcome with a 5-year survival rate higher by 20% to 40%. The use of HT in a neoadjuvant strategy before liver transplantation might increase the tolerance of the chemoradiation course avoiding an excessive adverse event which could interfere with the liver transplantation [47].

3.3. HT for Pancreatic Malignancies. The use of HT for *pancreatic adenocarcinoma*, whose prognosis and local control remains a challenging issue for oncologists, has been recently introduced [48]. Indeed, Ji et al. published the early results of a feasibility study as well as the early clinical outcome of concurrent administration of capecitabine with HT in 19 patients with advanced pancreatic cancer [49]. Another basis for offering radiotherapy to patients with pancreatic cancer is palliation of symptoms due to local invasion such as biliary and gastrointestinal obstruction. Because of its ability to restrict the dose to normal organs and minimize radiation toxicities, HT may be an ideal palliative option for challenging cases of pancreatic cancer.

3.4. Therapeutic Combinations. The use of high-precision external beam radiotherapy can be complementary or an alternative to other treatments. For example, radiation may be offered to patients with large tumors that exceed the size that can be treated by radiofrequency ablation or surgical resection. The shrinkage of these lesions could enable other local treatment. Moreover, a lesion that is treated by chemoembolization may be found to have an alternate vascular supply that cannot be occluded. Radiation can play a complementary role in these cases and be added to this modality. One study demonstrated that in HCC patients who had failed transarterial chemoembolization, local radiation induced an additional tumor response [50]. The collaboration of surgeons, medical oncologists, radiation oncologists, gastroenterologists, radiologists, and pathologists might offer better therapeutic indexes for challenging cases in a multidisciplinary approach.

4. Conclusion

We reported, here, our preliminary experience of the use of HT in various hepatobiliary malignant diseases as a way of understanding the perspectives offered by such a modern radiotherapeutic technique. Further investigations like comparative planning studies and longer followups are needed to confirm the dosimetric and clinical benefits offered by the HT over standard techniques or other new technique such dynamic arc therapy.

References

[1] J. M. Llovet, A. Burroughs, and J. Bruix, "Hepatocellular carcinoma: review," *The Lancet*, vol. 362, no. 9399, pp. 1907–1917, 2003.

[2] B. Nordlinger and P. Rougier, "Liver metastases from colorectal cancer: the turning point," *Journal of Clinical Oncology*, vol. 20, no. 6, pp. 1442–1445, 2002.

[3] B. Nordlinger and P. Rougier, "Nonsurgical methods for liver metastases including cryotherapy, radiofrequency ablation, and infusional treatment: what' s new in 2001?" *Current Opinion in Oncology*, vol. 14, no. 4, pp. 420–423, 2002.

[4] B. Emami, J. Lyman, A. Brown et al., "Tolerance of normal tissue to therapeutic irradiation," *International Journal of Radiation Oncology Biology Physics*, vol. 21, no. 1, pp. 109–122, 1991.

[5] G. B. Stillwagon, S. E. Order, C. Guse et al., "194 hepatocellular cancers treated by radiation and chemotherapy combinations: toxicity and response: a radiation therapy oncology group study," *International Journal of Radiation Oncology Biology Physics*, vol. 17, no. 6, pp. 1223–1229, 1989.

[6] M. A. Hawkins and L. A. Dawson, "Radiation therapy for hepatocellular carcinoma: from palliation to cure," *Cancer*, vol. 106, no. 8, pp. 1653–1663, 2006.

[7] J. C. Cheng, J. K. Wu, C. M. Huang et al., "Radiation-induced liver disease after three-dimensional conformal radiotherapy for patients with hepatocellular carcinoma: dosimetric analysis and implication," *International Journal of Radiation Oncology Biology Physics*, vol. 54, no. 1, pp. 156–162, 2002.

[8] L. A. Dawson, D. Normolle, J. M. Balter, C. J. McGinn, T. S. Lawrence, and R. K. Ten Haken, "Analysis of radiation-induced liver disease using the lyman NTCP model," *International Journal of Radiation Oncology Biology Physics*, vol. 53, no. 4, pp. 810–821, 2002.

[9] C. Greco, G. Catalano, A. Di Grazia, and R. Orecchia, "Radiotherapy of liver malignancies. From whole liver irradiation to stereotactic hypofractionated radiotherapy," *Tumori*, vol. 90, no. 1, pp. 73–79, 2004.

[10] J. C. Cheng, J. K. Wu, C. M. Huang et al., "Radiation-induced liver disease after radiotherapy for hepatocellular carcinoma: clinical manifestation and dosimetric description," *Radiotherapy and Oncology*, vol. 63, no. 1, pp. 41–45, 2002.

[11] C. Dejean, G. Kantor, B. Henriques de Figueiredo et al., "Helical tomotherapy: description and clinical applications," *Bulletin du Cancer*, vol. 97, no. 7, pp. 783–789, 2010.

[12] P. Giraud, M. Henni, and M. Housset, "Modern methods for cancer external radiation therapies," *Revue du Praticien*, vol. 58, no. 15, pp. 1637–1640, 2008.

[13] J. W. Jang, C. S. Kay, C. R. You et al., "Simultaneous multitarget irradiation using helical tomotherapy for advanced hepatocellular carcinoma with multiple extrahepatic metastases," *International Journal of Radiation Oncology Biology Physics*, vol. 74, no. 2, pp. 412–418, 2009.

[14] P. Das, R. A. Wolff, J. L. Abbruzzese et al., "Concurrent capecitabine and upper abdominal radiation therapy is well tolerated," *Radiation Oncology*, vol. 1, article 41, 2006.

[15] C. Pan, B. Kavanagh, and L. Dawson, "Radiation-associated liver injury," *International Journal of Radiation Oncology Biology Physics*, vol. 76, no. 3, supplement, pp. S94–S100, 2010.

[16] D. Azria, J. P. Gerard, G. Grehange et al., Société Française de Radiothérapie Oncologique-Guide des procédures de Radiothérapie Externe, 2007.

[17] V. S. Khoo and D. L. Joon, "New developments in MRI for target volume delineation in radiotherapy," *British Journal of Radiology*, vol. 79, pp. S2–S15, 2006.

[18] G. Kantor, M. A. Mahé, P. Giraud et al., "French national evaluation for helicoidal tomotherapy: description of indications, dose constraints and set-up margins," *Cancer Radiotherapie*, vol. 11, no. 6-7, pp. 331–337, 2007.

[19] K. K. Herfarth, J. Debus, F. Lohr et al., "Extracranial stereotactic radiation therapy: set-up accuracy of patients treated for liver metastases," *International Journal of Radiation Oncology Biology Physics*, vol. 46, no. 2, pp. 329–335, 2000.

[20] International Commission on Radiation Units and Measurements, "Prescribing, recording and reporting photon beam therapy," Report 62 (Supplement to ICRU Report 50), ICRU, Bethesda, Md, USA, 1999.

[21] A. Jackson, L. B. Marks, S. M. Bentzen et al., "The lessons of QUANTEC: recommendations for reporting and gathering data on dose-volume dependencies of treatment outcome," *International Journal of Radiation Oncology Biology Physics*, vol. 76, no. 3, supplement, pp. S155–S160, 2010.

[22] S. J. Shim, J. Seong, I. J. Lee, K. H. Han, C. Y. Chon, and S. H. Ahn, "Radiation-induced hepatic toxicity after radiotherapy

combined with chemotherapy for hepatocellular carcinoma," *Hepatology Research*, vol. 37, no. 11, pp. 906–913, 2007.

[23] Z. G. Ren, J. D. Zhao, K. Gu et al., "Three-dimensional conformal radiation therapy and intensity-modulated radiation therapy combined with transcatheter arterial chemoembolization for locally advanced hepatocellular carcinoma: an irradiation dose escalation study," *International Journal of Radiation Oncology Biology Physics*, vol. 79, no. 2, pp. 496–502, 2011.

[24] J. M. Baisden, A. G. Reish, K. Sheng, J. M. Larner, B. D. Kavanagh, and P. W. Read, "Dose as a function of liver volume and planning target volume in helical tomotherapy, intensity-modulated radiation therapy-based stereotactic body radiation therapy for hepatic metastasis," *International Journal of Radiation Oncology Biology Physics*, vol. 66, no. 2, pp. 620–625, 2006.

[25] M. Sherman and J. Bruix, "Management of hepatocellular carcinoma," *Hepatology*, vol. 42, no. 5, pp. 1208–1236, 2005.

[26] A. P. Venook, "Treatment of hepatocellular carcinoma: too many options?" *Journal of Clinical Oncology*, vol. 12, no. 6, pp. 1323–1334, 1994.

[27] M. A. Hawkins and L. A. Dawson, "Radiation therapy for hepatocellular carcinoma," *Cancer*, vol. 106, no. 8, pp. 1653–1663, 2006.

[28] L. A. Dawson, C. J. McGinn, D. Normolle et al., "Escalated focal liver radiation and concurrent hepatic artery fluorodeoxyuridine for unresectable intrahepatic malignancies," *Journal of Clinical Oncology*, vol. 18, no. 11, pp. 2210–2218, 2000.

[29] J. Seong, H. C. Park, K. H. Han, and C. Y. Chon, "Clinical results and prognostic factors in radiotherapy for unresectable hepatocellular carcinoma: a retrospective study of 158 patients," *International Journal of Radiation Oncology Biology Physics*, vol. 55, no. 2, pp. 329–336, 2003.

[30] K. Han, J. Seong, J. K. Kim et al., "Pilot clinical trial of localized concurrent chemoradiation therapy for locally advanced hepatocellular carcinoma with portal vein thrombosis," *Cancer*, vol. 113, no. 5, pp. 995–1003, 2008.

[31] E. Ben-Josef, D. Normolle, W. D. Ensminger et al., "Phase II trial of high-dose conformal radiation therapy with concurrent hepatic artery floxuridine for unresectable intrahepatic malignancies," *Journal of Clinical Oncology*, vol. 23, no. 34, pp. 8739–8747, 2005.

[32] A. McIntosh, K. D. Hagspiel, A. M. Al-Osaimi et al., "Accelerated treatment using intensity-modulated radiation therapy plus concurrent capecitabine for unresectable hepatocellular carcinoma," *Cancer*, vol. 115, no. 21, pp. 5117–5125, 2009.

[33] K. K. Herfarth, J. Debus, F. Lohr et al., "Stereotactic single-dose radiation therapy of liver tumors: results of a phase I/II trial," *Journal of Clinical Oncology*, vol. 19, no. 1, pp. 164–170, 2001.

[34] R. V. Tse, M. Hawkins, G. Lockwood et al., "Phase I study of individualized stereotactic body radiotherapy for hepatocellular carcinoma and intrahepatic cholangiocarcinoma," *Journal of Clinical Oncology*, vol. 26, no. 4, pp. 657–664, 2008.

[35] T. E. Schefter, B. D. Kavanagh, R. D. Timmerman, H. R. Cardenes, A. Baron, and L. E. Gaspar, "A Phase I trial of stereotactic body radiation therapy (SBRT) for liver metastases," *International Journal of Radiation Oncology Biology Physics*, vol. 62, no. 5, pp. 1371–1378, 2005.

[36] J. H. Kwon, S. H. Bae, J. Y. Kim et al., "Long-term effect of stereotactic body radiation therapy for primary hepatocellular

carcinoma ineligible for local ablation therapy or surgical resection. stereotactic radiotherapy for liver cancer," *BMC Cancer*, vol. 10, article 475, 2010.

[37] C. Louis, J. Dewas, X. Mirabel et al., "Stereotactic radiotherapy of hepatocellular carcinoma: preliminary results," *Technology in Cancer Research and Treatment*, vol. 9, no. 5, pp. 479–487, 2010.

[38] W. S. Koom, J. Seong, K. H. Han, D. Y. Lee, and J. T. Lee, "Is local radiotherapy still valuable for patients with multiple intrahepatic hepatocellular carcinomas?" *International Journal of Radiation Oncology Biology Physics*, vol. 77, no. 5, pp. 1433–1440, 2010.

[39] T. Ruers and R. P. Bleichrodt, "Treatment of liver metastases, an update on the possibilities and results," *European Journal of Cancer*, vol. 38, no. 7, pp. 1023–1033, 2002.

[40] J. K. Heimbach, G. J. Gores, M. G. Haddock et al., "Liver transplantation for unresectable perihilar cholangiocarcinoma," *Seminars in Liver Disease*, vol. 24, no. 2, pp. 201–207, 2004.

[41] F. Eckel and R. M. Schmid, "Chemotherapy in advanced biliary tract carcinoma: a pooled analysis of clinical trials," *British Journal of Cancer*, vol. 96, no. 6, pp. 896–902, 2007.

[42] T. A. Rich, D. B. Evans, S. A. Curley, and J. A. Ajani, "Adjuvant radiotherapy and chemotherapy for biliary and pancreatic cancer," *Annals of Oncology*, vol. 5, supplement 3, pp. 75–80, 1994.

[43] M. A. Ben-David, K. A. Griffith, E. Abu-Isa et al., "External-beam radiotherapy for localized extrahepatic cholangiocarcinoma," *International Journal of Radiation Oncology Biology Physics*, vol. 66, no. 3, pp. 772–779, 2006.

[44] M. F. Gerhards, T. M. van Gulik, D. González González, E. A. Rauws, and D. J. Gouma, "Results of postoperative radiotherapy for resectable hilar cholangiocarcinoma," *World Journal of Surgery*, vol. 27, no. 2, pp. 173–179, 2003.

[45] J. M. Baisden, M. Kahaleh, G. R. Weiss et al., "Capecitabine, and photodynamic therapy is feasible and well tolerated in patients with hilar cholangiocarcinom," *Gastrointestinal Cancer Research*, vol. 2, no. 5, pp. 219–224, 2008.

[46] D. J. Rea, J. K. Heimbach, C. B. Rosen et al., "Liver transplantation with neoadjuvant chemoradiation is more effective than resection for hilar cholangiocarcinoma," *Annals of Surgery*, vol. 242, no. 3, pp. 451–461, 2005.

[47] C. H. Crane, K. O. Macdonald, J. N. Vauthey et al., "Limitations of conventional doses of chemoradiation for unresectable biliary cancer," *International Journal of Radiation Oncology Biology Physics*, vol. 53, no. 4, pp. 969–974, 2002.

[48] C. Chargari, F. Campana, P. Beuzeboc, S. Zefkili, and Y. M. Kirova, "Preliminary experience of helical tomotherapy for locally advanced pancreatic cancer," *World Journal of Gastroenterology*, vol. 15, no. 35, pp. 4444–4445, 2009.

[49] J. S. Ji, C. W. Han, J. W. Jang et al., "Helical tomotherapy with concurrent capecitabine for the treatment of inoperable pancreatic cancer," *Radiation Oncology*, vol. 5, article 60, 2010.

[50] J. Seong, H. C. Park, K. H. Han et al., "Local radiotherapy for unresectable hepatocellular carcinoma patients who failed with transcatheter arterial chemoembolization," *International Journal of Radiation Oncology Biology Physics*, vol. 47, no. 5, pp. 1331–1335, 2000.

Acute Viral Hepatitis E Is Associated with the Development of Myocarditis

M. Premkumar,[1] Devraja Rangegowda,[1] Chitranshu Vashishtha,[1] Vikram Bhatia,[1] Jelen Singh Khumuckham,[2] and Badal Kumar[1]

[1]*Department of Hepatology, Institute of Liver and Biliary Sciences (ILBS), D-1 Vasant Kunj, New Delhi 110070, India*
[2]*Department of Cardiology, Institute of Liver and Biliary Sciences (ILBS), D-1 Vasant Kunj, New Delhi 110070, India*

Correspondence should be addressed to M. Premkumar; drmadhumitap@gmail.com

Academic Editor: Zu-Yau Lin

Myocarditis, an inflammatory disease of heart muscle, is an important cause of dilated cardiomyopathy worldwide. Viral infection is an important cause of myocarditis. This condition presents with various symptoms, ranging from minimally symptomatic cases to fatal arrhythmia and cardiogenic shock, and may develop chronic myocarditis and dilated cardiomyopathy in some patients. We report the case of a 26-year-old patient with acute viral hepatitis E who developed symptomatic myocarditis. As far as we could search, this is probably the 3rd case report of this rare association.

1. Introduction

Viral hepatitis associated with complications like cholestasis, arthritis, nephropathy, myocarditis, and peripheral neuropathy [1, 2]. Viral myocarditis presents with various symptoms, ranging from minimally symptomatic cases to fatal arrhythmia and cardiogenic shock, and may develop chronic myocarditis and dilated cardiomyopathy in some patients [3, 4]. Hepatitis E is endemic in India, and outbreaks occur following flooding and breakdown of sanitation barriers in monsoon [5, 6]. We report a case of probable myocarditis secondary to hepatitis E. As far as we could search, this is probably the 3rd case report of this rare association [7, 8]. We also report two similar cases with viral hepatitis E with suspected myocarditis.

2. Case 1

We report the case of a 26-year-old male who presented to us with the complaint of fever for 7 days which was insidious in onset, low grade without chills, and rigors. He also noted diarrhea for 5 days which was watery, 4-5 times per day associated with diffuse abdominal discomfort but not associated with the passage of blood or mucous. He then noticed jaundice and passage of dark urine for 3 days without any decrease in the frequency or volume of urine. There was no prior history of blood in urine or cola colored urine or burning micturition. There was no history of jaundice, pruritus, clay stools, melaena, hematemesis, abdominal distension, or altered sensorium. He reported only an occasional intake of ethanol. The patient denied intake of indigenous medications or intoxication. The patient did not report any past major surgeries, blood transfusions, or IV drug abuse prior to onset of the disease. He did not report any history of diabetes, hypertension, tuberculosis, thyroid disease, trauma, exposure to industrial toxins or radiation, blood or blood component therapy, bleeding disorders, promiscuity, or similar complaints in the family or neighbourhood. At the time of admission, he was conscious, was oriented, and was febrile. His blood pressure was 110/70 mm of Hg in the right arm, pulse-108/min. He was icteric and did not have pallor, clubbing, cyanosis, pedal edema, or lymphadenopathy. He did not have any skin rash or stigmata of chronic liver disease such as spider angioma, palmar erythema, and parotid enlargement. His initial lab data revealed a hemoglobin of 12 g/dL, total leucocyte counts 11330/dL, and INR (international normalized ratio) of 2.69. His serum bilirubin was 4.5 mg/dL with predominant direct fraction of 3 mg/dL

(a)

(b)

(c)

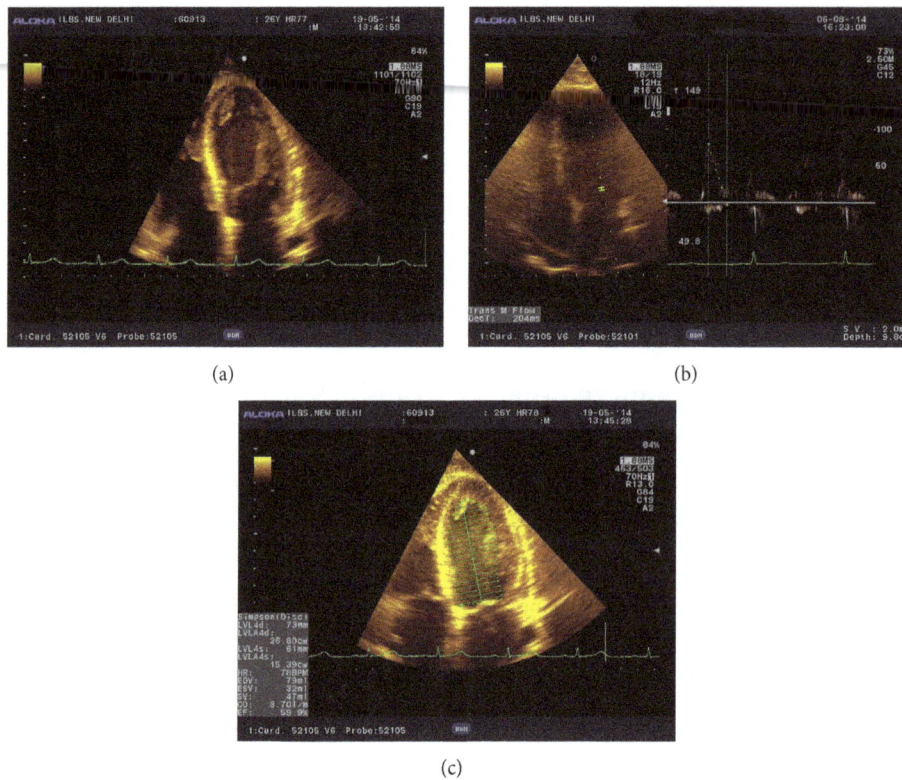

FIGURE 1: (a) ECHO images showing global hypokinesia in case 1. (b) and (c) ECHO image of patient 1.

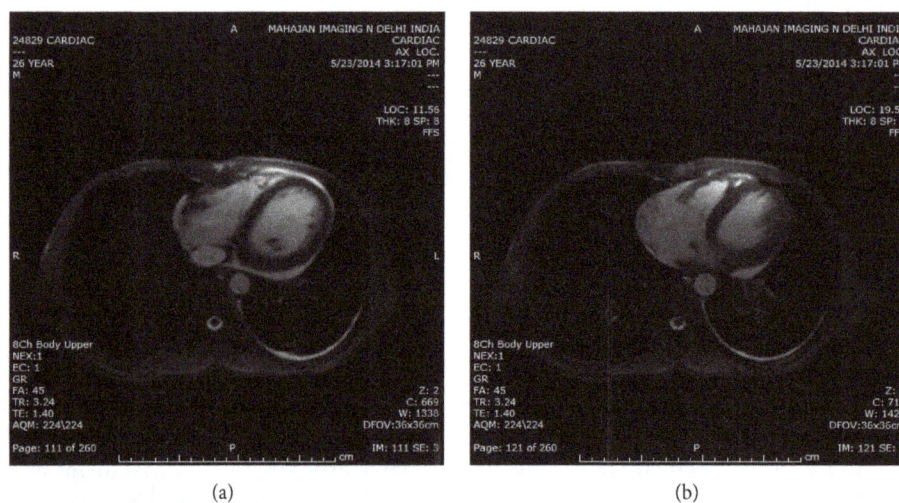

(a)

(b)

FIGURE 2: (a) and (b) Cardiac MRI of patient 1.

and indirect fraction of 1.5 mg/dL. Liver enzymes showed aspartate transaminase (AST) 452 IU/L, alanine transaminase (ALT) 2750 IU/L, alkaline phosphatase 254, and gamma glutamyl transferase (GGT) 169. Serum albumin was reduced at 2.2 g/dL with globulins 2.7 g/dL. His blood urea was 132 mg/dL with serum creatinine levels of 9.37 mg/dL with normal serum electrolytes suggestive of acute kidney injury. His IgM anti-HEV was positive and serology for hepatitis A, hepatitis B, hepatitis C, HIV, dengue, and *Leptospira*

was negative. His peripheral blood smear and rapid malaria test was negative. Due to his deranged renal functions, he was started on slow low efficiency dialysis (SLED) sessions and gradually his urine output improved over the next few days. He was managed conservatively with IV antibiotics, IV fluids, nutritional therapy, and other supportive measures. After two sessions of SLED, he progressed to a polyuric phase, so dialysis was stopped and patient was managed conservatively. On day 6 of presentation, he developed fever

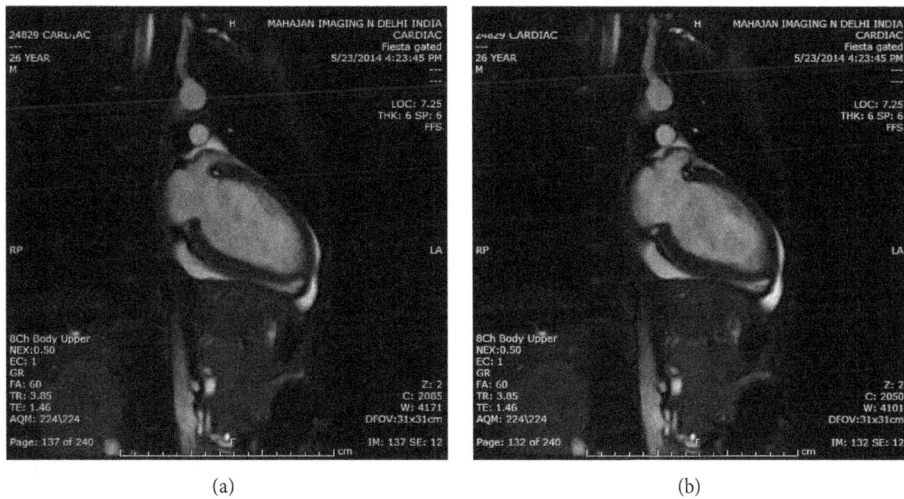

(a)   (b)

FIGURE 3: (a) Cardiac MRI of patient. (b) Coronal view cardiac MRI of patient 1.

again with left sided pleuritic pain and sudden onset of shortness of breath. He was found to be restless and dyspneic and on auscultation he had an S 3 gallop rhythm. Due to increasing respiratory distress, he was intubated and required mechanical ventilation for 3 days. Arterial blood gas analysis revealed type 1 respiratory failure with hypoxemia, and ECG showed sinus tachycardia and dynamic ST-T changes. Chest X-ray was suggestive of pulmonary congestion. Urgent 2D echocardiography revealed global hypokinesia, with normal LV and RV size, but ejection fraction was reduced to 25–30% with preserved right ventricular function. Troponin I was positive at 0.5 ng/mL and creatinine kinase-MB fraction levels were increased at 68 IU/L, 28% of total CK. This was suggestive of myocarditis. He was followed up by daily echocardiograms (see Figure 1). Over a period of 2 days, he gradually improved and was weaned off mechanical ventilation. His ejection fraction improved to 45% by day 3 and 60% with normal ventricular function by day 6. We performed a cardiac magnetic resonance imaging study on day 10 of myocarditis, but by then there was only marginal hypokinesia of the lateral left ventricular wall (see Figures 2 and 3). He was discharged on day 11 of hospital stay.

3. Case 2

The second case is that of a 22-year-old male with acute viral hepatitis E. He presented with a week long history of fever followed by jaundice and decreased urine output. At presentation, his total bilirubin level was 7.1 g/dL enzymes AST 945 U/L and ALT 268 U/L. This patient also had acute kidney injury; urea of 88 mg/dL; and creatinine of 3.1 mg/dL, which normalized on conservative management. He was found to have persistent bradycardia for 3 days and was dyspneic at rest, and cardiac enzymes (CK-MB) were elevated on day 3 of admission, and echocardiography revealed global hypokinesia with a reduced ejection fraction of 50%. However, he rapidly improved over the next two days and subsequent cardiac evaluation was normal by day 10 of his illness. Hence

he was screened only by serial echocardiography. Cardiac MRI was not done in this patient due to financial constraints.

4. Case 3

The third case is of a 24-year-old male patient with acute liver failure secondary to viral hepatitis E. He presented with fever, jaundice, and rapid progression to encephalopathy. This patient had elevated cardiac enzymes, that is, CK-MB, but his troponin I level was <1 ng/mL. ECG showed sinus tachycardia, nonspecific ST-T changes, and T inversions in the lateral leads. This patient was found to have global hypokinesia and LVEF of just 45%. He succumbed to his illness before further diagnostic evaluation could be done.

5. Discussion

Myocarditis, an inflammatory disease of heart muscle, is an important cause of dilated cardiomyopathy worldwide. Viral infection is also an important cause of myocarditis. The clinical spectrum of viral cardiomyopathy can be classified as fulminant, acute, or chronic [9, 10].

The progression of viral myocarditis involves three phases [11]. The first phase is characterized by an innate immune response including interferon gamma, natural killer cells, and nitric oxide. Antigen-presenting cells phagocytize released viral particles and cardiac proteins and migrate out of the heart to regional lymph nodes, causing virus-mediated cell lysis and the cardiomyocyte cell death [12]. Most patients recover, but a subset will progress to a second phase, consisting of a virus specific adaptive immune response. In this response, antibodies to viral proteins and to some cardiac proteins (including cardiac myosin, β_1, or muscarinic receptors) are produced, and CD 8+ T cells proliferate. In the third phase, commonly a few weeks after infection, the necrosed myocardium is replaced by diffuse fibrosis, resulting in progressive ventricular dilatation, resulting in chronic cardiac failure. The Dallas criteria [13] remain the standard for diagnosis, but a new clinicopathological staging system has been proposed.

Expanded Criteria for Diagnosis of Myocarditis [26]

> *Suggestive* of myocarditis: 2 positive categories;
>
> *compatible* with myocarditis: 3 positive categories;
>
> *high probability* of being myocarditis: all 4 positive categories.
>
> (Any matching feature in category = positive for category.)

Category I (Clinical Symptoms)

(1) Clinical heart failure,

(2) fever,

(3) viral prodrome,

(4) fatigue,

(5) dyspnea on exertion,

(6) chest pain,

(7) palpitations,

(8) presyncope or syncope.

Category II (Evidence of Cardiac Structural or Functional Perturbation in the Absence of Regional Coronary Ischemia)

(1) Echocardiography evidence:

    (a) regional wall motion abnormalities,

    (b) cardiac dilation,

    (c) regional cardiac hypertrophy;

(2) troponin release:

    (a) high sensitivity (>0.1 ng/mL);

(3) positive indium In 111 antimyosin scintigraphy;

(4) normal coronary angiography or

(5) absence of reversible ischemia by coronary distribution on perfusion scan.

Category III (Cardiac Magnetic Resonance Imaging)

(1) Increased myocardial T2 signal on inversion recovery sequence,

(2) delayed contrast enhancement after gadolinium-DTPA infusion.

Category IV (Myocardial Biopsy: Pathologic or Molecular Analysis)

(1) Pathology findings compatible with Dallas criteria,

(2) presence of viral genome by polymerase chain reaction or in situ hybridization.

The Dallas criteria have standardized the histopathological definition of myocarditis. Despite the EMB yield being only 10% to 20%, EMB findings remain the gold standard for unequivocally establishing the diagnosis. The largest case series of patients with an unexplained cardiomyopathy used biopsy findings to diagnose 111 of 1230 patients (9%) with myocarditis [14]. Notably, less than 10% of 2233 patients with dilated cardiomyopathy referred to the Myocarditis Treatment Trial had EMBs deemed positive by the Dallas criteria [15]. However, several studies have demonstrated strong clinical, echocardiographic, and laboratory evidence of myocarditis amongst patients with negative biopsies [16, 17].

Serum cardiac biomarkers (creatine kinase [CK], troponin I, and troponin T) are routinely measured when myocarditis is suspected. CK or its isoform (CK-MB) is not generally useful for noninvasive screening because of its low predictive value. Lauer et al. reported that only 28 of 80 patients (35%) with suspected myocarditis had elevated troponin levels. Using a serum troponin T cutoff >0.1 ng/mL, the sensitivity for detecting myocarditis is 53%, specificity is 94%, a positive predictive value is 93%, and a negative predictive value is 56% [18].

In our cases, myocarditis or Takotsubo cardiomyopathy was the main differential diagnosis. The first was a case of viral hepatitis E with acute kidney injury requiring dialysis, who developed symptomatic heart failure with pulmonary edema and evidence of cardiac hypokinesia. Takotsubo cardiomyopathy, induced by stress and excess catecholamines, shows a similar clinical course as myocarditis [19]. However, Takotsubo cardiomyopathy usually affects the apical and midventricular myocardium and does not cause diffuse hypokinesis as in our case. Secondly, the patchy diffuse distribution within the subepicardium on CMR is pathognomonic for myocarditis, whereas Takotsubo cardiomyopathy is generally not associated with late gadolinium enhancement [20]. We did not find changes on CMR suggestive of Takotsubo cardiomyopathy. On the basis of these findings, we diagnosed myocarditis. Therefore a combination of noninvasive imaging techniques may obviate the need for a myocardial biopsy to diagnose myocarditis. The second and third cases are only suspicious for myocarditis as though they meet clinical and echocardiographic criteria; we were unable to perform CMR tests in these cases. Neither were we able to perform endomyocardial biopsy in our patients, due to technical risks; all three had coagulopathy due to hepatitis, including one case with acute liver failure. However they further highlight the association of cardiac abnormalities like myocarditis with hepatitis E.

The evidence accumulated so far suggests that the onset of fulminant type 1 involves an immune reaction to an enterovirus. The viral infection would induce a self-perpetuating cycle of cytokine/chemokine overexpression in pancreatic beta cells, leading to apoptosis and destruction. Myocarditis is also commonly induced by viral infections, including the coxsackie virus B [21]. The viruses replicate in the gut and spleen and then spread to the heart. Their replication in the myocardium causes tissue damage amplified by an autoimmune response, leading to heart failure. Matsumori's study sought to detect HCV genomes in formalin-fixed paraffin sections of autopsied hearts from patients with myocarditis, dilated or hypertrophic cardiomyopathy. Among 106 hearts examined, beta-actin gene was amplified in 61 hearts (57.5%). Among the latter, HCV RNA was detected in 13 hearts (21.3%) and negative strands were detected in 4 hearts (6.6%). HCV RNA was found in 4 hearts (33.3%) with myocarditis, in 3 hearts (11.5%) with dilated cardiomyopathy, and in 6 hearts (26.0%) with hypertrophic cardiomyopathy [22, 23].

Several new diagnostic methods, such as cardiac magnetic resonance imaging, are useful for diagnosing myocarditis. Endomyocardial biopsy may be used for patients with acute dilated cardiomyopathy associated with hemodynamic compromise, those with life-threatening arrhythmia, and those whose condition does not respond to conventional supportive therapy. Important prognostic variables include the degree of left and right ventricular dysfunction, heart block, and specific histopathological forms of myocarditis [11, 12].

Therefore, the concomitant viral hepatitis and myocarditis exhibited by our patient may share a common etiology. We did not perform an endomyocardial biopsy in our patient as he had clinically improved, and CMR showed changes suggestive of myocarditis. However we feel that it is pertinent to report that our patient with clinical acute viral hepatitis E and renal dysfunction also developed myocarditis with acute pulmonary edema. Given the fact that viral hepatitis E is endemic in India, many more cases may have gone undetected because of lack of awareness of this association and also because in many cases hepatitis A and hepatitis E infection remain subclinical. Conversely, since we were unable to document myocarditis by means of a definite endomyocardial biopsy, our diagnosis remains clinical with imaging and biochemical supportive evidence. Nonetheless, with increasing number of case reports of association of viral hepatitis A with myocarditis [24, 25], we feel that hepatitis E should also be listed as a possible viral etiology of myocarditis.

References

[1] B. Xu, H. B. Yu, W. Hui et al., "Clinical features and risk factors of acute hepatitis E with severe jaundice," *World Journal of Gastroenterology*, vol. 18, no. 48, pp. 7279–7284, 2012.

[2] P. Jain, S. Prakash, S. Gupta et al., "Prevalence of hepatitis A virus, hepatitis B virus, hepatitis C virus, hepatitis D virus and hepatitis e virus as causes of acute viral hepatitis in North India: a hospital based study," *Indian Journal of Medical Microbiology*, vol. 31, no. 3, pp. 261–265, 2013.

[3] J. C. Schultz, A. A. Hilliard, L. T. Cooper Jr., and C. S. Rihal, "Diagnosis and treatment of viral myocarditis," *Mayo Clinic Proceedings*, vol. 84, no. 11, pp. 1001–1009, 2009.

[4] N. C. Sun and V. M. Smith, "Hepatitis associated with myocarditis. Unusual manifestation of infection with Coxsackie virus group B, type 3," *The New England Journal of Medicine*, vol. 274, no. 4, pp. 190–193, 1966.

[5] K. Das, A. Agarwal, R. Andrew, G. G. Frösner, and P. Kar, "Role of hepatitis E and other hepatotropic virus in aetiology of sporadic acute viral hepatitis: a hospital based study from urban Delhi," *European Journal of Epidemiology*, vol. 16, no. 10, pp. 937–940, 2000.

[6] P. Mathur, N. K. Arora, S. K. Panda, S. K. Kapoor, B. L. Jailkhani, and M. Irshad, "Sero-epidemiology of Hepatitis E virus (HEV) in urban and rural children of North India," *Indian Pediatrics*, vol. 38, no. 5, pp. 461–475, 2001.

[7] "Acute myopericarditis due to hepatitis E virus infection: a case report," Program P847, American College of Gastroenterology, Las Vegas, Nev, USA, 2012, ACG 2012 Annual Scientific Meeting Abstracts.

[8] B. K. Goyal, D. K. Mishra, R. Kawar, B. C. Kalmath, A. Sharma, and S. Gautam, "Hepatitis E associated myocarditis: an unusual entity," *Bombay Hospital Journal*, vol. 51, no. 3, pp. 361–362, 2009.

[9] JCS Joint Working Group, "Guidelines for diagnosis and treatment of myocarditis (JCS 2009): digest version," *Circulation Journal*, vol. 75, no. 3, pp. 734–743, 2011.

[10] H. T. Aretz, "Myocarditis: the Dallas criteria," *Human Pathology*, vol. 18, no. 6, pp. 619–624, 1987.

[11] L. T. Cooper Jr., "Myocarditis," *The New England Journal of Medicine*, vol. 360, no. 15, pp. 1526–1538, 2009.

[12] A. M. Feldman and D. McNamara, "Myocarditis," *The New England Journal of Medicine*, vol. 343, no. 19, pp. 1388–1398, 2000.

[13] H. T. Aretz, M. E. Billingham, W. D. Edwards et al., "Myocarditis: a histopathologic definition and classification," *The American Journal of Cardiovascular Pathology*, vol. 1, no. 1, pp. 3–14, 1987.

[14] G. M. Felker, R. E. Thompson, J. M. Hare et al., "Underlying causes and long-term survival in patients with initially unexplained cardiomyopathy," *The New England Journal of Medicine*, vol. 342, no. 15, pp. 1077–1084, 2000.

[15] J. W. Mason, J. B. O'Connell, A. Herskowitz et al., "A clinical trial of immunosuppressive therapy for myocarditis," *The New England Journal of Medicine*, vol. 333, no. 5, pp. 269–275, 1995.

[16] G. W. Dec Jr., I. F. Palacios, J. T. Fallon et al., "Active myocarditis in the spectrum of acute dilated cardiomyopathies. Clinical features, histologic corelates, and clinical outcome," *New England Journal of Medicine*, vol. 312, no. 14, pp. 885–890, 1985.

[17] A. Herskowitz, S. Campbell, J. Deckers et al., "Demographic features and prevalence of idiopathic myocarditis in patients undergoing endomyocardial biopsy," *The American Journal of Cardiology*, vol. 71, no. 11, pp. 982–986, 1993.

[18] B. Lauer, C. Niederau, U. Kühl et al., "Cardiac troponin T in patients with clinically suspected myocarditis," *Journal of the American College of Cardiology*, vol. 30, no. 5, pp. 1354–1359, 1997.

[19] S. W. Sharkey, J. R. Lesser, A. G. Zenovich et al., "Acute and reversible cardiomyopathy provoked by stress in women from the United States," *Circulation*, vol. 111, no. 4, pp. 472–479, 2005.

[20] L. Afonso, P. Hari, V. Pidlaoan, A. Kondur, S. Jacob, and V. Khetarpal, "Acute myocarditis: can novel echocardiographic techniques assist with diagnosis?" *European Journal of Echocardiography*, vol. 11, no. 3, p. E5, 2010.

[21] H. Mahrholdt, C. Goedecke, A. Wagner et al., "Cardiovascular magnetic resonance assessment of human myocarditis: a comparison to histology and molecular pathology," *Circulation*, vol. 109, no. 10, pp. 1250–1258, 2004.

[22] N. Akuzawa, N. Harada, T. Hatori et al., "Myocarditis, hepatitis, and pancreatitis in a patient with coxsackievirus A4 infection: a case report," *Virology Journal*, vol. 11, no. 1, article 3, 2014.

[23] A. Matsumori, T. Shimada, N. M. Chapman, S. M. Tracy, and J. W. Mason, "Myocarditis and heart failure associated with hepatitis C virus infection," *Journal of Cardiac Failure*, vol. 12, no. 4, pp. 293–298, 2006.

[24] T. Yazu, Y. Miyata, H. Matsuura, H. Kimura, and S. Koga, "A case of hepatitis A accompanied with acute myocarditis," *Nippon Shokakibyo Gakkai Zasshi*, vol. 85, pp. 1304–1307, 1988.

[25] C. Bosson, D. Q. Lim, J. Hadrami, and Y. Chotard, "Myoperi-carditis during hepatitis A," *Presse Médicale*, vol. 25, no. 21, pp. 995–996, 1996.

[26] P. P. Liu and H. P. Schultheiss, "Myocarditis," in *Braunwald's Heart Disease: A Textbook of Cardiovascular Medicine*, P. Libby and E. Braunwald, Eds., vol. 2, pp. 1784–1785, WB Saunders, Philadelphia, Pa, USA, 2008.

3

Fulminant Liver Failure Associated with Abdominal Crush Injury in an Eleven-Year Old

Erin Gordon and Sameer Kamath

Department of Pediatrics, Division of Critical Care, University of Iowa Children's Hospital, Iowa City, IA 52242, USA

Correspondence should be addressed to Sameer Kamath; sameer-kamath@uiowa.edu

Academic Editors: D. Lorenzin and H. Uchiyama

An 11-year-old obese male was involved in an all-terrain vehicle rollover accident. He had elevated transaminase levels along with a lactic acidosis. The imaging studies did not reveal any major intra-abdominal or thoracic injuries. The physical exam was unremarkable. The patient had an unremarkable PICU course and was transferred to the floor the next day. Within 24 hours of his transfer, he was noted to have interval worsening in liver function tests. He developed fulminant liver failure (FLF), renal failure, and encephalopathy. An ultrasound of the liver revealed increased echogenicity in the right lobe with focal sparing. Patient was listed for transplant. Investigations into any underlying medical cause of FLF were negative. Liver failure was presumed to be related to ischemia/reperfusion injury of the liver. The renal failure was due to rhabdomyolysis and was supported with renal replacement therapy. Patient received supportive care for FLF and was noted to have significant recovery of liver and renal function with time. He was discharged home after a 3-week hospitalization. Patients with crush abdominal injuries and elevated transaminase levels without evidence of parenchymal liver disruption may need to be closely monitored for liver failure related to ischemia reperfusion.

1. Introduction

Acute liver failure is characterized by the rapid development of severe liver injury with impaired synthetic function and hepatic encephalopathy in a patient without obvious, previous liver disease. Since the liver is capable of regeneration to a large extent, fulminant liver failure in principle may resolve with complete recovery. The decision for transplantation depends upon the likelihood of a spontaneous recovery. The indications for liver transplantation after trauma include uncontrolled hemorrhage, severe grade 4-5 injury resulting in liver parenchyma disruption, irreversible liver failure, and life-threatening postreperfusion injury. The requirement for liver transplantation after major liver trauma is rare with 19 cases reported in the literature with variable outcome [1]. FLF following abdominal trauma without hepatic parenchymal disruption has yet to be described in the pediatric population. In this case report, we describe an 11-year-old obese male with fulminant hepatic failure following a crush injury of the abdomen thought to be related to hepatic ischemia/reperfusion (I/R) injury.

2. Case Description

An 11-year-old obese boy (weight 84 kilograms, height 1.52 meters with BMI of 36.17 kg/m^2) was involved in an all-terrain vehicle (ATV) rollover accident. He was extricated by his grandfather and was taken by emergency medical services to the local emergency room. He received 2 liters of lactated ringers (LR) and underwent radiographic studies and laboratory tests. The laboratory evaluation at the local emergency room was remarkable for mild hypokalemia, elevated transaminase levels, and mild elevation in pancreatic enzymes. Head, chest, and Abdominal CT scans were unremarkable for major organ injury or bleeding. The patient was then transferred to our emergency room for further evaluation. The physical exam was remarkable for obesity, mild bruising over the abdomen, and an imprint from the ATV handle bar in the subcostal region. Outside laboratory results were reviewed and repeat laboratory tests at our center revealed a drop in hemoglobin from 15 to 10 g/dL with lactic acidosis. A repeat CT of the abdomen and chest was obtained to identify concealed blood loss, but again negative

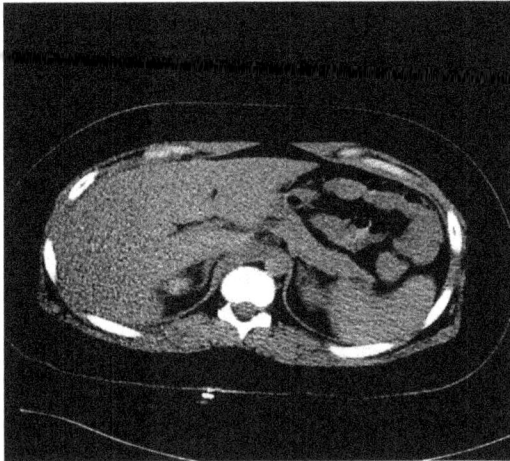

FIGURE 1: Abdominal CT scan showing no hepatic parenchymal injury.

TABLE 1: Laboratory results at time of readmission to PICU.

Laboratory test	Result	Normal range
Alanine transaminase	11275 U/L	5–30 U/L
Aspartate transaminase	13926 U/L	10–40 U/L
Blood urea nitrogen	26 mg/dL	10–20 mg/dL
Creatinine	1.5 mg/dL	0.3–0.9 mg/dL
Ammonia	112 mmol/L	7–42 mmol/L
Prothrombin time	90 seconds	9–12 seconds
INR	9.9	1.1–1.3
Partial thromboplastin time	40 seconds	23–31 seconds
Creatinine kinase	36399 U/L	40–200 U/L

(Figure 1). The patient was transferred to the Pediatric Intensive Care Unit (PICU) for serial monitoring of abdominal exams, hemoglobin/hematocrit, and hemodynamic status.

On admission to the PICU, he was noted to be hemodynamically stable. He had mild discomfort in the right upper quadrant of the abdomen with the imprint of the ATV handle bar and mild bruising. The cardiopulmonary exam was unremarkable. The patient was neurologically normal and denied any pain/tenderness along the spine. The patient's hemoglobin/hematocrit, hemodynamics, and liver enzymes remained stable overnight. His lactic acidosis had completely resolved with a peak venous lactate of 7 mEq/L. He was transferred to the floor on pediatric surgery service on hospital day (HD) 2 for further care until discharge from the hospital. He was transitioned to an enteral diet and intravenous fluids were discontinued. On HD 3, he was noted to have lethargy secondary to significant hypoglycemia (blood glucose level of 14 gm/dL). His mental status did not normalize, despite the correction of the hypoglycemia (blood glucose level of 78 gm/dL). His liver enzymes had worsened in the interim with worsening renal function and a decrease in urine output over the past 12–18 hours (Table 1). He was transferred back to the PICU urgently for monitoring of blood glucose and mental status.

On readmission, the patient was noted to have altered mental status with confusion and delirium consistent with stage 2 hepatic encephalopathy. The abdominal exam was unremarkable for any tenderness or distension and bowel sounds were audible. He was hemodynamically stable. Patient was noted to have rhabdomyolysis with an elevated creatine kinase level of 36,399 U/L (N = 40–200 U/L) with interval development of renal failure (blood urea nitrogen (BUN) 26 mg/dL and creatinine (Cr) 1.5 mg/dL). Liver enzymes were significantly worse on readmission with a 10-fold increase in aspartate transaminase (AST) and alanine transaminase (ALT) with interval reappearance of significant lactic acidosis (Table 1). The patient was noted to be severely coagulopathic with a prothrombin time (PT) of 90 seconds, international normalized ratio of 9.9, and partial thromboplastin time

(PTT) of 40 seconds. He received cryoprecipitate and fresh frozen plasma for severe coagulopathy due to FLF prior to the placement of a peripherally inserted central line for stable venous access. Hypoglycemia improved and stabilized with a glucose infusion rate of 6–8 mg/kg/min with gradual improvement in lactic acidosis (Figure 2(d)). Serum ammonia was noted to be 112 mmol/L. The pediatric gastroenterology, hepatology, and transplant consulting services were notified. A thorough evaluation of the potential causes of FLF was initiated based on recommendations made by the subspecialists. He had received acetaminophen during his hospital stay. The total dose administered was well below toxic range and the level obtained was therapeutic. In spite of this finding, intravenous N-acetylcysteine therapy was initiated after discussion with all specialists involved to replace hepatic glutathione stores in hopes of scavenging reactive oxygen species.

There was significant deterioration in his neurologic status with progression to stage III hepatic encephalopathy overnight (HD 4) along with respiratory distress due to fluid overload and renal failure. Urgently, he was intubated followed by placement of invasive lines for hemodynamic monitoring and initiation of renal replacement therapy. He received one dose of activated factor VII to limit any hemorrhagic complications from the invasive procedures (arterial line placement, central line insertion, and temporary hemodialysis catheter placement) given continued moderate-to-severe coagulopathy. He received aggressive supportive cares for his acute liver failure. The patient was listed for a liver transplant as a status 1 A.

The patient continued to receive supportive care over the course of the next week with stabilization of respiratory status, improvement in renal function, and improvement in his coagulopathy and liver failure (Figure 2). He was extubated on HD 10 and tolerated the same well. He was removed from the transplant list given continued improvement in liver synthetic function and was transferred to the floor on HD 12. His renal support was discontinued on HD 15 and the dialysis catheter was removed on HD 18. He was discharged home on HD 21 with scheduled followup arranged with gastroenterology, nephrology, and pediatric surgery. Peak abnormal laboratory values and values at the time of discharge for AST, ALT, bilirubin, BUN, and creatinine are listed in Table 2. Investigations to assess any underlying metabolic,

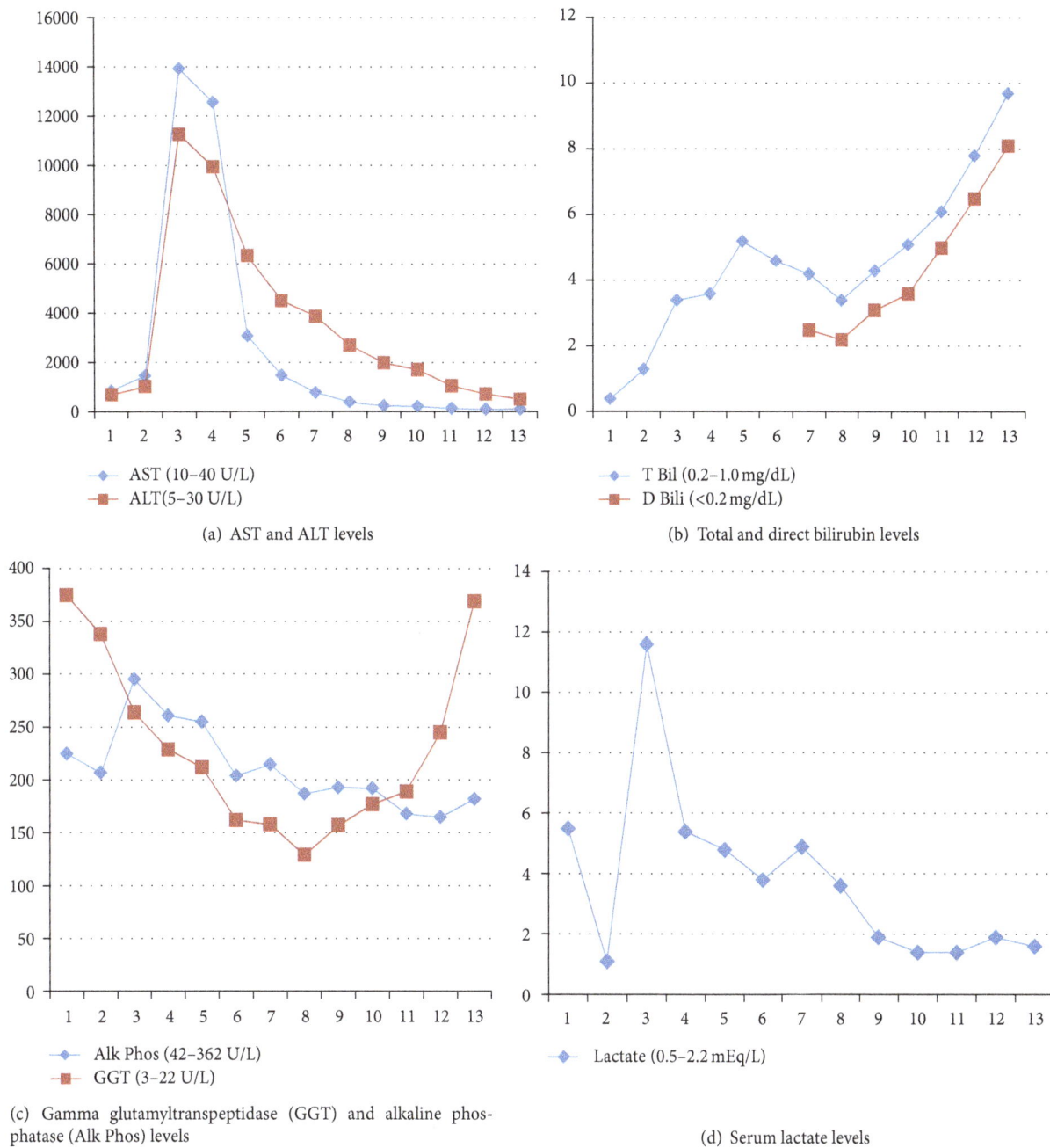

(a) AST and ALT levels

(b) Total and direct bilirubin levels

(c) Gamma glutamyltranspeptidase (GGT) and alkaline phosphatase (Alk Phos) levels

(d) Serum lactate levels

FIGURE 2: Laboratory trends from the emergency room to hospital day 13: Aspartate transaminase (AST) and alanine transaminase (ALT) (a); total and direct bilirubin (b), gamma glutamyltranspeptidase (GGT) and alkaline phosphatase (Alk Phos) (c), and serum lactate (d).

TABLE 2: Laboratory results: peak values and values at time of discharge.

Laboratory test	Peak value	Hospital day	Discharge value	Normal range
Total bilirubin	9.7 mg/dL	13	3.9 mg/dL	0.2–1 mg/dL
Direct bilirubin	8.1 mg/dL	13	2.7 mg/dL	<0.2 mg/dL
Aspartate transaminase	13926 U/L	3	98 U/L	10–40 U/L
Alanine transaminase	11275 U/L	3	129 U/L	5–30 U/L
Blood urea nitrogen	77 mg/dL	15	36 mg/dL	10–20 mg/dL
Creatinine	5.8 mg/dL	15	0.8 mg/dL	0.3–0.9 mg/dL

autoimmune, infectious, or genetic causes of liver failure were unremarkable. The patient's FLF was attributed to the abdominal crush injury that may have resulted in I/R of the liver.

At followup 2 weeks and 1 month from discharge, the liver and renal function tests were normal and patient was noted to be doing well without any sequelae from his injury and subsequent fulminant liver failure.

3. Discussion

3.1. Fulminant Liver Failure. Despite some degree of protection from the overlying rib cage, the liver is susceptible to injury from blunt abdominal trauma [2]. Liver trauma represents 1.2–4.6% of all trauma-related hospitalizations. It is more common in males and during the second and third decades of life. It is associated with 10–30% mortality. Nonoperative management of blunt liver injury is associated with lower hospital stay, transfusion needs, and rate of intra-abdominal infections [3].

Our patient had elevation in AST and ALT suggesting liver injury from the accident but no parenchymal lesion or vascular disruption was noted on CT scan (Figure 1). Clinically, he appeared well and denied significant abdominal pain on repeated evaluation in the emergency room and the PICU. He was transferred to the floor after a 24-hour period of observation in the PICU with stable vitals, reassuring exam, resolved lactic acidosis, and stable LFTs.

Our patient developed FLF and required readmission to the PICU about 48 hours after his injury. The mechanism of injury was noted to be crush from the ATV rollover. The ATV handlebar imprint was notably in the subcostal region. It is possible that the weight of the ATV resulted in hepatic ischemia caused by compression of the portal vein and hepatic artery, which resolved as soon as he was extricated. Further review of the abdominal CT scans did not reveal any vascular injury or thrombosis. Bedside ultrasound was done when the patent was readmitted and revealed increased echogenicity consistent with fatty infiltration in the right lobe with focal sparing with good flow in the portal vein and hepatic artery. However, on repeat evaluation, the patient has no radiographic evidence of fatty liver disease. The pediatric gastroenterologists have not diagnosed him with fatty liver disease at this time. The liver synthetic function recovered spontaneously and the patient needed supportive care for his FLF for about 2 weeks. The thorough evaluation into the cause of FLF (infection, autoimmune, and genetic/metabolic) was negative thus making I/R injury to be the most likely explanation of his clinical course.

I/R injury occurs when the liver is transiently deprived of oxygen and then is reoxygenated. When hepatic blood supply is temporarily interrupted, which is thought to be the case in this report of abdominal trauma, it results in warm ischemia. Warm I/R injury involves the activation of the immune system and is dominated by hepatocellular injury. The initial phase of injury (early phase) is marked by activation of immune cells and production of oxidant stress; this phase typically occurs within 2 hours following reperfusion. The late phase of injury is mediated by neutrophil accumulation and hepatocellular injury and typically occurs 6–48 hours after reperfusion. It has been associated with low flow states, surgical procedures, and during organ procurement for transplantation (cold ischemia) [4]. The pathogenesis of hepatic I/R injury is complex and includes activation of Kupffer cells, endothelial cells, leucocytes, and reactive oxygen species [5]. I/R injury is associated with histopathologic changes of cellular swelling, vacuolization, and leucocyte infiltration typically seen within 48 hours of reperfusion with normalization of liver architecture within 2 weeks of reperfusion [6]. Although several therapeutic interventions are suggested, none have been proven to be successful in humans.

3.2. Lactic Acidosis. Lactic acidosis following trauma may suggest inadequate tissue oxygen delivery and is often seen in association with severe hemorrhage. Clearance of lactate is decreased in patients with hepatic dysfunction [7]. LR contains sodium lactate. Our patient received 2 liters of LR at the outside emergency room and another 1 L in our institution. Lactic acidosis was noted despite any hemorrhage or evidence of inadequate tissue oxygen delivery which cleared after overnight observation in the PICU after his fluids were switched to 5% dextrose/half normal saline with potassium. In hindsight, his lactic acidosis was likely due to the exogenous lactate load in the setting of impaired lactate clearance secondary to hepatic dysfunction from ischemic injury sustained in the accident. The reappearance of lactic acidosis at readmission was likely representative of the degree of liver dysfunction from the I/R injury with inability to clear endogenous lactate. Significant lactic acidosis in the absence of inadequate tissue oxygen delivery following administration of LR may suggest liver dysfunction and should be appropriately monitored.

3.3. Renal Failure. We believe that the renal failure in our patient was due to a combination of rhabdomyolysis and contrast exposure. Crush injury is associated with rhabdomyolysis and renal failure due to acute tubular necrosis (ATN). Our patient had an abdominal crush injury. His clinical exam was very benign without any clinical signs of significant abdominal muscle injury. Patient's clinical wellness in the first 48 hours of hospitalization may have falsely reassured the team. It was only after he was re-admitted to the PICU with oliguria that a creatinine kinase level was obtained and found to be markedly elevated.

Intravenous contrast agents are a well-known cause of renal failure especially when other contributing factors coexist. Abdominal CT scan is the standard of care when intra-abdominal injury is suspected based on mechanism of injury and screening laboratory tests [2, 3]. Although our patient received intravenous fluids before intravenous contrast agents were administered, he may have been relatively intravascularly depleted contributing to contrast-induced renal injury.

The patient tolerated continuous renal replacement therapy very well and was transitioned to intermittent hemodialysis. He was noted to have adequate recovery of renal function in 2 weeks and at followup 1 month from his hospitalization he was noted to have normal renal function. Thus, obtaining a creatinine kinase level earlier in his course may have allowed therapies aimed at preventing acute tubular necrosis.

4. Conclusion

Abnormal AST and ALT in the absence of hepatic parenchymal disruption in abdominal crush injury may be related to transient hepatic ischemia. These patients may be at risk of FLF from reperfusion injuries. Lactic acidosis in the absence of inadequate tissue oxygen delivery following LR administration may suggest significant hepatic dysfunction. LR should be avoided in the setting of significant liver dysfunction to prevent development of lactic acidosis. Creatinine kinase should be obtained in trauma patients with a crush mechanism of injury to enable possible prevention of ATN. FLF due to ischemia/reperfusion injury often resolves spontaneously with supportive care, and liver transplantation is rarely needed.

Abbreviations

ATV: All-terrain vehicle
FLF: Fulminant liver failure
CT: Computed tomogram
PICU: Pediatric intensive care unit
I/R: Ischemia/reperfusion
HD: Hospital day
LFT: Liver function test
LR: Lactated ringers
AST: Aspartate transaminase
ALT: Alanine transaminase
BUN: Blood urea nitrogen
Cr: Creatinine.

References

[1] O. N. Tucker, P. Marriott, M. Rela, and N. Heaton, "Emergency liver transplantation following severe liver trauma," *Liver Transplantation*, vol. 14, no. 8, pp. 1204–1210, 2008.

[2] D. V. Feliciano, "Surgery for liver trauma," *Surgical Clinics of North America*, vol. 69, no. 2, pp. 273–284, 1989.

[3] A. K. Malhotra, T. C. Fabian, M. A. Croce et al., "Blunt hepatic injury: a paradigm shift from operative to nonoperative management in the 1990s," *Annals of Surgery*, vol. 231, no. 6, pp. 804–813, 2000.

[4] C. Fondevila, R. W. Busuttil, and J. W. Kupiec-Weglinski, "Hepatic ischemia/reperfusion injury—a fresh look," *Experimental and Molecular Pathology*, vol. 74, no. 2, pp. 86–93, 2003.

[5] D. G. Farmer, F. Amersi, J. Kupiec-Weglinski, and R. W. Busuttil, "Current status of ischemia and reperfusion injury in the liver," *Transplantation Reviews*, vol. 14, no. 2, pp. 106–126, 2000.

[6] T. Ikeda, K. Yanaga, K. Kishikawa, S. Kakizoe, M. Shimada, and K. Sugimachi, "Ischemic injury in liver transplantation: difference in injury sites between warm and cold ischemia in rats," *Hepatology*, vol. 16, no. 2, pp. 454–461, 1992.

[7] P. L. Almenoff, J. Leavy, M. H. Weil, N. B. Goldberg, D. Vega, and E. C. Rackow, "Prolongation of the half-life of lactate after maximal exercise in patients with hepatic dysfunction," *Critical Care Medicine*, vol. 17, no. 9, pp. 870–873, 1989.

4

Severe Aplastic Anemia following Acute Hepatitis from Toxic Liver Injury: Literature Review and Case Report of a Successful Outcome

Kamran Qureshi,[1] Usman Sarwar,[2] and Hicham Khallafi[3]

[1] Section of Gastroenterology and Hepatology, Division of Hepatology, Department of Medicine, Temple University School of Medicine, Temple University Health System, 3440 N Broad Street, Kresge Building West No. 209, Philadelphia, PA 19140, USA
[2] Temple University Hospital, 3401 North Broad Street, Philadelphia, PA 19140, USA
[3] Division of Gastroenterology and Hepatology, Department of Medicine, Case Western Reserve University School of Medicine, MetroHealth System, Medical Center, 2500 MetroHealth Drive, Cleveland, OH 44109, USA

Correspondence should be addressed to Kamran Qureshi; kamran.qureshi@temple.edu

Academic Editor: Melanie Deutsch

Hepatitis associated aplastic anemia (HAAA) is a rare syndrome in which severe aplastic anemia (SAA) complicates the recovery of acute hepatitis (AH). HAAA is described to occur with AH caused by viral infections and also with idiopathic cases of AH and no clear etiology of liver injury. Clinically, AH can be mild to fulminant and transient to persistent and precedes the onset SAA. It is assumed that immunologic dysregulation following AH leads to the development of SAA. Several observations have been made to elucidate the immune mediated injury mechanisms, ensuing from liver injury and progressing to trigger bone marrow failure with the involvement of activated lymphocytes and severe T-cell imbalance. HAAA has a very poor outcome and often requires bone marrow transplant (BMT). The findings of immune related myeloid injury implied the use of immunosuppressive therapy (IST) and led to improved survival from HAAA. We report a case of young male who presented with AH resulting from the intake of muscle building protein supplements and anabolic steroids. The liver injury slowly resolved with supportive care and after 4 months of attack of AH, he developed SAA. He was treated with IST with successful outcome without the need for a BMT.

1. Introduction

Hematologic abnormalities are commonly seen in the patients with acute or chronic liver disease. These derangements are mostly due to nutritional deficiencies, concurrent autoimmune diseases, hypersplenism, or portal hypertension. Severe aplastic anemia (SAA) is defined as severe pancytopenia with at least two of the following abnormalities: an absolute neutrophil count (ANC) of <500/mm^3, a platelet count of $<20 \times 10^3$/mm^3, and a reticulocyte count of $<60 \times 10^3$/mm^3 in the presence of bone marrow cellularity of <30% [1]. SAA can rarely complicate the course of acute hepatitis (AH) and presents as an acute bone marrow failure within a few weeks to months of an episode of acute liver injury [2]. A few studies have described the occurrence of SAA following 0.03–0.2% of cases of AH [3]. Looking at its prevalence

from the hematological standpoint, 2–5% of cases of SAA in Western studies [4], 10% of adults, and as high as 25% of children with SAA in Asian studies have AH documented to be present prior to SAA [5]. This association is labelled as hepatitis associated aplastic anemia (HAAA) in literature and is considered one of the causes of secondary SAA in young population. SAA is mostly seen to occur in adolescent males and presents with the clinical picture of pancytopenia within 1 week to 6 months after an episode of clinical AH [6]. HAAA was first described in 1955 [7], and since then the syndrome has been well defined and several pathogenesis mechanisms have been suggested. It has been reported in association with viral hepatitis related to hepatitis A, B, C, and G infections. Also, Parvovirus, Epstein Barr virus (EBV), transfusion transmitted virus (TTV), and echovirus have been implicated as causative agents [8]. However, in

TABLE 1: Laboratory test flow chart.

Lab	Day 1	Day 8	Day 35	Day 142	Day 160	Day 180	2 years	3 years
WBC	6		5.45	0.11	0.22	1.58	3.9	4.1
RBC	5.18		5.29	2.81	2.99	3.61	4.28	4.92
Hgb	15.7		15.2	8.4	8.7	10.8	13.7	14.9
Platelets	146		117	6	22	34	97	92
ANC	3.53		4.23	0.05	0.15	0.75	2.2	2.2
Bands				0.02	0.03	0.11		
INR	1		1.1		1.1			
Glucose	93	98	94	142	97	99	14	16
Blood urea	12	13	10	30	16	19		
Creatinine	0.88	0.85	0.86	0.78	1.03	0.91	0.99	0.97
Protein	7	5.9	4.6	4.6	5.7	5.9	6.9	7.1
Albumin	4.3	3.7	3.3	3.3	3.7	4.3	4.5	4.5
Globulin	2.7	2.2	1.3	1.0	2.0	2	2.4	2.6
T bilirubin	12.2	30.5	20	9.2	4.4	1.4	0.8	0.7
AlkP	272	231	319	119	234	126	130	114
ALT	2112	1747	922	381	43	17	31	24
AST	1055	1251	827	75	27	23	25	20

WBC: white blood count × 1000/mm^3; RBC: red blood cells × million/mm^3; Hgb: hemoglobin × g/dL; ANC: absolute neutrophil count × 1000/mm^3; INR: international normalized ratio; AlkP: alkaline phosphatase IU/dL; ALT: alanine aminotransferase IU/dL; AST: aspartate aminotransferase IU/dL.

most of the cases, no specific etiology of AH could be identified on clinical and serologic basis. Recently, a case of HAAA was reported in the literature and an anabolic steroid methasterone was linked to the development of transient cholestatic hepatitis and subsequently aplastic anemia [9]. Untreated HAAA has high mortality and survival of initially described cases was dismal [6]. Frequently, patient died from the complications of SAA and bone marrow transplant (BMT) was later used to treat HAAA. More recently, HAAA is being treated with immunosuppression and BMT is done only in cases of refractory SAA.

We illustrate the case of an adult male who was initially managed for a probable DILI and resultant AH in our hospital and whose clinical course of recovery from AH was complicated with development of SAA. With prompt identification and management, his HAAA was successfully treated with IST along with our hematology colleagues and patient recovered without needing a BMT. This review summarizes the literature on this rare and often fatal syndrome and suggests the extension of the spectrum of etiologic definition of HAAA.

2. Case Report

We describe a case of a 26-year-old Hispanic male, who presented (Day 1) to his primary care physician (PCP) office after he noticed progressively worsening yellowish discoloration of his eyes and skin for 10 days' duration. In addition, he had noticed dark urine for 2-3 weeks and pale colored stools for 5–7 days. He complained of nausea, generalized fatigue, and malaise but did not have any abdominal pain, fever, chills, diarrhea, or any skin rash. He was noted to have diffuse jaundice, hepatomegaly, and mild epigastric tenderness on

examination. The laboratory evaluation revealed abnormalities in liver panel, with total bilirubin (TBili) of 12.2 mg/dL, alkaline phosphatase (AlkP) 272 IU/dL, alanine aminotransferase (ALT), and aspartate aminotransferase (AST) of 2112 and 1055 IU/dL, respectively (Table 1). The complete blood count (CBC) and coagulation panel (INR) were normal at that time. He was admitted to our hospital where he underwent initial workup for painless jaundice. Upon initial evaluation by hepatology service, he informed us that he was originally from Puerto Rico and was living in the US for 17 years. He denied any history of significant illness as a child or any known history of liver disease in any family member. He denied any episodes of mental confusion and excessive sleepiness, as well as hematemesis, hematochezia, melena, or poor appetite. He also denied pruritus at any time and lower extremity edema or increased abdominal girth. He denied any recent sick contacts, animal exposure, or travel outside the US. He denied any history of incarceration, tattoos, or blood transfusions. He denied any history of tobacco use, illicit drug usage such as marijuana, cocaine, and heroin, or abuse of amphetamines. He reported drinking alcohol only on occasions and his last drink was approximately 7 months prior to this admission. However, he did report that he had been using over-the-counter anabolic steroids and a supplement from a vitamin store as a muscle-building high performance protein supplement (the ingredients are indicated in Table 3) on a daily basis for approximately 6 months. On examination, he appeared comfortable with diffuse jaundice and somewhat tender hepatomegaly. No clinical stigmata of advanced liver disease were identified on examination. The baseline serologic workup is shown in Table 2 which ruled out any infectious, autoimmune, or metabolic causes of his liver disease. The radiological

TABLE 2: Initial acute hepatitis workup.

Antinuclear antibodies	Negative	Ferritin	829
Antimitochondrial antibodies	Negative	Iron	173
Smooth muscle antibody	Negative	TIBC	337
Liver kidney microsomal antibody	Negative	% sat.	51
Cytokeratin antibody	Negative	IgG	414
Anti-Smith antibody	Negative	IgA	44
Hepatitis A IgM	Nonreactive	IgM	63
Hepatitis B core IgM	Nonreactive	Alpha1AT	327
Hepatitis B surface antigen	Nonreactive	AFP tumor marker	22.8
Hepatitis C IgG antibody	Nonreactive	Ceruloplasmin	35
HIV 1 & 2 antibody	Nonreactive	Adenovirus IgG antibody	1.5
CMV IgG antibody	Positive	Adenovirus IgM antibody	0.15
CMV IgM antibody	Negative	Adenovirus PCR quantitative	No DNA detected
CMV PCR quantitative	<100	Ethanol level	<10
Herpes 1 IgG antibody	Negative	Ur amphetamine screen	Negative
Herpes 2 IgG antibody	Negative	Ur barbiturate screen	Negative
HSV IgM antibody	Negative	Ur benzodiazepine screen	Negative
HSV PCR qualitative	Not detected	Ur cocaine screen	Negative
EBV IgG antibody	Positive	Ur methadone screen	Negative
EBV IgM antibody	Negative	Ur opiate screen	Negative
EBV ultraquantitative	<100	Ur PCP screen	Negative
Parvovirus B19 IgG antibody	Positive	Ur THC screen	Negative
Parvovirus B19 IgM antibody	Negative	Ur Tricyclics screen	Negative
Parvovirus B19 DNA PCR	Not detected	Hemochromatosis mutation	Negative

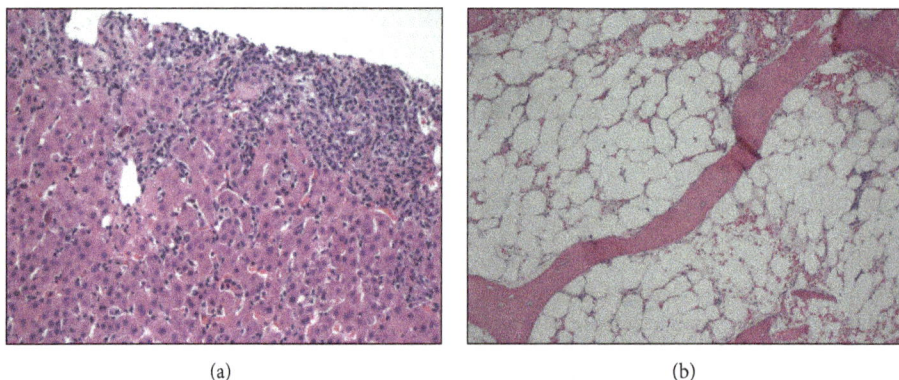

(a)   (b)

FIGURE 1: (a) Liver biopsy demonstrating features of active hepatitis, impressive inflammatory process involving both portal areas, and the lobules displaying also a pattern of sinusoidal lymphocytosis. (b) Bone marrow biopsy showing severe marrow hypocellularity.

workup with ultrasound, and a Magnetic Resonance Cholangiopancreatography did not reveal any biliary obstruction. He was suspected to have probable DILI with significant hyperbilirubinemia based on the negative etiologic workup. For further confirmation, he underwent a liver biopsy (Day 5) which revealed quite an impressive inflammatory process involving both portal areas and the lobules displaying also a pattern of sinusoidal lymphocytosis (Figure 1). The hepatocytic injury was identified and was more prominent in centrilobular (zone 3) location. Trichrome stain revealed only mild portal and periportal fibrosis and some perisinusoidal fibrosis especially in centrilobular location where the majority of the hepatocytic damage was identified along with mild collapse of the reticulin framework and likely was the result of hepatocytic dropout. Within the lobules, there was prominent "spotty necrosis," highlighted with the PAS positive, diastase resistant stain, revealing macrophages loaded with phagocytic debris. Iron stores were not increased and immunostain for adenovirus, cytomegalovirus (CMV), herpes virus, and hepatitis B surface antigen were also negative on the histologic tissue. Iron stain was negative and copper stain showed no increased copper deposition in the hepatocytes. Based on the above findings, he was started on a short course of oral prednisone and ursodiol (Day 8) as the treatment for severe AH with cholestasis. His laboratory tests showed gradual improvement in hepatitis and subsequently

TABLE 3: Ingredient description of the used muscle building supplement.

Amount per serving		
Calories	140	
Calories from fat	35	
Total fat	3.00 g	
Saturated fat	3.00 g	
Cholesterol	5.00 mg	
Sodium	230.00 mg	
Potassium	490.00 mg	
Total carbohydrate	2.00 g	
Dietary fiber	0.00 g	
Sugars	0.00 g	
Protein	20.00 g	
Phosphorus	490.00 mg	
Calcium	670.00 mg	
Iron	3.50 mg	
Alanine	4230.00 mg	
Arginine	7040.00 mg	
Aspartic acid	11130.00 mg	
Cysteine	1250.00 mg	
Glutamine (as glutamic acid)	21710.00 mg	
Glycine	3830.00 mg	
Histidine	2600.00 mg	
Isoleucine	5950.00 mg	
Leucine	7650.00 mg	
Lysine	6500.00 mg	
Methionine	1380.00 mg	
Phenylalanine	5100.00 mg	
Proline	5430.00 mg	
Serine	5180.00 mg	
Threonine	3890.00 mg	
Tryptophan	1280.00 mg	
Tyrosine	3860.00 mg	
Valine	6010.00 mg	
Total amino acids	104020.00 mg	
Total fat	65 g	80 g
Sat. fat	20 g	25 g
Cholesterol	300 mg	300 mg
Sodium	2400 mg	2400 mg
Total carbohydrate	300 g	375 g
Dietary fiber	25 g	30 g

Other Ingredients. Sustained release amino acid enhanced protein matrix (whey peptides, whey protein concentrate, Supro brand and regular brand soy protein isolate, branched chain amino acid blend (*L*-isoleucine, *L*-leucine, valine (as *L*-valine))), Lipobolic & trade; advanced lipid complex (evening primrose oil (*Oenothera biennis*), conjugated linoleic acid (CLA) (80%), medium chain triglycerides, flax seed powder, borage seed oil powder, and omega-3 complex), natural and artificial flavors, stearic acid, gum blend (carrageenan, xanthan gum, and cellulose gum), beet color, silica, lecithin, malic acid, acesulfame potassium, sucralose, and citric acid

he was discharged to be followed up as outpatient. He was seen in the clinic for monitoring (Day 35) and reported over

all symptomatic improvement and he had started back his job as a residential painter. His follow-up monitoring laboratory testing 6 weeks later showed continued improvement in AH (Figure 2) while he stayed on low dose ursodiol.

On his next set of monitoring laboratory testing (Day 142), new onset severe pancytopenia (Table 1) was identified which prompted urgent hospital admission for evaluation and management of his pancytopenia. All viral etiologies of acute pancytopenia were ruled out by serologic analysis. He did not have any family history of AA. Extensive hematological workup was performed and all other causes of primary SAA were ruled (negative anti-CD55 and anti-CD59 antibodies, negative urinary collections for lead and arsenic, and negative flow cytometry). Peripheral blood smear analysis revealed severe neutropenia and normocytic anemia with frequent target cells, consistent with clinical history of liver disease along with severe thrombocytopenia. He underwent a bone marrow biopsy and flow cytometry analysis which showed severe hypocellular bone marrow (less than 5%) with dyserythropoiesis (Figure 1). The cytogenetic study showed normal karyotype. Immunostain with CD3 and PAX5 stains showed no involvement of lymphoma. CD34, TdT, and CD117 stains confirmed no significant increase of blasts. D31 and Factor-VIII stains show virtual absence of megakaryocytes. In view of the patient's age, gender, and his presentation with initial AH, the diagnosis of HAAA was made. The patient did not have any full siblings and in view of the absence of matched HLA siblings, the decision was made to immediately initiate IST. He initially received thymoglobulin (ATG) along with methylprednisolone treatment for a total of 5 days. He received prophylactic antimicrobials, in addition to filgrastim daily and platelet transfusions as needed to support his peripheral cell count. He responded to the induction therapy with the improvement in cell counts and significant reduction in his liver enzymes. Later, he was kept on cyclosporine (Cys) and prednisone was tapered off. This resulted in stable cell counts and partial recovery of bone marrow (Day 160). IST was continued as cyclosporine monotherapy and further improvement in cell counts was seen (Figure 2). He continues on cyclosporine with complete recovery of HAAA (Table 1) after 3 years of initial presentation.

3. Discussion

The unique aspect of our case is the etiology of AH, which has not been widely reported in the past as a specific cause of AH leading to HAAA. Hepatotoxicity in the form of cholestasis and hepatitis has been well described in the literature resulting from anabolic steroids and also occasionally with protein supplements [10, 11]. These agents are not specifically considered myelotoxic. Our patient was taking these over-the-counter products for more than 3 months prior to the initiation of symptoms and subsequent diagnosis of AH. After the diagnosis of AH and the cessation of those products, the hepatocellular injury pattern improved with ALT decreasing to > 50% in a month. Extensive evaluation was undertaken and it ruled out presence of any concomitant toxic, viral, autoimmune, or metabolic causes of AH (Table 3). Also,

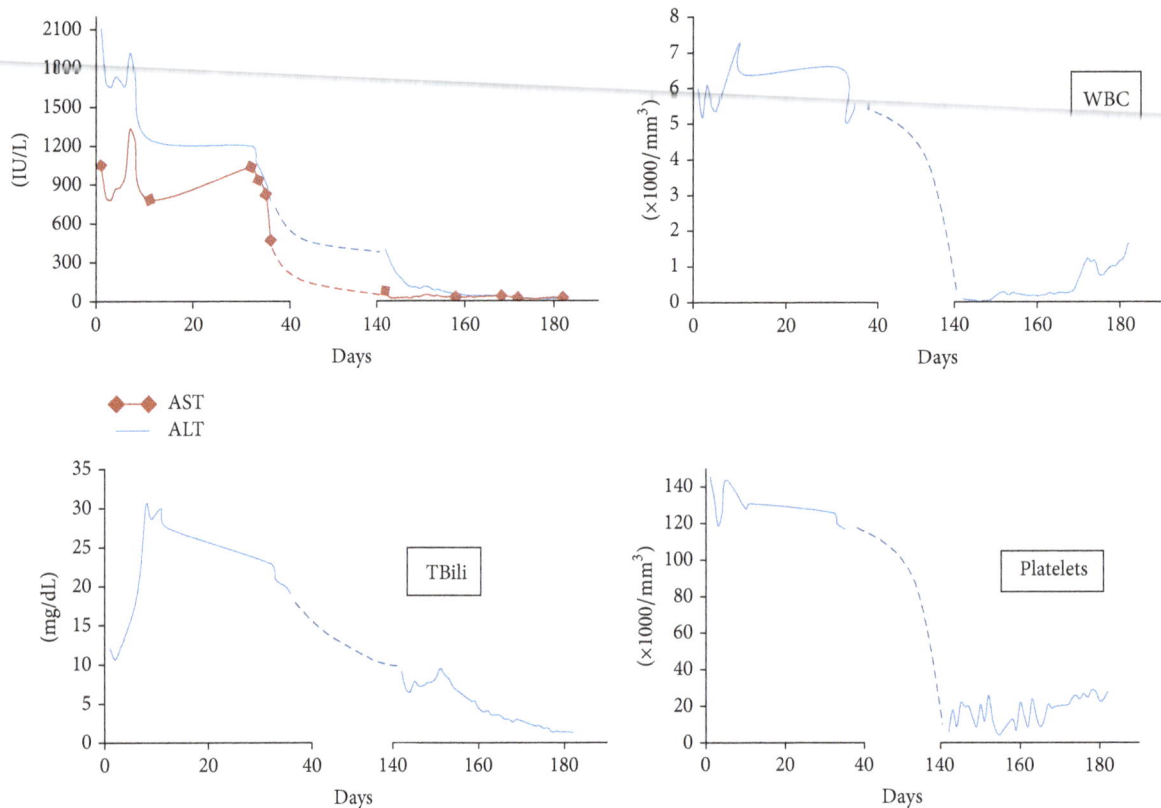

FIGURE 2: Graphical trends of the laboratory parameters of HAAA over six months.

there were no other clinical risk factors, high risk behavior, sick contact, or a recent travel identified in this case which could contribute to unidentifiable cause of his AH. Based on this data and by using Roussel Uclaf Causality Assessment Method (RUCAM) [12], we calculated the score of 7, which suggested that those products are the "probable" cause of his liver injury and AH. We did not check for hepatitis E and G viruses, GB virus C, or TTV viruses which have been implicated as etiologic agents leading to HAAA. The clinical suspicion for these viral infections was low and also laboratory assays were not available for clinical use.

Our patient followed the typical stereotypic presentation of HAAA which most often develops in male adolescents or young men. Our patient showed evidence of bone marrow failure 4 months after the onset of AH. There is currently no clear determination of the duration of the onset of hepatitis and a diagnosis of HAAA; it varies from less than a year to less than 3 months [13, 14]. HAAA most often occurs in the recovery period after AH. In one study, AH completely resolved in only 60% of cases [15] while the rest of the patients had mild persistent hepatitis, as was the case with our patient. The typical hepatitis viruses including A, B, C, D, E, and G and other viruses such as Parvovirus B-19, CMV, Epstein-Barr virus, TTV, and non-A-E hepatitis virus have been implicated as a cause of AH and subsequent development of HAAA [16]. We screened our patient with all of the available serologic assays. Our clinical suspicion for the rare forms of viral hepatitis was low. The symptoms of hepatitis

have been reported to be ranging from mild to fulminant liver failure requiring liver transplantation (LT). Our patient presented with insidious onset of cholestasis and liver injury typical for anabolic steroids hepatotoxicity [17, 18]. HAAA is reported to arise even after LT in up to 30% of children who underwent LT for non-A, non-B, and non-C hepatitis related liver failure [19] suggesting continuum of underlying pathogenic mechanism even after the curative treatment of inciting event. Our patient was given a short course of prednisone for treatment of drug induced liver injury based on the past experience [20], although it is widely believed to be ineffective in such drug induced liver injury. The clinical presentation of SAA after AH is variable and oftentimes it is diagnosed on routine laboratory testing as the new onset pancytopenia. The clinical symptoms of SAA include spontaneous bleeding (mucosal or cutaneous) related to thrombocytopenia, fatigue, and pallor caused by progressive anemia, fever, mucosal ulcerations, and infections secondary to neutropenia. Intracranial bleeding and severe sepsis are identified as the most common fatal complications of HAAA [6]. Our patient was lucky to be identified on the routine monitoring laboratory testing before he developed any complications of pancytopenia. He underwent an extensive workup to rule out primary aplastic anemia or other causes of acquired SAA. His bone marrow biopsy showing severe hypocellularity (<5%) and hematologic evaluation suggested SAA and the history of proceeding AH; in view of his age, gender, and timeline of events, HAAA was a strongly considered diagnosis. Curiously, the globulin levels were noted to be normal at the onset and gradually decreased to low levels in our patient. Severe hepatitis with features similar to autoimmune hepatitis has been reported in patient with common variable immunodeficiency (CVID) [21]. CVID is a syndrome which is characterized by various degrees of primary hypogammaglobulinemia and is frequently associated with autoimmune diseases [22]. Our patient did not have any history of recurrent sinopulmonary or gastrointestinal infections. While CVID remains an interesting differential in the diagnosis of our patient, clinical resolution of AH after avoiding the offending supplements and normalization of globulin levels after complete recovery of HAAA would favor a toxic etiology. CVID is diagnosed by excluding the causes of acquired immunodeficiency and that workup was not performed in our patient.

In the mechanistic studies of patients with HAAA, several immunological abnormalities have been described and a favorable response to IST has suggested immunologic dysregulation as the main pathogenic mechanism leading to HAAA. Patients with HAA were found to have a decreased ratio of CD4/CD8 cells in peripheral blood, which is associated with activated cytotoxic T cells and an increase in the proportion of CD8 cells that are HLA-DR positive [2, 23]. Activated CD8-positive lymphocytes have been implicated to be cytotoxic to myelopoietic cells in the bone marrow in patients with aplastic anemia [24]. In addition, interferon-gamma is found to be a marrow suppressing cytokine [25] and is secreted by activated T cells. Intense lymphocytic infiltrate is seen on histologic evaluation of AH from viral hepatitis and predominantly consists of T cells. CD-8 expressing Kupffer cells could be important mediators of HAAA [23]. The liver biopsy of our patient showed significant sinusoidal lymphocytosis. The time interval between the occurrence of hepatitis and the onset of bone marrow failure in HAAA suggests that the initial target organ of the immunological response is the liver [26]. A recent study suggested that T-lymphocytes clones are formed in the early stage of AH which recognize similar target antigens against both hepatocytes and myeloid cells. Subsequent selective expansion of the clones that are highly tropic to bone marrow could lead to HAAA [27].

The major curative options which are evaluated for treating severe HAAA are BMT and IST [28]. Supportive care is provided by prompt treatment and prophylaxis of possible infectious complications, antiviral prophylaxis of hepatitis B carriers, institution of hematopoietic growth factors, and blood products transfusion as needed [29]. Overall BMT has better survival (up to 82%) [8, 30] and a search for a Human Leucocyte Antigen identical sibling as a donor of bone marrow, to enable BMT to be undertaken promptly. Our patient did not have a matching family member. IST is an alternative first line treatment for a patient without an option of BMT [30] with a mean response rate of 70% [8]. Initial induction regimens when tested as ATG alone or Cys alone were associated with response rates of about 50% [31]. This led to the use of combination regimens of ATG, Cys, corticosteroids, and hematopoietic growth factors with the response rates of 75–80% [31]. Those patients who do not respond to the initial IST either can be managed by different

IST regimens [32] or can be offered a matched unrelated donor, but overall prognosis is dismal is such cases [2, 33]. Successful treatment with IST is usually associated with rapid resolution of AH in patients with persistent hepatitis. Cytotoxic T-lymphocytes are thought to cause ongoing hepatic damage ATG and Cys may suppress those cells and improve hepatitis as well as bone marrow failure.

In conclusion, HAAA is a well-defined clinical syndrome in which an attack of hepatitis leads to bone marrow failure through immunologic mechanisms. Overall prognosis of unrecognized and thus untreated cases is very poor. HAAA mostly affects young male population who present with illness of viral or nonviral AH and later progress to SAA. Our report suggests extending the etiologic spectrum of HAAA to involve DILI as the inciting cause. Prompt identification and referral to BMT centers are imperative. We were able to identify our patient and coordinate his care of HAAA in a timely manner, which resulted in the recovery of liver injury and bone marrow failure with institution of IST. He is being followed in our clinic for over 3 years and has shown a successful recovery from HAAA following a toxic liver injury.

References

[1] "Incidence of aplastic anemia: the relevance of diagnostic criteria. By the International Agranulocytosis and Aplastic Anemia Study," *Blood*, vol. 70, pp. 1718–1721, 1987.

[2] K. E. Brown, J. Tisdale, A. J. Barrett, C. E. Dunbar, and N. S. Young, "Hepatitis-associated aplastic anemia," *The New England Journal of Medicine*, vol. 336, no. 15, pp. 1059–1064, 1997.

[3] H. Wang, M. Tu, R. Fu et al., "The clinical and immune characteristics of patients with hepatitis-associated aplastic anemia in China," *PLoS ONE*, vol. 9, no. 5, Article ID e98142, 2014.

[4] A. Locasciulli, A. Bacigalupo, B. Bruno et al., "Hepatitis-associated aplastic anaemia: epidemiology and treatment results obtained in Europe. A report of the EBMT aplastic anaemia working party," *British Journal of Haematology*, vol. 149, no. 6, pp. 890–895, 2010.

[5] S. Issaragrisil, C. Sriratanasatavorn, A. Piankijagum et al., "Incidence of aplastic anemia in Bangkok. The Aplastic Anemia Study Group," *Blood*, vol. 77, pp. 2166–2168, 1991.

[6] L. Hagler, R. A. Pastore, and J. J. Bergin, "Aplastic anemia following viral hepatitis. Report of two fatal cases and literature review," *Medicine*, vol. 54, no. 2, pp. 139–164, 1975.

[7] E. Lorenz and K. Quaiser, "Panmyelopathy following epidemic hepatitis," *Wiener Medizinische Wochenschrift*, vol. 105, no. 1, pp. 19–22, 1955.

[8] R. Gonzalez-Casas, L. Garcia-Buey, E. A. Jones, J. P. Gisbert, and R. Moreno-Otero, "Systematic review: hepatitis-associated aplastic anaemia—a syndrome associated with abnormal immunological function," *Alimentary Pharmacology & Therapeutics*, vol. 30, no. 5, pp. 436–443, 2009.

[9] A. Khurana and C. A. Dasanu, "Hepatitis associated aplastic anemia: case report and discussion," *Connecticut Medicine*, vol. 78, pp. 493–495, 2014.

[10] H. Zimmerman, "Hormonal derivatives and related drugs," in *Hepatotoxicity: The Adverse Effects of Drugs and Other Chemicals on the Liver*, H. J. Zimmerman, Ed., pp. 555–588, Lippincott, Philadelphia, PA, USA, 2nd edition, 1999.

[11] A. L. Vilella, C. Limsuwat, D. R. Williams, and C. F. Seifert, "Cholestatic jaundice as a result of combination designer supplement ingestion," *Annals of Pharmacotherapy*, vol. 47, no. 7-8, article e33, 2013.

[12] G. Danan and C. Benichou, "Causality assessment of adverse reactions to drugs—I: a novel method based on the conclusions of international consensus meetings: application to drug-induced liver injuries," *Journal of Clinical Epidemiology*, vol. 46, no. 11, pp. 1323–1330, 1993.

[13] J. R. Hibbs, N. Frickhofen, S. J. Rosenfeld et al., "Aplastic anemia and viral hepatitis. Non-A, Non-B, Non-C?" *JAMA*, vol. 267, no. 15, pp. 2051–2054, 1992.

[14] E. Baumelou, M. Guiguet, and J. Y. Mary, "Epidemiology of aplastic anemia in France: a case-control study. I. Medical history and medication use," *Blood*, vol. 81, no. 6, pp. 1471–1478, 1993.

[15] R. Safadi, R. Or, Y. Ilan et al., "Lack of known hepatitis virus in hepatitis-associated aplastic anemia and outcome after bone marrow transplantation," *Bone Marrow Transplantation*, vol. 27, no. 2, pp. 183–190, 2001.

[16] B. Rauff, M. Idrees, S. A. R. Shah et al., "Hepatitis associated aplastic anemia: a review," *Virology Journal*, vol. 8, article 87, 2011.

[17] K. G. Ishak and H. J. Zimmerman, "Hepatotoxic effects of the anabolic/androgenic steroids," *Seminars in Liver Disease*, vol. 7, no. 3, pp. 230–236, 1987.

[18] A. Timcheh-Hariri, M. Balali-Mood, E. Aryan, M. Sadeghi, and B. Riahi-Zanjani, "Toxic hepatitis in a group of 20 male body-builders taking dietary supplements," *Food and Chemical Toxicology*, vol. 50, no. 10, pp. 3826–3832, 2012.

[19] A. G. Tzakis, M. Arditi, P. F. Whitington et al., "Aplastic anemia complicating orthotopic liver transplantation for non-A, non-B hepatitis," *The New England Journal of Medicine*, vol. 319, no. 7, pp. 393–396, 1988.

[20] R. J. Veneri and S. C. Gordon, "Anabolic steroid-induced cholestasis: choleretic response to corticosteroids," *Journal of Clinical Gastroenterology*, vol. 10, no. 4, pp. 467–468, 1988.

[21] K. Fukushima, Y. Ueno, H. Kanegane et al., "A case of severe recurrent hepatitis with common variable immunodeficiency," *Hepatology Research*, vol. 38, no. 4, pp. 415–420, 2008.

[22] L. D. Notarangelo, A. Fischer, R. S. Geha et al., "Primary immunodeficiencies: 2009 update," *Journal of Allergy and Clinical Immunology*, vol. 124, no. 6, pp. 1161–1178, 2009.

[23] C. Cengiz, N. Turhan, O. F. Yolcu, and S. Yilmaz, "Hepatitis associated with aplastic anemia: do CD8(+) Kupffer cells have a role in the pathogenesis?" *Digestive Diseases and Sciences*, vol. 52, no. 9, pp. 2438–2443, 2007.

[24] W. A. Kagan, J. A. Ascensão, R. N. Pahwa et al., "Aplastic anemia: presence in human bone marrow of cells that suppress myelopoiesis," *Proceedings of the National Academy of Sciences of the United States of America*, vol. 73, no. 8, pp. 2890–2894, 1976.

[25] E. E. Solomou, K. Keyvanfar, and N. S. Young, "T-bet, a Th1 transcription factor, is up-regulated in T cells from patients with aplastic anemia," *Blood*, vol. 107, no. 10, pp. 3983–3991, 2006.

[26] J. Lu, A. Basu, J. J. Melenhorst, N. S. Young, and K. E. Brown, "Analysis of T-cell repertoire in hepatitis-associated aplastic anemia," *Blood*, vol. 103, no. 12, pp. 4588–4593, 2004.

[27] Y. Ikawa, R. Nishimura, R. Kuroda et al., "Expansion of a liver-infiltrating cytotoxic T-lymphocyte clone in concert with the development of hepatitis-associated aplastic anaemia," *British Journal of Haematology*, vol. 161, no. 4, pp. 599–602, 2013.

[28] K. Doney, W. Leisenring, R. Storb, and F. R. Appelbaum, "Primary treatment of acquired aplastic anemia: outcomes with bone marrow transplantation and immunosuppressive therapy," *Annals of Internal Medicine*, vol. 126, no. 2, pp. 107–115, 1997.

[29] B. Pongtanakul, P. K. Das, K. Charpentier, and Y. Dror, "Outcome of children with aplastic anemia treated with immunosuppressive therapy," *Pediatric Blood and Cancer*, vol. 50, no. 1, pp. 52–57, 2008.

[30] N. S. Young, P. Scheinberg, and R. T. Calado, "Aplastic anemia," *Current Opinion in Hematology*, vol. 15, no. 3, pp. 162–168, 2008.

[31] J. K. Davies and E. C. Guinan, "An update on the management of severe idiopathic aplastic anaemia in children," *British Journal of Haematology*, vol. 136, no. 4, pp. 549–564, 2007.

[32] W. J. Savage, P. A. DeRusso, L. M. Resar et al., "Treatment of hepatitis-associated aplastic anemia with high-dose cyclophosphamide," *Pediatric Blood and Cancer*, vol. 49, no. 7, pp. 947–951, 2007.

[33] Y. Osugi, H. Yagasaki, M. Sako et al., "Antithymocyte globulin and cyclosporine for treatment of 44 children with hepatitis associated aplastic anemia," *Haematologica*, vol. 92, no. 12, pp. 1687–1690, 2007.

5

A Case of Hepatic Angiomyolipoma Which Was Misdiagnosed as Hepatocellular Carcinoma in a Hepatitis B Carrier

Jin Yeon Hwang,[1] Sung Wook Lee,[1] Yang Hyun Baek,[1] Jong Han Kim,[1] Ha Yeon Kim,[1] Suck Hyang Bae,[1] Jin Han Cho,[2] Hee Jin Kwon,[2] Jin Sook Jeong,[3] Young Hoon Roh,[4] and Sang Young Han[1]

[1] Department of Internal Medicine, Dong-A University College of Medicine, Busan 602-715, Republic of Korea
[2] Department of Radiology, Dong-A University College of Medicine, Busan, Republic of Korea
[3] Department of Pathology, Dong-A University College of Medicine, Busan, Republic of Korea
[4] Department of Surgery, Dong-A University College of Medicine, Busan, Republic of Korea

Correspondence should be addressed to Sang Young Han, syhan@dau.ac.kr

Academic Editors: F. Kondo and Z.-Y. Lin

We report a rare case of resected hepatic AML, which was misdiagnosed as hepatocellular carcinoma in a chronic hepatitis B carrier. A 45-year-old woman who was a carrier of hepatitis B virus infection presented with a hepatic tumor. Her serum alpha-fetoprotein level was normal. Ultrasonography revealed a round and well-circumscribed echogenic hepatic tumor measuring 2.5 cm in the segment VI. On contrast-enhanced computed tomography, a hypervascular tumor was observed in the arterial phase and washing-out of the contrast medium in the portal phase and delayed phase. On MR T1-weighted in-phase images, the mass showed low signal intensity, and on out-of-phase images, the mass showed signal drop and dark signal intensity. On MR T2-weighted images, the mass showed high signal intensity. The mass demonstrated high signal intensity on arterial phase after contrast injection, suggestive of hepatocellular carcinoma. The patient underwent hepatic wedge resection and histopathological diagnosis was a hepatic angiomyolipoma.

1. Introduction

Angiomyolipoma (AML) typically occurs in the kidney and rarely in liver [1]. Hepatic AML is a rare, primarily benign mesenchymal tumor, composed of blood vessels, fat tissue, and smooth muscle cells [2]. Ishak reported the first hepatic AML in 1976 [3] and since then, there have been about 200 cases reported in the literature and they have been increasing with improvement in imaging modalities, including ultrasonography (US), computed tomography (CT), magnetic resonance imaging (MRI), and fine-needle aspiration biopsy (FNAB) [4]. The hepatic AML may pose a diagnostic challenge clinically, radiologically, and pathologically because of its wide variation due to the different proportions of the three cell types which make up the tumor. In particular, in a region endemic for hepatocellular carcinoma, the diagnosis of AML by imaging modality can be difficult and frequently misdiagnosed as hepatocellular carcinoma. The definitive diagnostic study remains the histological examination coupled with immunohistochemical stains. Among the components of hepatic AML, homatropine methyl bromide 45 (HMB-45) positive smooth muscle cell is the only specific and definitive criterion for diagnosis [5]. Hepatocellular carcinoma and liver hemangioma are negative for this marker. We report a case of resected hepatic AML, which was misdiagnosed as hepatocellular carcinoma in a hepatitis B carrier.

2. Case Report

A 45-year-old woman, a chronic hepatitis B carrier, was admitted to our hospital for further evaluation and treatment

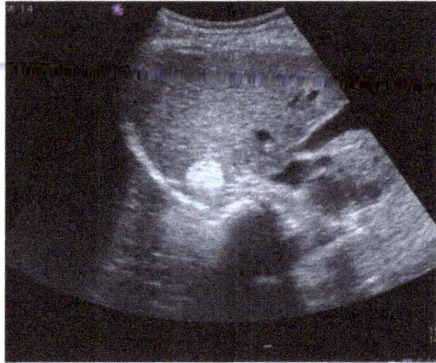

FIGURE 1: Ultrasonographic findings of the liver mass. Ultrasonogram demonstrates a 2.5 cm sized round, well-marginating hyperechoic mass.

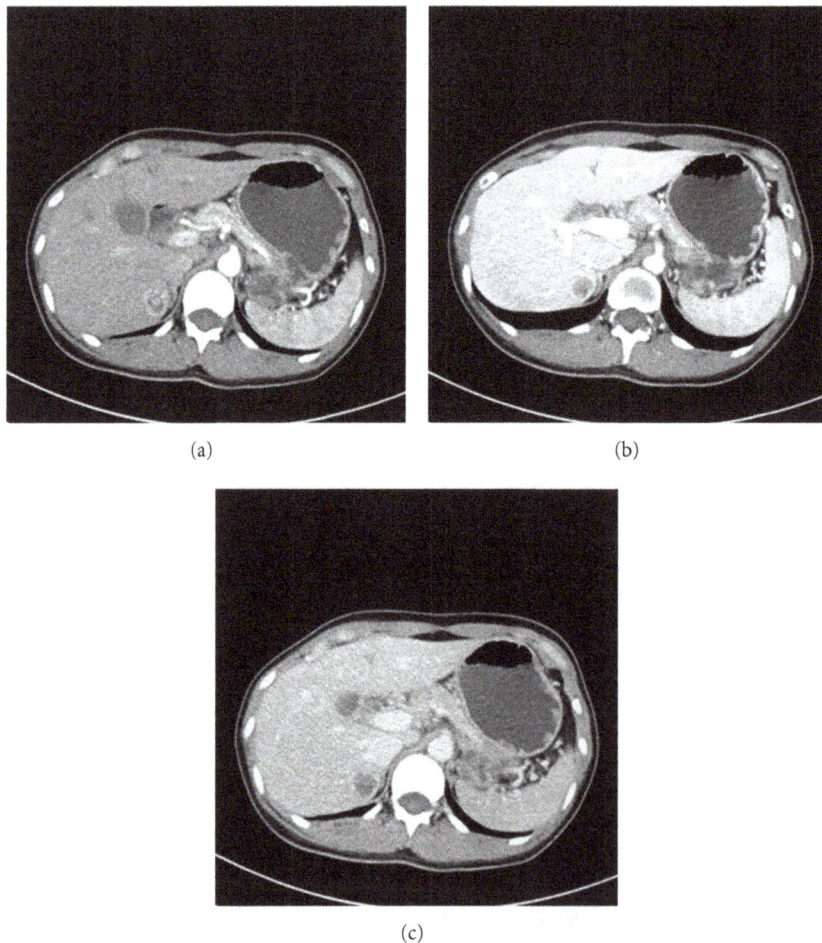

(a)

(b)

(c)

FIGURE 2: CT findings of the liver mass. Contrast-enhanced CT revealed a heterogeneous hypervascular mass in the arterial phase (a) and washing-out of the medium in the portal (b) and delayed phases (c).

of a liver mass that had been found on abdominal US at regular medical checkup in November 11, 2011. Clinically, no pathologic findings were observed during physical examination. All routine blood investigations, including liver function tests, were normal. The serologic studies for viral hepatitis B showed only positive hepatitis B surface antigen (HBs Ag) test result. The serologic markers for hepatitis

C were nonreactive. The hepatitis B virus DNA titer was 438 IU/mL (1,495 copies/mL) and serum alpha-fetoprotein level was 2.01 ng/mL (normal <20 ng/mL).

Abdominal US showed a well-defined, hyperechoic mass, with maximal diameter of 2.5 cm in the segment VI of the liver (Figure 1). On contrast-enhanced computed tomography (CT), a hypervascular tumor was observed in the arterial

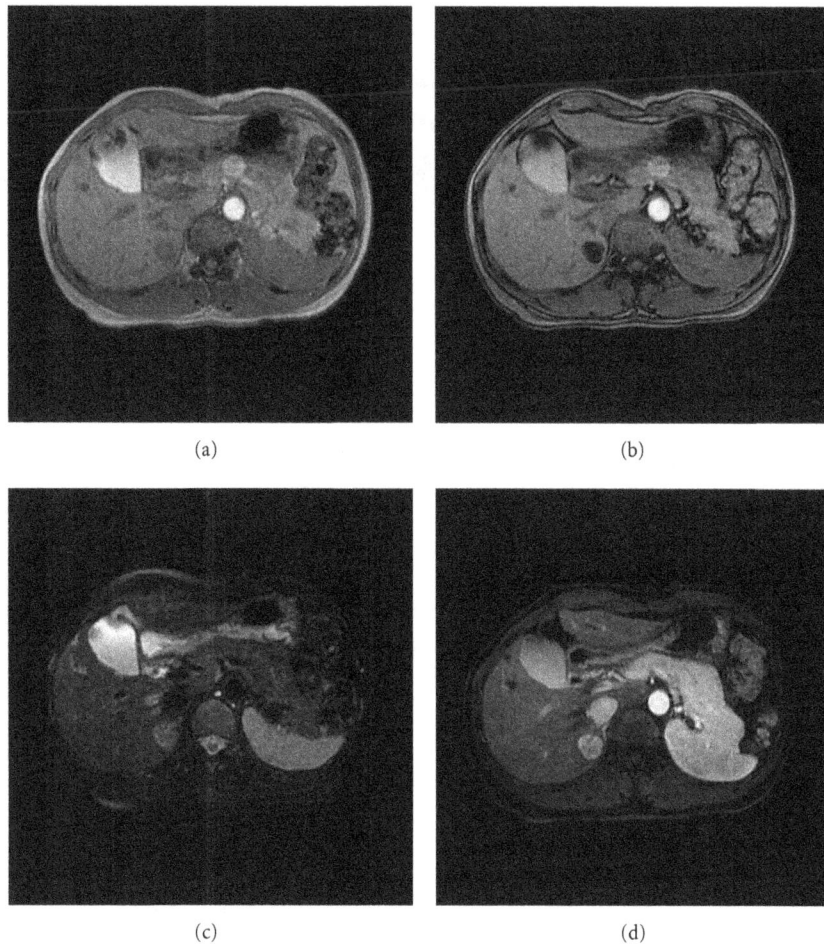

(a)

(b)

(c)

(d)

FIGURE 3: MR findings of the liver mass. On MR T1-weighted in-phase images, the mass shows low signal intensity (a), and on out-of-phase images, the mass shows signal drop and dark signal intensity (b). On MR T2-weighted images, the mass shows high signal intensity (c). The mass demonstrates high signal intensity on arterial phase after contrast injection (d).

phase (Figure 2(a)) and washing-out of the contrast medium in the portal phase and delayed phase (Figures 2(b) and 2(c)). On abdominal magnetic resonance (MR) images, the lesion showed low signal intensity on the T1-weighted in-phase images (Figure 3(a)) and showed signal drop and dark signal intensity on the T1-weighted out-of-phase images (Figure 3(b)). On MR T2-weighted images, the mass shows high signal intensity (Figure 3(c)). The mass demonstrates high signal intensity on arterial phase after contrast injection (Figure 3(d)), suspicious for fat containing hepatocellular carcinoma.

As hepatocellular carcinoma was highly suspected from preoperative image studies with her medical history, hepatic wedge-resection with tumor in the segment VI was performed. Wedge resected liver showed a well-demarcated but nonencapsulated soft mass, representing variegated cut surface with yellowish fat tissue, multifocal hemorrhage, and no necrosis (Figure 4(a)). The mass composed of blood vessels, fat tissue and areas of epithelioid cells, and some inflammatory cells (Figures 4(b)–4(d)). The epithelioid cells showed monotonous round nuclei and clear cytoplasm and anti-CK8/18 (−) and anti-HSA (−), which were recognized

as nonliver cells (Figures 2(e), and 2(f)). The epithelioid cells were anti-smooth muscle antibody (SMA) (+) (Figure 4(g)), anti-vimentin (+), and anti-S100 (−), representing smooth muscle cell. Furthermore, the epithelioid cells show strong anti-HMB45 (+) (Figure 4(h)), which has been known as a unique marker for AML. Pathologically, the tumor was diagnosed as an AML of the liver, benign. The patient recovered uneventfully and was discharged 1 week after operation.

3. Discussion

Angiomyolipoma (AML) is an uncommon mesenchymal tumor that occurred more frequently in kidney than in liver [1]. Most of the patients have no symptoms or signs; the majorities were found incidentally on routine medical examination using ultrasound. Preoperative diagnosis of hepatic AML mostly relies on imaging studies and the radiological characteristics of the lesion have been described in some of the reported cases [2, 6, 7]. It is typically echogenic on ultrasound, hypodense on precontrast CT scans, markedly enhanced on arterial phase, and remained

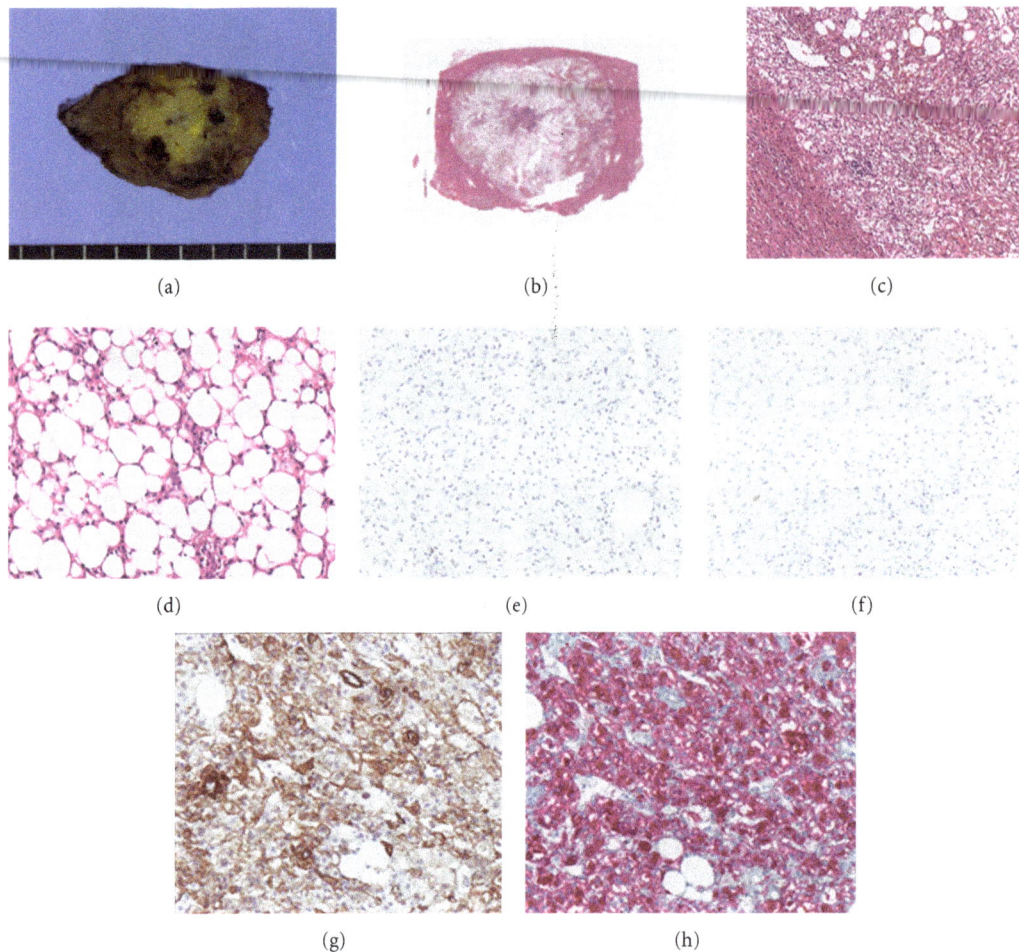

FIGURE 4: Pathologic findings of the liver mass ((a) Gross, (b)–(d); Hematoxylin & eosin stain, (e)-(f); Immnuohistochemistry ((e) anti-CK8/18, (f) anti-HSA, (g) anti-SMA, (h) anti-HMB45, (e)–(g) brown chromogen, (h) red chromogen), (b) ×1, (c) and (d) ×40, (e)–(h) ×200). The liver shows a well-demarcated mass with yellowish cut surface and hemorrhage. Microscopically, the mass composes of fat cells, vessels and epithelioid cells. The epithelioid cells exhibit non-epithelial origin (negative CK8/18 and negative HSA), SMA (+) and HMB45 (+).

in enhancement with portal venous phase. MR imaging characteristics vary depending on the proportion of intratumoral fat [6]. Commonly, AML has a high fat content, with high signal intensity on T1-weighted images and a significant drop in signal intensity on fat-suppressed images. However, the imaging feature of hepatic AML varies because of variations in the proportion of adipose cells, smooth muscle cells, and vessels. In particular, the number of adipose cells varies between 10% and 90% [7]. This heterogeneity makes the preoperative diagnosis by imaging quite difficult, and it is possible to misdiagnose hepatic AML as a number of entities, both benign and malignant [7–13]. Commonly confused entities include lipoma, hepatocellular adenoma, hepatocellular carcinoma with fatty metamorphosis, sarcoma, or other metastatic neoplasm. Notably, hepatic AML has been misdiagnosed as hepatocellular carcinoma with a frequency more than 50% due to a significant overlap of the imaging features [8, 9, 13]. Some studies place emphasis on the differentiation of hepatic AML and fat-containing hepatocellular carcinoma that usually arise from the cirrhotic liver [8, 10].

The definitive diagnostic study remains the histological examination coupled with immunohistochemical stains. Among the components of hepatic AML, HMB-45 positive smooth muscle cell is the only specific and definitive criterions for diagnosis [5]. Hepatocellular carcinoma and liver hemangioma are negative for this marker.

In the present case, the preoperative radiological image was quite difficult to distinguish from fat-containing hepatocellular carcinoma. Although her serum alpha-fetoprotein was normal, the radiological findings and her clinical history are compatible with hepatocellular carcinoma. Under the above impression, these lesions were resected and the histological examination coupled with immunohistochemical stains made the final diagnosis of hepatic AML. Because the preoperative images showed atypical findings for AML, we did not make a accurate diagnosis of hepatic AML at that time.

The management of hepatic AML sometimes remains controversial. Several authors have suggested that this disease can be managed with conservative treatment with followup after fine-needle aspiration biopsy in previous series [1, 14, 15]. Some reports recommended that surgical intervention may be needed in selected cases to alleviate the mass effect on the neighboring organs [1, 16], and very few cases of AML with concomitant hepatocellular carcinoma, malignant transformation, and its spontaneous rupture have been reported [16–20]. No surgical treatment of AML in an endemic area for hepatocellular carcinoma should proceed with caution because cases of fat-contained hepatocellular carcinoma will make the diagnosis difficult. Given the high prevalence of hepatocellular carcinoma in Korea, the decision for surgical intervention is straightforward if imaging and laboratory studies are equivocal.

In conclusion, preoperative diagnosis of hepatic AML by image is sometimes quite difficult particularly in endemic areas of hepatocellular carcinoma, and in the patients who have risk factors of hepatocellular carcinoma with suggested malignancy by image but showing normal laboratory findings, repeated studies with different diagnostic modalities, such as biopsy or angiography, and careful interpretation are recommended.

References

[1] C. N. Yeh, M. F. Chen, C. F. Hung, T. C. Chen, and T. C. Chao, "Angiomyolipoma of the liver," *Journal of Surgical Oncology*, vol. 77, no. 3, pp. 195–200, 2001.

[2] S. R. Prasad, H. Wang, H. Rosas et al., "Fat-containing lesions of the liver: radiologic-pathologic correlation," *Radiographics*, vol. 25, no. 2, pp. 321–331, 2005.

[3] K. G. Ishak, "Mesenchymal tumors of the liver," in *Hepatocellular carcinoma*, K. Okuda and R. L. Peters, Eds., pp. 247–307, Wiley Medical, New York, NY, USA, 1976.

[4] T. A. Jiang, Q. Y. Zhao, M. Y. Chen, L. J. Wang, and J. Y. Ao, "Diagnostic analysis of hepatic angiomyolipoma," *Hepatobiliary and Pancreatic Diseases International*, vol. 4, no. 1, pp. 152–155, 2005.

[5] Y. De Bruecker, F. Ballaux, S. Allewaert et al., "A solitary hepatic lesion: MRI-pathological correlation of an hepatic angiomyolipoma (2004:4b)," *European Radiology*, vol. 14, no. 7, pp. 1324–1326, 2004.

[6] F. Yan, M. Zeng, K. Zhou et al., "Hepatic angiomyolipoma: various appearances on two-phase contrast scanning of spiral CT," *European Journal of Radiology*, vol. 41, no. 1, pp. 12–18, 2002.

[7] C. Basaran, M. Karcaaltincaba, D. Akata et al., "Fat-containing lesions of the liver: cross-sectional imaging findings with emphasis on MRI," *American Journal of Roentgenology*, vol. 184, no. 4, pp. 1103–1110, 2005.

[8] T. Ahmadi, Y. Itai, M. Takahashi et al., "Angiomyolipoma of the liver: significance of CT and MR dynamic study," *Abdominal Imaging*, vol. 23, no. 5, pp. 520–526, 1998.

[9] R. Ning, L. X. Qin, Z. Y. Tang, Z. Q. Wu, and J. Fan, "Diagnosis and treatment of hepatic angiomyolipoma in 26 cases," *World Journal of Gastroenterology*, vol. 9, no. 8, pp. 1856–1858, 2003.

[10] W. M. S. Tsui, R. Colombari, B. C. Portmann et al., "Hepatic angiomyolipoma: a clinicopathologic study of 30 cases and delineation of unusual morphologic variants," *American Journal of Surgical Pathology*, vol. 23, no. 1, pp. 34–48, 1999.

[11] P. Bergeron, V. L. Oliva, L. Lalonde et al., "Liver angiomyolipoma: classic and unusual presentations," *Abdominal Imaging*, vol. 19, no. 6, pp. 543–545, 1994.

[12] S. Worawattanakul, R. C. Semelka, N. L. Kelekis, and J. T. Woosley, "Hepatic angiomyolipoma with minimal fat content: MR demonstration," *Magnetic Resonance Imaging*, vol. 14, no. 6, pp. 687–689, 1996.

[13] D. R. Zhong and X. L. Ji, "Hepatic angiomyolipoma-misdiagnosis as hepatocellular carcinoma: a report of 14 cases," *World Journal of Gastroenterology*, vol. 6, no. 4, pp. 608–612, 2000.

[14] T. K. F. Ma, M. K. Tse, W. M. S. Tsui, and K. T. Yuen, "Fine needle aspiration diagnosis of angiomyolipoma of the liver using a cell block with immunohistochemical study: a case report," *Acta Cytologica*, vol. 38, no. 2, pp. 257–260, 1994.

[15] I. Cha, D. Cartwright, M. Guis et al., "Angiomyolipoma of the liver in fine-needle aspiration biopsies: its distinction from hepatocellular carcinoma," *Cancer*, vol. 87, no. 1, pp. 25–30, 1999.

[16] C. Y. Yang, M. C. Ho, Y. M. Jeng, R. H. Hu, Y. M. Wu, and P. H. Lee, "Management of hepatic angiomyolipoma," *Journal of Gastrointestinal Surgery*, vol. 11, no. 4, pp. 452–457, 2007.

[17] A. Nonomura, Y. Enomoto, M. Takeda et al., "Invasive growth of hepatic angiomyolipoma; a hitherto unreported ominous histological feature," *Histopathology*, vol. 48, no. 7, pp. 831–835, 2006.

[18] I. Dalle, R. Sciot, R. De Vos et al., "Malignant angiomyolipoma of the liver: a hitherto unreported variant," *Histopathology*, vol. 36, no. 5, pp. 443–450, 2000.

[19] Y. C. Chang, H. M. Tsai, and N. H. Chow, "Hepatic angiomyolipoma with concomitant hepatocellular carcinomas," *Hepato-Gastroenterology*, vol. 48, no. 37, pp. 253–255, 2001.

[20] G. Guidi, O. Catalano, and A. Rotondo, "Spontaneous rupture of a hepatic angiomyolipoma: CT findings and literature review," *European Radiology*, vol. 7, no. 3, pp. 335–337, 1997.

6

Death from Liver Failure despite Lamivudine Prophylaxis during R-CHOP Chemotherapy due to Rapid Emergence M204 Mutations

Lay Lay Win,[1] Jeff Powis,[2] Hemant Shah,[1] Jordan J. Feld,[1] and David K. Wong[1]

[1] *Hepatology, Toronto Western Hospital, University of Toronto, 399 Bathurst Street, 6b-176, Toronto, ON, Canada M5T 2S8*
[2] *Infectious Diseases, Toronto East General Hospital, 825 Coxwell Avenue, East York, ON, Canada M4C 3E7*

Correspondence should be addressed to Lay Lay Win; laylay.win@gmail.com

Academic Editors: N. Koike, H. Nagahara, and N. Snyder

Background. Rapid and early emergence of clinically significant LAM resistance is thought to be unlikely during the first year of treatment, and as a result LAM is thought to be a reasonable choice as a first line agent for prophylaxis during chemotherapy. *Aim*. To report fatal HBV reactivation despite appropriate LAM prophylaxis in two previously treatment-naive individuals undergoing R-CHOP chemotherapy. *Case Presentation*. Case 1 is a 65-year-old man with chronic HBV infection: HBeAg-negative, HBV DNA 6.65E5 IU/mL, ALT 43 IU/L, and Fibroscan 4.4 kPa, consistent with F0, who was diagnosed with lymphoma that was treated with R-CHOP and LAM prophylaxis. HBV DNA fell to 2.18E1 IU/mL within 2 months of starting LAM. Four months after chemotherapy, despite ongoing LAM of 7-month duration with confirmed adherence, severe asymptomatic hepatitis was noted during routine monitoring with ALT 1019 IU/L, HBeAg negative, HBV DNA 1.43E7 IU/mL, and genotyping confirmed L80I and M204I mutations. He died 14 days after flare diagnosis despite a switch to tenofovir (HBV DNA had fallen to 1.94E5 IU/mL 2 weeks after starting tenofovir). Case 2 is a 50-year-old man who was found to have HBeAg-negative hepatitis B, ALT 37 IU/L, and no clinical features of cirrhosis (platelets 283, APRI 0.19) after lymphoma diagnosis. Lymphoma was treated with R-CHOP and LAM prophylaxis. Pretreatment HBV DNA was not done but was 8.90E4 IU/mL 3 weeks after starting LAM and 3.96E3 IU/mL 3 months after starting LAM. Two months after chemotherapy, despite ongoing LAM of 7-month duration with confirmed adherence, severe symptomatic hepatitis presenting with jaundice, abdominal pain, and confusion was noted. ALT 902 IU/L, HBeAg negative, HBV DNA 1.02E8 IU/mL, and genotyping confirmed L80I, M80V, and M204V/S mutations. He died 3 days after flare diagnosis despite the addition of tenofovir. *Conclusion*. Lamivudine should not be used for prophylaxis of patients with chronic hepatitis B with detectable HBV DNA undergoing chemotherapy with rituximab containing cytotoxic chemotherapy even if they have never had exposure to lamivudine in the past. In this setting, lamivudine failure due to resistance can develop quickly leading to liver failure that cannot be salvaged with tenofovir. Whether LAM is safe for prophylaxis with rituximab-based cytotoxic chemotherapy for patients with undetectable HBV DNA is unknown, but agents with a high barrier to resistance may be preferable.

1. Introduction

Reactivation of hepatitis B infection has been reported in 20%–50% of patients during conventional chemotherapy and up to 80% of patients during rituximab-containing chemotherapy [1]. Chemotherapy-induced reactivation occurs in not only hepatitis B surface antigen- (HBsAg-) positive patients but also in HBsAg-negative/anti-hepatitis B core antibody- (anti-HBc-) positive patients, particularly when rituximab is used [2]. Reactivation is thought to

reflect a loss of immune control resulting in abrupt increase in viral replication with or without ALT flare that can be asymptomatic or lead to jaundice in 26%, nonfatal liver failure in 3.7%, and even death in 7% of those with positive HBsAg [3].

The Centers for Disease Control and Prevention (CDC) recommends testing for HBsAg, anti-HBc, and anti-hepatitis B surface Ab (anti-HBs) in persons needing immunosuppressive therapy, including cancer chemotherapy, immunosuppression related to organ transplantation, and immunosuppression for rheumatological, dermatological, or gastroenterological disorders [4].

Many studies have shown the effectiveness of lamivudine to prevent chemotherapy-associated hepatitis B reactivation, with 2 meta-analyses showing a survival benefit to this approach [5, 6]. Katz et al. performed a systematic review and meta-analysis of the effectiveness of lamivudine for all chemoprophylaxis including rituximab-based chemotherapy and found a marked reduction in both clinical and virological reactivations compared to no treatment (OR 0.09; 95% confidence interval (CI) 0.05–0.14 and OR 0.04; 95% CI 0.01–0.20, resp.). All-cause mortality was significantly reduced in the patients who received lamivudine (OR 0.39; 95% CI 0.24–0.62), and prophylaxis also reduced HBV-related mortality (OR 0.20; 95% CI 0.09–0.45) and discontinuation or disruptions of the immunosuppressive treatment [5]. Loomba et al. showed a similar finding that the relative risk for both HBV reactivation and HBV-related hepatitis ranged from 0.00 to 0.21 with preventive lamivudine and none of the patients in the preventive lamivudine group developed HBV-related hepatic failure [6].

The American Association for the Study of Liver Diseases (AASLD) guidelines recommend prophylactic antiviral therapy for HBsAg-positive patients at the onset of immunosuppressive treatment and to continue for 6 months afterwards [7]. Clear guidelines on how to manage patients who are HBsAg negative/anti-HBc positive are lacking, but monitoring is required and it is recommended to start antiviral therapy if HBV DNA becomes detectable (AASLD guidelines Hepatology 2008).

Currently, lamivudine is still used as the first line antiviral agent for prophylaxis to prevent hepatitis B reactivation during immunosuppressive therapy, as it is cheap, safe, and well tolerated. However, the long-term efficacy of lamivudine is limited by the frequent emergence of lamivudine-resistant hepatitis B virus [8]. The incidence of resistance has been reported to be approximately 20% annually in immunocompetent patients receiving long-term treatment [9]. Pelizzari et al. analysed 32 cases of primary lamivudine prophylaxis given to HBV carriers with hematologic malignancies for median followup of 19.5 months and found that the HBV YMMD mutant occurred in only 3.1% of patients with no clinical relevance [10]. Rapid and early emergence of clinically significant resistance is thought to be unlikely during the first year of treatment, particularly for patients with low HBV DNA levels at baseline, and as a result, lamivudine is thought to be a reasonable choice as prophylaxis for most patients during chemotherapy, particularly those scheduled to require prophylaxis for less than one year (AASLD guidelines). This premise is challenged by our recent experience where fatal HBV reactivation was observed despite appropriate lamivudine prophylaxis in two previously treatment-naive individuals undergoing R-CHOP chemotherapy.

2. Case Report

2.1. Case 1. A 65-year-old Chinese man was diagnosed with stage IIA diffuse, large B-cell lymphoma in April 2011 after

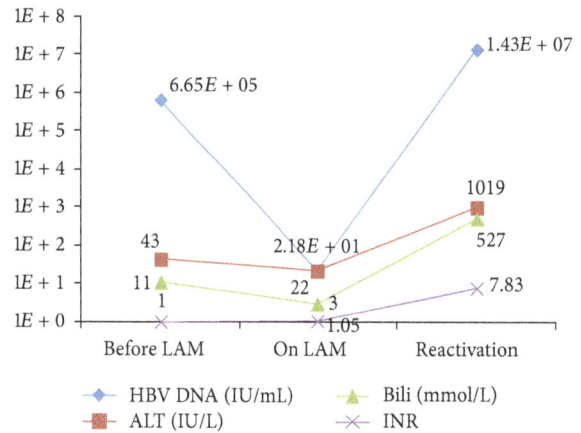

FIGURE 1: : Biochemical and HBV DNA VL changes in Case 1.

presenting with cervical lymphadenopathy. His past medical history was significant for hypertension, thyroidectomy in 2008 for papillary cancer, thalassemia trait, and right inguinal hernia. He was known to have chronic HBV infection but had been told he was an "inactive carrier" and did not receive regular followup and had never received antiviral therapy. He was taking levothyroxine 0.112 mg, valsartan 160 mg, and hydrochlorothiazide 12.5 mg daily. He was also found to have latent TB during screening before R-CHOP chemotherapy. He received the first cycle of R-CHOP on June 2, 2011. He was evaluated by the hepatology service the same week, and lamivudine 100 mg daily was started immediately, on June 10, 2011. Isoniazid 300 mg daily and pyridoxine 25 mg daily were started for latent TB on July 24, 2011, at the recommendation of the infectious disease consultant. Chemotherapy was complicated by febrile neutropenia after the second cycle of R-CHOP, treated with piperacillin-tazobactam (Tazocin) and filgrastim (neupogen), and he subsequently received levofloxacin prophylaxis for the fifth and sixth cycles of chemotherapy. Metformin was also started after the fifth cycle for hyperglycemia. He finished a total of 6 cycles of R-CHOP on September 16, 2011.

Evaluation of the hepatitis B status prechemotherapy showed that he was HBeAg negative and anti-HBe positive with an HBV DNA of 6.65E5 IU/mL and ALT of 43 IU/L. Fibroscan was 4.4 KPa, suggesting F0 (no) liver fibrosis. There was a good initial response to lamivudine, as HBV DNA fell to 2.18E1 IU/mL after 2 months of therapy. His ALT was 36 IU/L after two months, 22 IU/L after three months, and 23 IU/L after 4 months (October 2011) of treatment.

On January 18, 2012, ALT was found to be increased to 79 IU/L on routine bloodwork. Repeated bloodwork on February 2, 2012, 4 months after completing chemotherapy, showed ALT 877 IU/L, AST 1188 IU/L, ALP 118 IU/L, total bilirubin 226 mmol/L, INR 3.21, and HBV DNA 1.34E7 IU/mL (Figure 1). The patient was notably jaundiced but otherwise asymptomatic. He and his family confirmed adherence to lamivudine during and after completing chemotherapy. He was admitted to hospital, despite feeling well, and ALT peaked at ALT 1019 IU/L. INH was also discontinued; however the marked rise in HBV DNA was strongly suggestive of HBV-reactivation-associated hepatitis rather than INH hepatotoxicity. HBeAg remained negative, and genotyping with the INNO-LIPA assay confirmed L80I and M204I mutations, conferring lamivudine resistance. Tenofovir was started on presentation; however there was continued deterioration with investigations showing ALT 578 IU/L, AST 619 IU/L, ALP 121 IU/L, total bilirubin 534 mmol/L, INR 7.05, and HBV DNA 1.94E5 IU/mL. With the continued deterioration despite potent antiviral therapy, a decision was made to add prednisone therapy for a possible anti-inflammatory effect with continuation of tenofovir. Unfortunately there was no clinical response to prednisone, and the patient died on February 17, 2012, from progressive liver failure.

2.2. Case 2. A 50-year-old Canadian man of Chinese ancestry was diagnosed with stage III diffuse and large B-cell lymphoma in June 2011 after presenting with cervical lymphadenopathy. His past medical history was significant for gout and psoriasis for which he was using betamethasone/calcipotriol ointment (Dovobet) topically. Hepatitis B was diagnosed during screening for chemotherapy. He received the first cycle of R-CHOP on August 18, 2011, and lamivudine 100 mg daily was started on August 22, 2011. After the first cycle of R-CHOP chemotherapy, he had a significant ALT flare and the second cycle was postponed for 2 weeks with a subsequent 50% dose reduction during the second and third cycles of chemotherapy. He received full dose of chemotherapy after the third cycle. He finished 6 cycles of R-CHOP in February 2012.

Evaluation of the hepatitis B status prechemotherapy showed that he was HBeAg negative. Unfortunately, HBV DNA was not tested, but ALT was 37 IU/L. He did not have clinical evidence of advanced liver fibrosis (platelets 283 × 10E9/mL, AST 21 IU/L, APRI 0.19, suggesting F0 (no) liver fibrosis). After the first cycle of R-CHOP, 24 days after starting lamivudine, his ALT went up to 440 IU/L and AST to 115 IU/L. With the ALT flare, the HBV DNA was measured and found to be 8.90E4 IU/mL. He continued on lamivudine. His ALT subsequently normalized and remained normal during the next 5 cycles of chemotherapy. The HBV DNA was repeated in mid-October 2011 and had declined to 3.96E3 IU/mL, indicating at least a 1.4 log drop with 2 months of lamivudine therapy. The ALT was normal on subsequent testing in January 2012 (30 IU/L) and was found to be slightly elevated at 43 IU/L on March 19, 2012.

At the end of March 2012, he became unwell with fatigue, nausea, and vomiting. On April 10, 2012, two months after completing chemotherapy, while still on lamivudine, he became jaundiced and was admitted to the hospital with acute liver failure. At the time of admission, he had been taking lamivudine for a total of 7 months with confirmed adherence. Investigations revealed a peak ALT of 902 IU/L, AST 612 IU/L, total bilirubin 249 mmol/L, INR 7.3 (Figure 2). HBeAg status was not done, but HBV DNA was found to have risen to 1.02E8 IU/mL. Genotyping with the INNO-LIPA assay confirmed L80I, M80V, and M204V/S mutations,

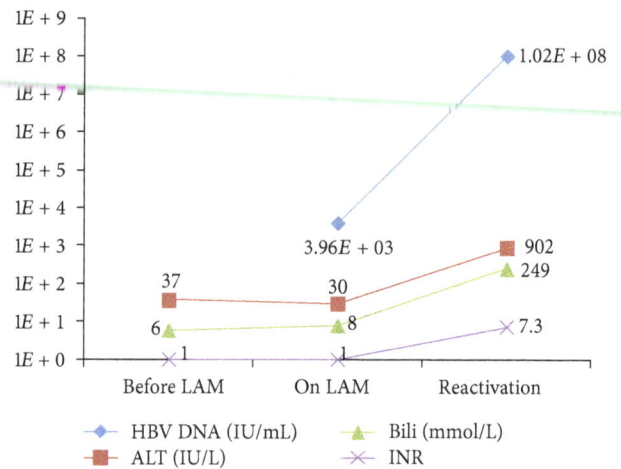

FIGURE 2: Biochemical and HBV DNA VL changes in Case 2.

conferring lamivudine resistance. Despite immediate addition of tenofovir, the patient died 3 days later.

3. Discussion

Hepatitis B reactivation due to chemotherapy is thought to occur from loss of HBV immune control allowing high-level HBV replication in hepatocytes. The subsequent immune reconstitution after chemotherapy can result in a severe inflammatory syndrome resulting in massive destruction of infected hepatocytes, hepatitis, and liver failure. Loss of HBV-specific immunity seems more likely if rituximab or steroid therapy is combined with standard cytotoxic chemotherapy [11, 12]. Rituximab is a monoclonal anti-CD20 antibody that causes long-lasting B-cell depletion that may last as long as 3 years after stopping the medication [13]. Why rituximab specifically leads to more frequent and potentially more severe HBV-reactivation is unknown but suggests the importance of B cells in HBV immune control.

The two cases presented were very similar (Table 1). Both patients had relatively inactive HBV infection with detectable HBV DNA but normal ALT and no evidence of advanced liver fibrosis. Importantly both patients were treatment-naïve. Both patients reported adherence with medication but neither adhered perfectly to the required monitoring for lamivudine therapy. HBV DNA monitoring is recommended every 3 months during lamivudine treatment. However patient 1 missed his November 2011 visit, which may have identified the presence of genotypic resistance before he presented with clinical liver failure 2 months later. Patient 2 did not have HBV DNA viral load before starting chemotherapy, he missed his March 2012 visit, and he presented with clinical symptoms 1 month later. As has been previously well described, both patients presented with HBV reactivation after completing chemotherapy, presumably due to immune reconstitution leading to hepatitis. Despite taking lamivudine for only 7 months with relatively low viral loads at baseline, both patients developed mutations conferring

TABLE 1: Basic characteristics and summary of cases.

Characteristics	Case 1	Case 2
Age (years)	65	50
Sex	Male	Male
Ethnicity	Chinese	Chinese
HBV status before chemotherapy	HBeAg negative, Anti-HBe positive, HBV DNA 6.65E5 IU/mL, ALT 43 IU/L	HBeAg negative, Anti-HBe positive, HBV DNA 8.90E4 IU/mL*, ALT 37 IU/L
Prior hepatitis B treatment	No	No
Clinical evidence of advanced liver fibrosis	Absent	Absent
Fibrosis stage	Fibroscan 4.4 KPa (F0)	APRI 0.19 (F0-1)
Comorbidities	Hypothyroid, hypertension, latent tuberculosis infection	Gout, psoriasis
Medications used	Levothyroxine, valsartan, isoniazid, pyridoxine, metformin	Calcipotriol/betamethasone ointment, Chinese herbal tea
Diffuse, large B-cell lymphoma stage	Stage IIA	Stage III
Lymphoma treatment	R-CHOP x 6	R-CHOP x 6
Lamivudine start date	8 days after first chemotherapy	4 days after first chemotherapy
HBV DNA after 2 months of LAM treatment	2.18E1 IU/mL	3.96E3 IU/mL
Time of HBV reactivation diagnosis	18 weeks after R-CHOP number 6	7 weeks after R-CHOP number 6
Duration of LAM at HBV reactivation	7 months	7 months
Lamivudine resistance pattern	L80I, M204I	L80I, M80V, M204V/S
HBV status at reactivation	HBeAg negative, anti-HBe positive, HBV DNA 1.43E7 IU/mL, ALT 1019 IU/L	HBV DNA 1.02E8 IU/mL, ALT 902 IU/L
Time to death despite tenofovir treatment	14 days	3 days

*HBV DNA at 24 days after starting lamivudine. No baseline HBV DNA was done before lamivudine treatment.

high-level lamivudine resistance, which ultimately led to HBV reactivation, liver failure, and rapid demise.

Although both patients started lamivudine after starting chemotherapy, the short delay in institution of antiviral therapy was unlikely to have affected their outcome. HBV reactivation typically occurs after the third cycle of rituximab-based chemotherapy [3]. The use of prednisone in the first patient was also somewhat atypical; however this was only added after the patient presented with liver failure and had no response to tenofovir. Antiviral therapy does not work immediately, and the liver dysfunction in the acute setting is due primarily to overwhelming hepatic inflammation. Therefore it was felt that the anti-inflammatory effect of prednisone may be helpful, recognizing that with or without steroids the mortality in this setting was likely to be extremely high.

AASLD guidelines recommend that tenofovir or entecavir could be used as an alternative to lamivudine, particularly in patients who are anticipated to require more than 12 months of therapy in whom there is a higher risk of developing lamivudine resistance. Li et al. compared entecavir and lamivudine in preventing hepatitis B reactivation in lymphoma patients during chemotherapy and found significantly lower rates of hepatitis (5.9 versus 27.0%,

$P = 0.007$), hepatitis B reactivation (0 versus 12.4%, $P = 0.024$), and disruption of chemotherapy (5.9 versus 20.2%, $P = 0.042$) in the entecavir-treated patients [14]. There are no specific data comparing tenofovir with other agents in this setting; however its potency, very high barrier to resistance and good safety profile make it a reasonable alternative.

Although only 2 cases, this report highlights that resistance to lamivudine may emerge quickly during immunosuppressive therapy with potentially severe consequences. The use of a more potent agent with a higher barrier to resistance (entecavir or tenofovir) would likely significantly reduce the risk of HBV reactivation due to antiviral resistance. Arguably had both patients adhered strictly to recommended followup, lamivudine resistance may have been recognized before significant hepatitis occurred, which may have led to improved outcomes. However, particularly during cancer chemotherapy with the many potential unforeseen eventualities, followup with scheduled HBV DNA testing may not be strictly followed. Use of an antiviral agent with a lower risk of resistance would reduce the risk that lapses in scheduled followup and would have significant clinical consequences. A trial to compare the efficacy of different antiviral agents to prevent HBV-reactivation during immunosuppressive therapy is unlikely to be performed, and hence inferences may have to be drawn from case reports, case series, and existing data in other clinical settings.

4. Conclusion

Lamivudine should not be used for prophylaxis of patients with chronic hepatitis B, especially with detectable HBV DNA, undergoing chemotherapy with rituximab-based chemotherapy even if lamivudine treatment-naive. In this setting, lamivudine resistance may develop quickly with the risk of severe HBV reactivation and subsequent liver failure that cannot be salvaged with tenofovir. If lamivudine is used initially for chemoprophylaxis, close monitoring of HBV DNA is required with consideration of a switch to a more potent agent with a higher genetic barrier to resistance if HBV DNA is not suppressed to undetectable levels within 3 months.

References

[1] S. Kusumoto, Y. Tanaka, R. Ueda, and M. Mizokami, "Reactivation of hepatitis B virus following rituximab-plus-steroid combination chemotherapy," *Journal of Gastroenterology*, vol. 46, no. 1, pp. 9–16, 2011.

[2] A. M. Evens, B. D. Jovanovic, Y.-C. Su et al., "Rituximab-associated hepatitis B virus (HBV) reactivation in lymphoproliferative diseases: metaanalysis and examination of FDA safety reports," *Annals of Oncology*, vol. 22, no. 5, pp. 1170–1180, 2011.

[3] U. Zurawska, L. Hicks, G. Woo, C. Bell, M. Krahn et al., "Hepatitis B virus screening before chemotherapy for lymphoma: a cost-effectiveness analysis," *Journal of Clinical Oncology*, vol. 30, no. 26, pp. 3167–3173, 2012.

[4] C. M. Weinbaum, E. E. Mast, and J. W. Ward, "Recommendations for identification and public health management of persons with chronic hepatitis B virus infection," *Hepatology*, vol. 49, no. 5, pp. S35–S44, 2009.

[5] L. H. Katz, A. Fraser, A. Gafter-Gvili, L. Leibovici, and R. Tur-Kaspa, "Lamivudine prevents reactivation of hepatitis B and reduces mortality in immunosuppressed patients: systematic review and meta-analysis," *Journal of Viral Hepatitis*, vol. 15, no. 2, pp. 89–102, 2008.

[6] R. Loomba, A. Rowley, R. Wesley et al., "Systematic review: the effect of preventive lamivudine on hepatitis B reactivation during chemotherapy," *Annals of Internal Medicine*, vol. 148, no. 7, pp. 519–528, 2008.

[7] A. S. F. Lok and B. J. McMahon, "Chronic hepatitis B: update 2009," *Hepatology*, vol. 50, no. 3, pp. 661–662, 2009.

[8] N. Leung, "Clinical experience with lamivudine," *Seminars in Liver Disease*, vol. 22, no. 1, pp. 15–21, 2002.

[9] F. Von Weizsäcker, "Management of chronic hepatitis B," *Praxis*, vol. 94, no. 16, pp. 649–652, 2005.

[10] A. M. Pelizzari, M. Motta, E. Cariani, P. Turconi, E. Borlenghi, and G. Rossi, "Frequency of hepatitis B virus mutant in asymptomatic hepatitis B virus carriers receiving prophylactic lamivudine during chemotherapy for hematologic malignancies," *Hematology Journal*, vol. 5, no. 4, pp. 325–328, 2004.

[11] A.-L. Cheng, C. A. Hsiung, I.-J. Su et al., "Steroid-free chemotherapy decreases risk of hepatitis B virus (HBV) reactivation in HBV-carriers with lymphoma," *Hepatology*, vol. 37, no. 6, pp. 1320–1328, 2003.

[12] W. Yeo, T. C. Chan, N. W. Y. Leung et al., "Hepatitis B virus reactivation in lymphoma patients with prior resolved hepatitis B undergoing anticancer therapy with or without rituximab," *Journal of Clinical Oncology*, vol. 27, no. 4, pp. 605–611, 2009.

[13] M. J. Arin, A. Engert, T. Krieg, and N. Hunzelmann, "Anti-CD20 monoclonal antibody (rituximab) in the treatment of pemphigus," *British Journal of Dermatology*, vol. 153, no. 3, pp. 620–625, 2005.

[14] H.-R. Li, J.-J. Huang, H.-Q. Guo et al., "Comparison of entecavir and lamivudine in preventing hepatitis B reactivation in lymphoma patients during chemotherapy," *Journal of Viral Hepatitis*, vol. 18, no. 12, pp. 877–883, 2011.

7

Systemic Mastocytosis: A Rare Case of Increased Liver Stiffness

Stefanie Adolf,[1] Gunda Millonig,[1] Helmut Karl Seitz,[1] Andreas Reiter,[2] Peter Schirmacher,[3] Thomas Longerich,[3] and Sebastian Mueller[1]

[1] *Department of Medicine, Salem Medical Center and Alcohol Research Center, University of Heidelberg, Zeppelinstraße 11-33, 69121 Heidelberg, Germany*
[2] *Department of Medicine III, Mannheim Hospital, University of Heidelberg, Wiesbadener Straße 7-11, 68305 Mannheim, Germany*
[3] *Institute of Pathology, University of Heidelberg, Im Neuenheimer Feld 220/221, 69120 Heidelberg, Germany*

Correspondence should be addressed to Sebastian Mueller, sebastian.mueller@urz.uni-heidelberg.de

Academic Editors: D. Y. Kim, D. Lorenzin, V. Lorenzo-Zúñiga, and C. Miyabayashi

Assessment of liver stiffness (LS) by transient elastography (Fibroscan) has significantly improved the noninvasive diagnosis of liver fibrosis. We here report on a 55-year-old patient with drastically increased LS due to previously unknown systemic mastocytosis. The patient initially presented with increased weight loss, nocturnal pruritus, increased transaminases, bilirubinemia, and thrombocytopenia. Abdominal ultrasound showed ascites, hepatomegaly, and splenomegaly. In addition, LS was 75 kPa (IQR 0 kPa) clearly exceeding the cut-off value for F4 cirrhosis of 12.5 kPa. However, histological analysis of the liver specimen indicated liver involvement by systemic mastocytosis and excluded liver cirrhosis. An additional CT scan detected disseminated bone lesions. After three months of treatment with Midostaurin, LS slightly decreased down to 31.9 kPa (IQR 8.3 kPa). This case illustrates that diffused sinusoidal neoplastic infiltrates are a pitfall in the non-invasive diagnosis of liver cirrhosis. In conclusion, refined clinical algorithms for increased LS should also include mastocytosis in addition to inflammation, congestion, and biliary obstruction.

1. Introduction

In the last six years, transient elastography [TE, Fibroscan] has become an established key tool for the rapid and non-invasive assessment of liver fibrosis and cirrhosis [1]. TE determines liver stiffness (LS) with high reproducibility in about 95% of all patients and LS has been shown to be in excellent agreement with the degree of fibrosis stage in patients with various liver diseases [2–5]. On the basis of these studies, a cut-off value of above 12.5 kPa has been elaborated for the discrimination of liver cirrhosis (F4) while LS values below 6 kPa are considered as normal [6, 7]. Liver biopsy which is the gold standard for assessing hepatic fibrosis or cirrhosis is an invasive procedure, with rare but potentially severe complications. In addition, the accuracy of liver biopsy in assessing fibrosis has limitations because of well-known sampling errors and interobserver variability [8–12]. Nevertheless, liver biopsy and measurement of LS should be regarded as synergistic diagnostic approaches. Thus, while the sampling error of TE is significantly less with regard to fibrosis assessment as compared to biopsy, histology

provides many valuable diagnostic information. In addition, factors have been identified that increase LS irrespective of fibrosis. Such factors include hepatic congestion [13], inflammation [14, 15], or cholestasis [16]. To avoid potential misinterpretations of increased LS, the precise knowledge of these factors has an important impact on the usage of TE for fibrosis assessment. Recently, new refined algorithms have been developed to increase the diagnostic accuracy [7, 17] of LS that include a timely abdominal ultrasound and laboratory tests. Here we describe a case of hepatic involvement in systemic mastocytosis with drastically elevated LS in the absence of cirrhosis. Thus, a further clinical entity is added to the differential diagnosis of increased LS underscoring the necessity of accurate disease typing for LS assessment.

2. Case Presentation

A 55-year-old man was admitted to our hospital with weight loss of 20 kg in 6 months, fatigue, and increasing nocturnal pruritus mainly in lower extremities. The remaining patient's history was uneventful. The physical examination was normal except for slightly enlarged painless submandibular lymph nodes. Chest X-ray and electrocardiogram were normal. Initial laboratory tests showed anemia (Hb 9.6 g/dl) and significant thrombocytopenia (65/nl). White blood count was elevated (15.8/nl) as was the C-reactive protein with 21.7 mg/l (normal <0.5). Liver enzymes were elevated (GOT 65 U/l, GPT 74 U/l, GGT 329, AP 830 U/l, bilirubin 2.4 mg/dl) while synthesis parameters such as albumin and INR were normal. Serum ferritin was also elevated (581 ng/ml).

Abdominal ultrasound showed ascites and an enlarged liver (craniocaudal diameter of 19 cm) and spleen (16.3 cm). Liver echogenicity was homogenous and there were no classical signs of liver cirrhosis detectable such as nodular aspect of the liver surface or collaterals such as a revascularized umbilical vein. LS assessed by Fibroscan (XL probe) was drastically increased with 75 kPa (IQR 0 kPa, success rate 100%). This value represents the upper detection limit of the Fibroscan device and exceeds by far the cut-off value of cirrhosis (F4; 12.5 kPa). An additional CT scan revealed disseminated bone metastasis and was suspicious of peritoneal carcinomatosis. Endoscopy of the upper and lower gastrointestinal tract was normal.

A liver biopsy was performed that revealed a mild portal fibrosis but excluded liver cirrhosis (Figure 1). In contrast, there were portal, sinusoidal, and micronodular infiltrates of spindle cells with round to oval nuclei with dense chromatin and moderately developed pale cytoplasm. These cells were positive for CD117 (c-kit) and CD68 and negative for CD1a by immunohistochemistry and were thus identified as mast cells.

A cutaneous manifestation of the mastocytosis was evident by reddening of body and lower extremities and red papules pretibially and was confirmed by a skin biopsy. During staging a bone marrow biopsy was taken which demonstrated an extensive bone marrow infiltration by atypical mast cells and a significantly reduced haematopoiesis (Figure 2). Genetic analysis of the bone marrow allowed the identification of a point mutation (D816V) within the kit gene (c-Kit) which is known to be responsible for hyperactivation of the growth receptor Kit (tyrosine kinase) on the mast cell surface [18]. Thus, the diagnosis of systemic mastocytosis was established in this patient. Accordingly, serum tryptase levels were found to be elevated with 200 ng/l (normal 1–11.3 ng/ml).

The excessive infiltration of the bone marrow and other extracutaneous organs with mast cells suggested that the patient suffered from aggressive systemic mastocytosis. This was confirmed by the presence of several additional key criteria for the aggressive form (so-called c-findings) such as cytopenia, enlarged liver and spleen, ascites, malabsorption, and weight loss. Consequently, immediate treatment with a tyrosine kinase inhibitor was initiated. Dasatinib was used since Kit-D816V positive patients are known to be resistant against Imatinib. In addition, the patients pruritus was treated with H-1 blockers. Proton pump inhibitors were administered to prevent gastric ulcer development. Since the patient did not respond to Dasatinib within 6

weeks and diarrhea deteriorated, he was enrolled in the PKC412 study with Midostaurin. Restaging after 6 weeks also showed progressive disease including a further enlargement of spleen, liver as well as cervical, axillar, and inguinal lymph nodes, an increase of tryptase levels to 410 µg/l, an increasing diffuse sclerosis of the skeleton, and an increased bone density. At the moment, the patient has slightly improved after three months of treatment with Midostaurin and liver stiffness decreased down to 31.9 kPa (IQR 8.3 kPa, success rate 100%).

3. Discussion

3.1. Systemic Mastocytosis. Mastocytosis is defined as clonal expansion and accumulation of mast cells in at least one organ [19]. Incidence is low with five cases per 1 million people; most of the cases occur in children. According to the WHO, major manifestations include cutaneous or systemic forms [20]. The D816V point mutation within the tyrosine kinase Kit (*c-Kit*) that is detected in 80% of cases is considered a driver mutation causing the permanent receptor activation and consequent proliferation, and thus neoplastic expansion of the mutated mast cell clone. The activation of several additional oncogenes and other mutations probably contributes to the development of the more aggressive form present in our patient [21]. General symptoms such as hypotension, flush, and dyspnea are directly caused by mast cell activation while local symptoms are due to organ infiltration. Bone marrow involvement is present in most patients (90%) followed by involvement of gastrointestinal tract, liver, spleen, and lymph nodes. Gastrointestinal manifestations are unspecific and include abdominal pain, nausea, vomiting, and diarrhea [22, 23]. For complete staging of systemic mastocytosis, a bone marrow biopsy is required. At present, tyrosine kinase inhibitors are the major treatment strategy. Imatinib is rarely used since 80% of patients have the D816V genotype and are therefore resistant to this drug. Dasatinib is more potent and well tolerated [24]. Novel drugs include Nilotinib (BCR-ABL tyrosine kinase inhibitor) and Midostaurin [25]. Midostaurin is a potent inhibitor of the tyrosine kinase FTL3 (Fetal-Liver-Tyrosine-Kinase 3), a receptor of the hematopoetic precursor cell. A recent phase II study on 20 patients with refractory AML or high-grade myelodysplastic syndrome showed a significant reduction of peripheral blasts [26]. At the moment, Midostaurin is studied in phase III for the treatment of acute myeloid leukemia and aggressive form of systemic mastocytosis [27].

3.2. Increased Liver Stiffness by Systemic Mastocytosis. The present case is remarkable for two reasons. First, it is the first description of a drastically increased LS in a patient with hepatic involvement by systemic mastocytosis. Second, it adds a further if not rare clinical entity to the differential diagnoses of increased LS. Although LS is now well established as excellent non-invasive parameter for the assessment of liver cirrhosis, other clinical conditions such as hepatic congestion [13], inflammation [14, 15], or cholestasis [16] are known to drastically increase LS independent of fibrosis

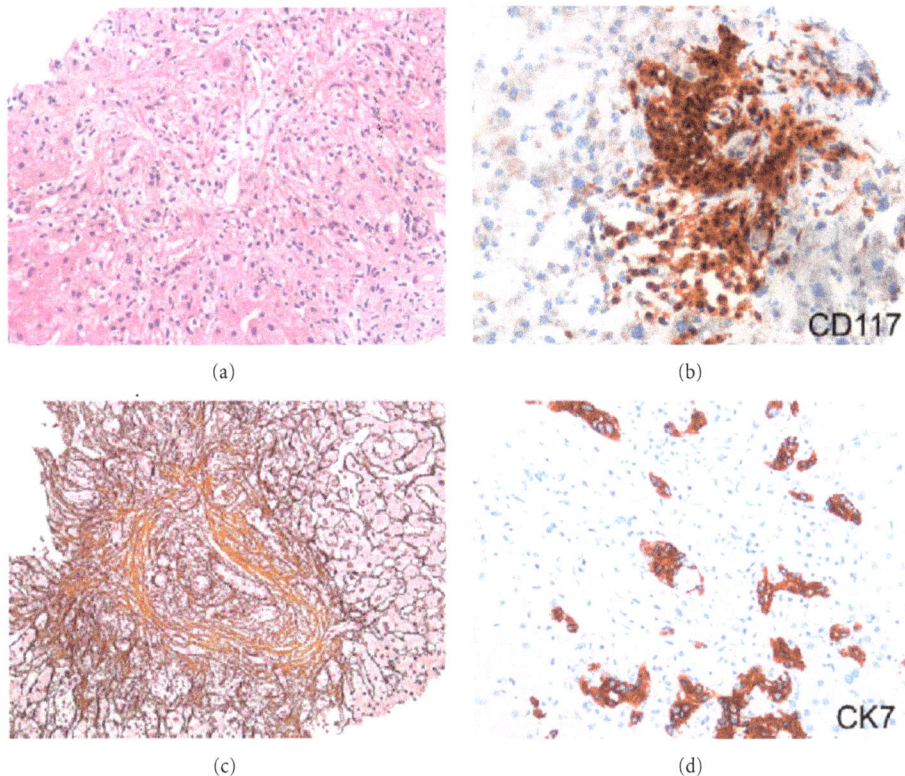

FIGURE 1: Liver biopsy of the patient with drastically increased liver stiffness due to mast cell infiltrates. (a) Infiltration of portal tract and liver sinusoids with neoplastic mast cell like cells (HE). (b) CD117 immunostaining shows nodular infiltration with mast cells. (c) Portal, periportal, and perisinusoidal fibrosis (modified Gomori stain. 200×). (d) CK7 immunostain identifies neoplastic mast cells that infiltrate the portal bile ducts and ductular structures 200×.

stage. In addition, deposition of hepatic amyloid was shown to increase LS in the absence of cirrhosis [28, 29].

We have recently suggested that these LS interfering conditions can be separated in two major categories [7, 17]: either they are caused by deposition of matrix such as collagen during fibrogenesis or they are associated with an increase in intrahepatic pressure such as in mechanic cholestasis or liver congestion (Figure 3). Inflammation-dependent increase of LS is also predominantly pressure driven since it is accompanied by infiltration with inflammatory cells, increase of interstitial fluid, and increase of cellular size (ballooning). The major goal for an optimal diagnostic interpretation of LS, therefore, is exact disease typing to clearly discriminate in a patient between matrix- and pressure-associated conditions. For these reasons, we consider abdominal ultrasound and laboratory tests mandatory for the correct interpretation of LS by TE [7]. Ultrasound imaging is a very robust and rapid way to exclude manifest cholestasis, nodular liver masses, or congestion.

Our present case of systemic mastocytosis in which diagnosis was primarily established by liver biopsy fits within this concept. Under these conditions, the liver was massively infiltrated by mast cells which, in turn, caused an increase of liver volume and LS, consequently. Since the patient also showed increased transaminases, bilirubin levels, thrombocytopenia, and ascites, he could have been easily mistaken for

having cirrhosis by superficial screening although some of his complaints were atypical for liver cirrhosis such as the rapid weight loss and nocturnal pruritus. From the basic exams, normal liver synthesis parameters and the absence of classical sonographic signs of cirrhosis are highly indicative that liver cirrhosis might not be the correct diagnosis. The increased LS seems to be predominantly due to mast cell infiltration since transaminase levels were only mildly increased and below 100 U/l. Moreover, during treatment, LS decreased by 50% in the absence of increased transaminases. False positive elevation of LS due to ascites can also be ruled out although ascites had been previously regarded as an exclusion criterion for transient elastography. Recently, we could demonstrated that (a) TE can be performed in the presence of ascites using the XL or sometimes even the M probe (b) consequent increased intra-abdominal pressure does not affect LS and (c) a normal LS allows to exclude hepatic causes of ascites [30].

Figure 4 shows an updated diagnostic algorithms for the interpretation of LS. At present, with the use of the available probes (S, M, and XL probe), 95% of all patients can be measured by TE. While a normal LS rules out any severe chronic liver disease [7], abdominal ultrasound and lab tests should be performed in the case of increased LS to exclude congestion, cholestasis, or, as shown here, infiltration with mast cells. In cases of elevated transaminases higher than 100 U/l, diagnosis of cirrhosis is also uncertain

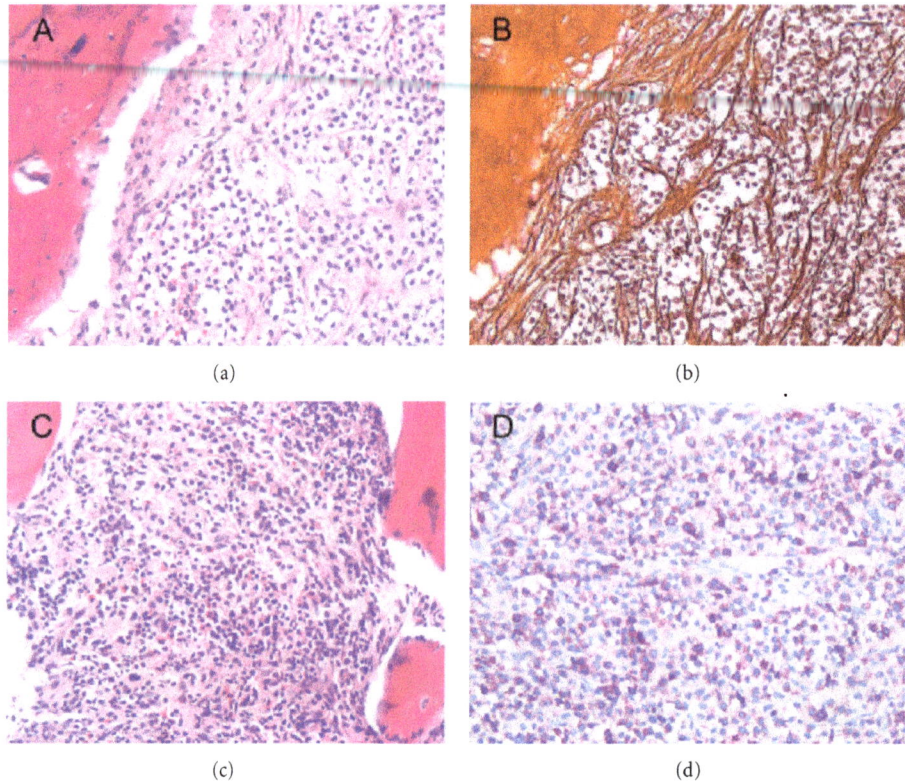

(a)

(b)

(c)

(d)

FIGURE 2: Bone marrow specimen of the patient with systemic mastocytosis. (a) Diffuse infiltration of the bone marrow with neoplastic mast cells and massive displacement of hematopoetic cells (HE). (b) Induction of myelofibrosis by neoplastic cells (modified Gomori stain). (c) Residual hematopoiesis besides neoplastic infiltrates (HE). (d) Giemsa staining shows cytoplasmatic granules of neoplastic mast cells 200×.

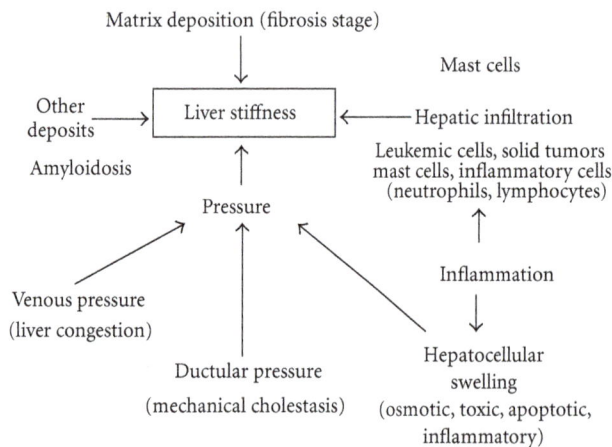

FIGURE 3: Factors that affect liver stiffness including mast cell infiltration.

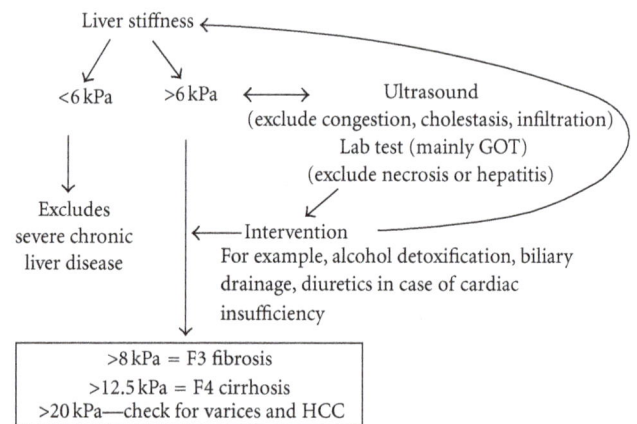

FIGURE 4: Present clinical algorithms for the interpretation of increased liver stiffness.

unless LS exceeds 30 kPa. To discriminate between cirrhosis and these interfering factors, interventions are necessary such as antidiuretic therapy, decompression of the bile duct, for example, by biliary drainage, or treatment of the underlying hepatitis, for example, alcohol detoxification [13, 16, 17]. These interventions will eventually remove the "pressure associated component" of increased LS. We recently demonstrated that reassessment of LS after such

interventions correlated much better with fibrosis stage [17]. Our case also shows that LS may actually prompt in some cases to a liver biopsy. Previously, there had been the fear that LS measurements will spare most patients from liver biopsies [5, 31] and indeed there are certainly situations now where liver biopsies can be omitted or postponed. However, as shown in our case, increased LS in the context of conflicting clinical findings is indicative that further histological evaluation may be necessary to finally settle the diagnosis.

In our opinion, the case further demonstrates that increased LS cannot be interpreted as liver cirrhosis automatically. Instead, exact disease typing supported by additional information such as ultrasound imaging, laboratory tests, and other clinical findings is critical for the correct interpretation of LS. In some cases, the pathologically elevated LS may even prompt the patient to further histological analysis. Therefore, we add mast cell infiltration as additional LS increasing condition.

Abbreviations

LS: Liver stiffness
TE: Transient elastography.

Acknowledgments

This study was supported by a grant from the Dietmar Hopp and the Dietmar Lautenschläger Foundation.

References

[1] L. Sandrin, B. Fourquet, J. M. Hasquenoph et al., "Transient elastography: a new noninvasive method for assessment of hepatic fibrosis," *Ultrasound in Medicine and Biology*, vol. 29, no. 12, pp. 1705–1713, 2003.

[2] J. Foucher, L. Castéra, P. H. Bernard et al., "Prevalence and factors associated with failure of liver stiffness measurement using FibroScan in a prospective study of 2114 examinations," *European Journal of Gastroenterology and Hepatology*, vol. 18, no. 4, pp. 411–412, 2006.

[3] L. Castéra, J. Vergniol, J. Foucher et al., "Prospective comparison of transient elastography, Fibrotest, APRI, and liver biopsy for the assessment of fibrosis in chronic hepatitis C," *Gastroenterology*, vol. 128, no. 2, pp. 343–350, 2005.

[4] N. Ganne-Carrié, M. Ziol, V. de Ledinghen et al., "Accuracy of liver stiffness measurement for the diagnosis of cirrhosis in patients with chronic liver diseases," *Hepatology*, vol. 44, no. 6, pp. 1511–1517, 2006.

[5] M. Friedrich-Rust, M. F. Ong, S. Martens et al., "Performance of transient elastography for the staging of liver fibrosis: a meta-analysis," *Gastroenterology*, vol. 134, no. 4, pp. 960–974, 2008.

[6] L. Castera and M. Pinzani, "Biopsy and non-invasive methods for the diagnosis of liver fibrosis: does it take two to tango?" *Gut*, vol. 59, no. 7, pp. 861–866, 2010.

[7] S. Mueller and L. Sandrin, "Liver stiffness: a novel parameter for the diagnosis of liver disease," *Hepatic Medicine*, vol. 2, pp. 49–67, 2010.

[8] W. Abdi, J. C. Millan, and E. Mezey, "Sampling variability on percutaneous liver biopsy," *Archives of Internal Medicine*, vol. 139, no. 6, pp. 667–669, 1979.

[9] P. Bedossa, D. Dargère, and V. Paradis, "Sampling variability of liver fibrosis in chronic hepatitis C," *Hepatology*, vol. 38, no. 6, pp. 1449–1457, 2003.

[10] J. F. Cadranel, P. Rufat, and F. Degos, "Practices of liver biopsy in France: results of a prospective nationwide survey," *Hepatology*, vol. 32, no. 3, pp. 477–481, 2000.

[11] B. Maharaj, R. J. Maharaj, W. P. Leary et al., "Sampling variability and its influence on the diagnostic yield of percutaneous needle biopsy of the liver," *The Lancet*, vol. 1, no. 8480, pp. 523–525, 1986.

[12] A. Regev, M. Berho, L. J. Jeffers et al., "Sampling error and intraobserver variation in liver biopsy in patients with chronic HCV infection," *American Journal of Gastroenterology*, vol. 97, no. 10, pp. 2614–2618, 2002.

[13] G. Millonig, S. Friedrich, S. Adolf et al., "Liver stiffness is directly influenced by central venous pressure," *Journal of Hepatology*, vol. 52, no. 2, pp. 206–210, 2010.

[14] U. Arena, F. Vizzutti, G. Corti et al., "Acute viral hepatitis increases liver stiffness values measured by transient elastography," *Hepatology*, vol. 47, no. 2, pp. 380–384, 2008.

[15] A. Sagir, A. Erhardt, M. Schmitt, and D. Häussinger, "Transient elastography is unreliable for detection of cirrhosis in patients with acute liver damage," *Hepatology*, vol. 47, no. 2, pp. 592–595, 2008.

[16] G. Millonig, F. M. Reimann, S. Friedrich et al., "Extrahepatic cholestasis increases liver stiffness (fibroScan) irrespective of fibrosis," *Hepatology*, vol. 48, no. 5, pp. 1718–1723, 2008.

[17] S. Mueller, G. Millonig, L. Sarovska et al., "Increased liver stiffness in alcoholic liver disease: differentiating fibrosis from steatohepatitis," *World Journal of Gastroenterology*, vol. 16, no. 8, pp. 966–972, 2010.

[18] S. Schnittger, T. M. Kohl, T. Haferlach et al., "KIT-D816 mutations in AML1-ETO-positive AML are associated with impaired event-free and overall survival," *Blood*, vol. 107, no. 5, pp. 1791–1799, 2006.

[19] M. R. Johnson, S. Verstovsek, J. L. Jorgensen et al., "Utility of the World Heath Organization classification criteria for the diagnosis of systemic mastocytosis in bone marrow," *Modern Pathology*, vol. 22, no. 1, pp. 50–57, 2009.

[20] H. P. Horny, K. Sotlar, and P. Valent, "Mastocytosis: state of the art," *Pathobiology*, vol. 74, no. 2, pp. 121–132, 2007.

[21] P. Valent, C. Akin, W. R. Sperr et al., "Mastocytosis: pathology, genetics, and current options for therapy," *Leukemia and Lymphoma*, vol. 46, no. 1, pp. 35–48, 2005.

[22] R. T. Jensen, "Gastrointestinal abnormalities and involvement in systemic mastocytosis," *Hematology/Oncology Clinics of North America*, vol. 14, no. 3, pp. 579–623, 2000.

[23] U. Mickys, A. Barakauskiene, C. De Wolf-Peeters, K. Geboes, and G. De Hertogh, "Aggressive systemic mastocytosis complicated by protein-losing enteropathy," *Digestive and Liver Disease*, vol. 39, no. 7, pp. 693–697, 2007.

[24] N. P. Shah, F. Y. Lee, R. Luo, Y. Jiang, M. Donker, and C. Akin, "Dasatinib (BMS-354825) inhibits KITD816V, an imatinib-resistant activating mutation that triggers neoplastic growth in most patients with systemic mastocytosis," *Blood*, vol. 108, no. 1, pp. 286–291, 2006.

[25] E. Weisberg, P. Manley, J. Mestan, S. Cowan-Jacob, A. Ray, and J. D. Griffin, "AMN107 (nilotinib): a novel and selective inhibitor of BCR-ABL," *British Journal of Cancer*, vol. 94, no. 12, pp. 1765–1769, 2006.

[26] R. M. Stone, D. J. DeAngelo, V. Klimek et al., "Patients with acute myeloid leukemia and an activating mutation in FLT3 respond to a small-molecule FLT3 tyrosine kinase inhibitor, PKC412," *Blood*, vol. 105, no. 1, pp. 54–60, 2005.

[27] M. Sanz, A. Burnett, F. Lo-Coco, and B. Lowenoerg, "FLT3 inhibition as a targeted therapy for acute myeloid leukemia," *Current Opinion in Oncology*, vol. 21, no. 6, pp. 594–600, 2009.

[28] A. Cypierre, A. Jaccard, A. Rousseau et al., "Fibroscan is a non-invasive tool for detecting hepatic amyloidosis," *Hepatology*, vol. 50, article 921, 2009.

[29] A. Lanzi, A. Gianstefani, M. G. Mirarchi, P. Pini, F. Conti, and L. Bolondi, "Liver AL amyloidosis as a possible cause of high liver stiffness values," *European Journal of Gastroenterology and Hepatology*, vol. 22, no. 7, pp. 895–897, 2010.

[30] A. Kohlhaas, E. Durango, G. Millonig et al., "Transient elastography with the XL probe rapidly identifies patients with non-hepatic ascites," *Hepatic Medicine*, vol. 4, pp. 11–18, 2012.

[31] G. Sebastiani, P. Halfon, L. Castera et al., "SAFE biopsy: a validated method for large-scale staging of liver fibrosis in chronic hepatitis C," *Hepatology*, vol. 49, no. 6, pp. 1821–1827, 2009.

8

Asymptomatic Liver Abscesses Mimicking Metastases in Patients after Whipple Surgery: Infectious Complications following Percutaneous Biopsy—A Report of Two Cases

Kan K. Zhang,[1] **Majid Mayody,**[1] **Rajesh P. Shah,**[2] **Efsevia Vakiani,**[1]
George I. Getrajdman,[1] **Lynn A. Brody,**[1] **and Stephen B. Solomon**[1]

[1] Division of Interventional Radiology, Department of Radiology, Memorial Sloan-Kettering Cancer Center (MSKCC),
 1275 York Avenue, M276C, New York, NY 10065, USA
[2] Stanford Hospital and Clinics, Stanford, CA 94305, USA

Correspondence should be addressed to Majid Mayody, maybodym@mskcc.org

Academic Editors: A. Grasso, A. Irisawa, and C. Miyabayashi

We present two cases of hepatic abscesses that mimicked metastases in patients having undergone Whipple surgery. Both patients had similar imaging features on computed tomographic (CT) scan and ultrasound, and at the time of referral for biopsy neither patient was clinically suspected to have liver abscess. Both patients underwent biopsy of liver lesions and developed postprocedural infectious complications.

1. Introduction

Cancer patients require frequent cross-sectional imaging to assess for progression of disease. The liver is a common site of metastasis for many cancers. New liver lesions in cancer patients are likely to be metastases and biopsy is commonly performed to confirm the diagnosis.

Less frequently, new liver lesions in cancer patients can have an infectious etiology. In patients with biliary, duodenal, or pancreatic cancer, Whipple surgery (pancreaticoduodenectomy) and other biliary interventions which remove or disrupt the sphincter of Oddi and allow bacterial colonization of the biliary tree increase the risk of hepatic abscess formation [1]. Liver-directed therapies can exacerbate infection in these high-risk patients [2].

Liver abscess typically is the result of a pyogenic or amoebic infection and generally cause symptoms including fever and leukocytosis. It is possible, however, that the episode of infection that preceded liver abscess formation either remains subclinical or coincides with other postoperative issues. So when new liver lesions are found on surveillance cross-sectional imaging studies, infection is rarely considered, particularly in the absence of suggestive clinical history and laboratory abnormalities. We present two cases of hepatic abscesses that mimicked metastases in patients having undergone Whipple surgery. Both patients had similar imaging features on computed tomographic (CT) scan and ultrasound, and at the time of referral for biopsy neither patient was clinically suspected to have liver abscess. Both patients underwent biopsy of liver lesions and developed postprocedural infectious complications.

2. Case Report

2.1. Case 1. A 73-year-old woman with history of Crohn's disease and cholangiocarcinoma invading the duodenum and pancreas underwent pancreaticoduodenectomy (PD). A surveillance CT scan performed several weeks after the surgery revealed two new hepatic lesions (Figure 1(a)). She had no clinical symptoms. She was referred to the interventional radiology service for biopsy of a liver lesion and for placement of a venous infusion port. Complete blood count, liver function tests, coagulation profile, and basic metabolic profile were all within normal limits. The liver biopsy was performed under moderate sedation with the patient in the supine position. Under CT guidance, a 2.5 cm

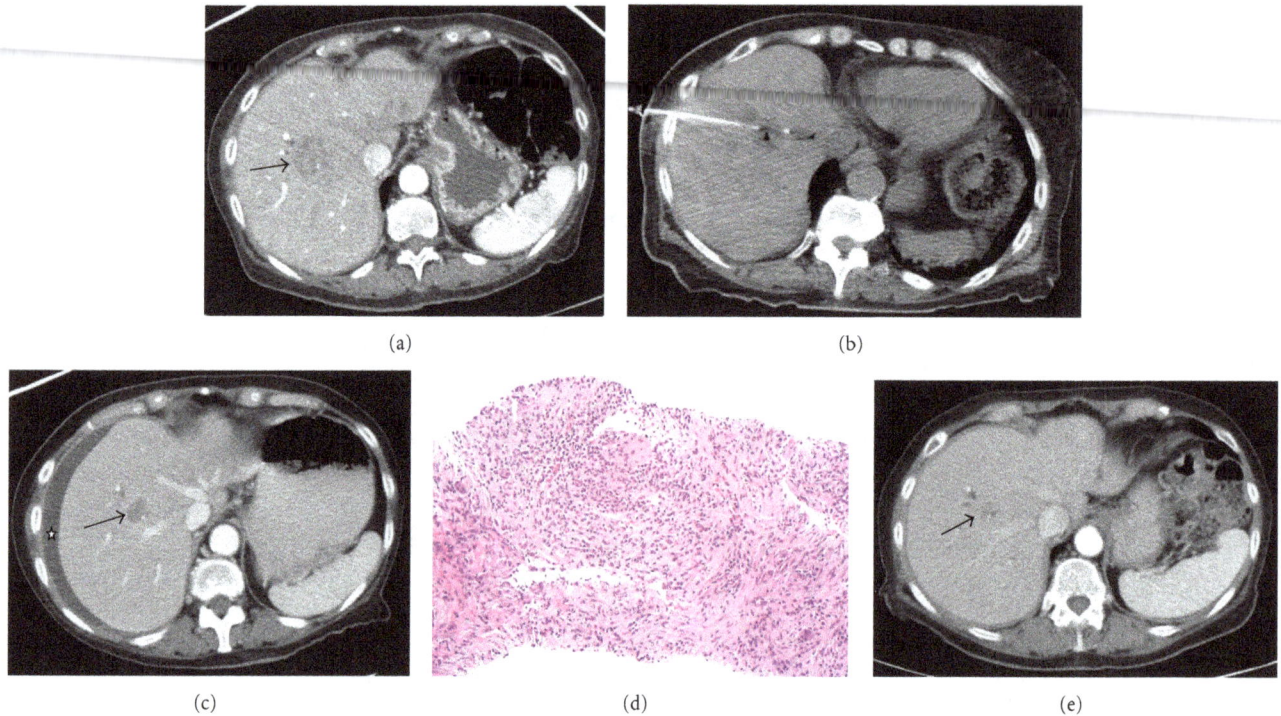

(a)

(b)

(c)

(d)

(e)

FIGURE 1: (a) Patient with history of cholangiocarcinoma status after pancreaticoduodenectomy. Axial contrast-enhanced CT image obtained a few weeks after surgery demonstrates one of the two new hepatic lesions in segment 8 (arrow). (b) Axial image from CT guided needle biopsy of the same lesion. The biopsy needle is placed within the lesion to obtain one of core samples. (c) Axial contrast-enhanced CT image one day after biopsy demonstrates new right perihepatic/subdiaphragmatic collection (asterix), which cultured positive for *E. coli*. The biopsied lesion is visible (arrow). (d) Histologic examination of core specimens shows a granuloma along with a mixed inflammatory infiltrate composed of lymphocyte, eosinophils, and neutrophils. (e) Contrast-enhanced CT image three months after biopsy shows resolution of liver lesions. The area of the biopsied segment 8 lesion is marked by an arrow.

lesion in segment 8 was accessed with a 19-gauge/20-gauge automatic core biopsy gun (Temno, CareFusion, Waukegan, IL) via a lateral intercostal approach (Figure 1(b)). A good core of tissue was obtained. A touch preparation was made by placing the core of tissue on a glass slide and rolling the specimen gently around the slide. The sample was immediately evaluated for adequacy by an on-site cytotechnologist. No neoplastic cells were seen on the initial touch preparation. Ultimately five core samples were obtained from different areas of the lesion; each appeared visually adequate, but none of the touch preparation samples contained neoplastic cells on the on-site evaluation. The biopsy was terminated based on CT imaging confirmation of adequate sampling of the lesion. The specimens were submitted for both cytopathologic and surgical pathologic evaluations, which revealed liver parenchyma with chronic active inflammation, granulomas, and a reactive bile ductule proliferation (Figure 1(d)). No carcinoma was seen. Special stains for mycobacteria and fungal organisms were negative. No microbiology specimens were sent due to lack of clinical suspicion for infectious etiology.

The patient developed right upper quadrant pain in the recovery area. She did not have any clinical signs of hemorrhage or sepsis. The pain was controlled with 50 micrograms of intravenous fentanyl. She remained hemodynamically stable throughout a three-hour postbiopsy observation period.

The pain was attributed to minimal blood or bile leaking from the puncture site irritating the diaphragm. She was sent home on oral pain medications. The day after the biopsy, the patient continued to complain of right upper quadrant pain. She also developed fever and was brought back to the hospital for further evaluation. She had an elevated white blood cell count of 13.6 K/mcL, increased from prebiopsy value of 5.1 K/mcL. CT scan showed a new right perihepatic/subcapsular fluid collection. This was aspirated under CT guidance and yielded 600 mL of serosanguineous fluid (Figure 1(c)). The patient was discharged home with instructions regarding signs of hemorrhage and infection. No drainage catheter was placed due to the benign gross character of the fluid. Culture results returned positive for *Escherichia coli*. The patient was placed on oral ciprofloxacin. In the following 2 weeks, the patient's pain persisted and she developed dyspnea; a CT scan of chest was performed to rule out pulmonary embolism. This showed subsegmental bilateral pulmonary artery embolism and also enlarging, recurrent right perihepatic/subdiaphragmatic collection with new loculations. It was drained with an all-purpose drainage catheter and intracavitary alteplase instillation. Culture showed *Escherichia coli*. Pulmonary embolism was treated with anticoagulation therapy. The patient was treated and discharged with ciprofloxacin for her perihepatic infection. The collection resolved and the catheter was removed three

(a)

(b)

(c)

(d)

(e)

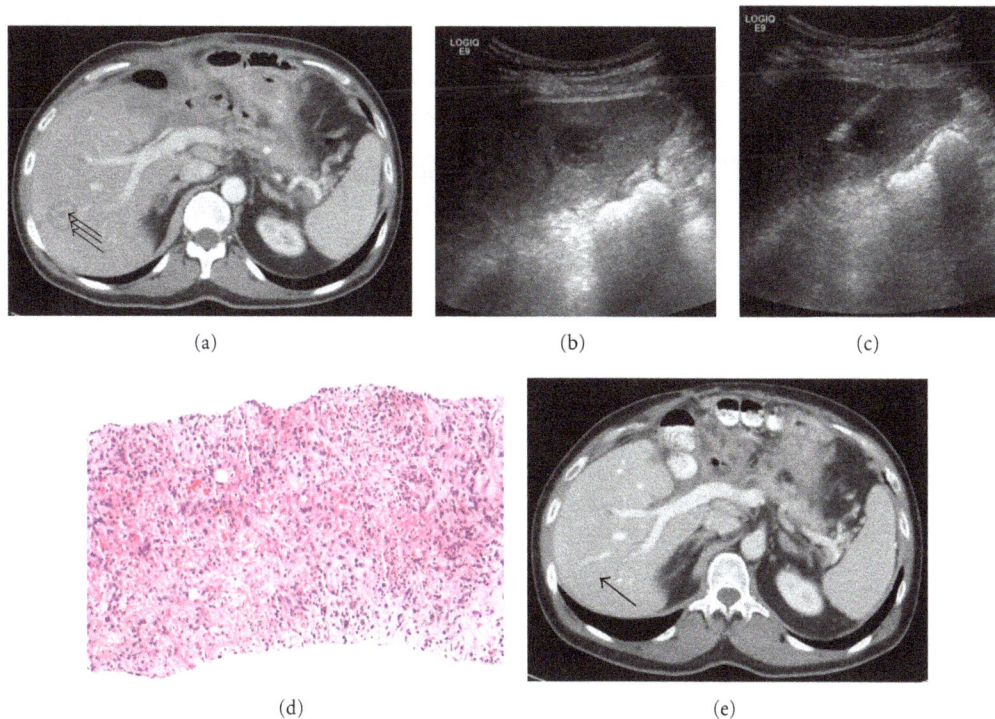

FIGURE 2: (a) Patient with history of pancreatic adenocarcinoma status after pancreaticoduodenectomy. Axial contrast-enhanced CT image obtained a few weeks after surgery showed three new liver lesions. This lesion in segment 8 has "double target sign" with three discrete layers (arrows). (b) Oblique image from ultrasound guided needle biopsy demonstrates another "double target sign" lesion in segment 6. (c) Biopsy needle within the segment 6 lesion. (d) Histologic examination of core specimens shows abundant neutrophils admixed with reactive fibroblasts. (e) Contrast-enhanced CT image three months after biopsy shows resolution of liver lesions. The area of the segment 8 lesion shown on (a) is marked by an arrow.

weeks after placement. CT scan of the abdomen was repeated 3 months after the biopsy, which showed resolution of the hepatic lesions, including the lesion that was biopsied (Figure 1(e)). The patient had not received any chemotherapy since biopsy.

2.2. Case 2. A 61-year-old man 2 months after Whipple surgery for pancreatic head adenocarcinoma developed three new hepatic lesions on CT scan (Figure 2(a)). He had an episode of postoperative abdominal infection which had resolved by the time of surveillance CT scan. He was referred to the interventional radiology service for biopsy of a liver lesion to confirm metastatic disease. Complete blood count, coagulation profile, and basic metabolic profile were all within normal limits. Liver function tests were unremarkable except for mild elevation of alkaline phosphatase to 176 Units/L (normal range 45–129 Units/L) and ALT to 56 Units/L (normal range 5–37 Units/L).

Core biopsy was performed under ultrasound guidance with conscious sedation. Gray scale ultrasound images revealed an approximately 2.5 cm segment 6 liver lesion with "double target sign" appearance, similar to CT findings (Figure 2(b)). A 19-gauge/20-gauge automatic core biopsy gun (Temno, CareFusion, Waukegan, IL) was used to ultimately obtain 4 samples via a lateral intercostal approach (Figures 2(c) and 2(d)). None of the touch preparation slides of the core specimens revealed neoplastic cell on the on-site

microscopic examination. The biopsy was terminated based on ultrasound imaging confirmation of adequate sampling of the lesion. Specimens were submitted for cytopathologic, microbiologic, and surgical pathologic evaluations which revealed a benign fibroinflammatory infiltrate consistent with organizing abscess and positive culture for *Escherichia coli* (Figure 2(d)).

The patient developed rigors in the recovery area after biopsy and was admitted for intravenous antibiotic treatment. Blood cultures were negative and blood chemistries remained within normal limits during his hospital stay. The patient was discharged after five days to complete a 4-week course of intravenous ceftriaxone treatment. All liver lesions near-completely resolved on follow up CT scan three months after biopsy (Figure 2(e)). The patient did not receive any chemotherapy since biopsy.

3. Discussion

Liver abscess does not have any pathognomonic imaging appearance. Infectious etiology is generally suspected based on a combination of clinical symptoms, laboratory abnormalities, medical history, and corresponding imaging findings.

Liver abscesses may appear as a unilocular central hypodense area with a hypovascular or hypervascular rim [3, 4]. A common appearance is a multiloculated cystic cavity with thin or thick enhancing walls [5]. They may contain gas or air-fluid levels [6]. A "cluster" sign is when small abscesses appear to cluster or aggregate together suggesting coalescence into a single large cavity [6]. A "double target" sign is caused by addition of perilesional edema or parenchymal hyperemia where there are at least three discernible layers including the central cavity [3, 4]. On ultrasound, a similar pattern is sometimes referred to as a "bull's eye" lesion [3, 7]. The double target sign is not specific to abscess. It is seen in 50% of abscesses but can be seen in up to 30% of hepatic malignancies [8–10].

However, when the infection and inflammation is more chronic, a central pus filled cavity may not form in such a lesion. Granulation tissues may organize into layers instead. Histologically, authors have described these lesions with central necrotic components containing polymorphonuclear leukocytes, surrounded by layers of granulation tissue [6] and possible edema in the outer periphery. This explanation seems appropriate for both of our patients where chronic ascending biliary infection is more likely due to removal of the Sphincter of Oddi during pancreaticoduodenectomy (PD). The liver lesions in both patients were proven to be infectious by lack of neoplastic histology, positive cultures, and improvement with antibiotic therapy.

Liver abscesses are almost always symptomatic and are almost always associated with laboratory abnormalities [6, 11]. Among the most common presentations of liver abscesses are fever, chills, right upper quadrant pain, jaundice, leukocytosis, and abnormal liver functions tests. Asymptomatic liver abscess in a nonimmune compromised patient is extremely rare. A patient with asymptomatic pyogenic liver abscess had abnormal liver function and ultimately succumbed to fulminating sepsis [12]. Four patients with liver abscesses and pylephlebitis who were thought to have hepatocellular carcinoma were all febrile and had abnormal liver function [13].

Liver abscesses are often a result of amoebic, or bacterial infections [7, 11, 14]. Escherichia coli, likely from gastrointestinal origin, was the organism responsible for the infection in both of our patients.

The mortality of PD has decreased drastically in the past decade, but morbidity remains steady [15]. One of the most serious and common complications is formation of liver abscess [1]. Post-PD patients are more prone to liver parenchymal infection due to removal of Sphincter of Oddi, which normally prevents gastrointestinal tract bacteria from entering the sterile biliary tree. After PD, the biliary tract is colonized with gastrointestinal flora, which can more easily cause liver abscess formation, especially after liver-directed therapies [1, 2]. Therefore, post-PD patients who have a high risk for liver metastases due to the nature and location of their primary tumors are also at high risk for hepatic abscess formation.

Biopsy of infectious lesions in our patients likely caused dissemination manifested by infected perihepatic fluid collection in one and rigors in the other. The biopsy needle likely contracted bacteria from the abscess and seeded the organism in the surrounding parenchyma and blood stream during needle manipulation and withdrawal. While infections caused by more invasive liver directed therapies have been widely reported [2], those caused by biopsy have not been reported.

Proper awareness on the part of the referring physician and the interventional radiologist about the possibility of an infectious etiology for new liver lesions helps setting an appropriate endpoint for a biopsy procedure. It also facilitates addressing of the potential postbiopsy infectious complications more effectively.

Our cases may serve as precautionary examples that asymptomatic liver abscesses can mimic metastases, especially in patients after Whipple surgery who are more prone to both liver metastases and liver infections. Biopsy of these lesions may cause spread of infection. It may be wise to monitor these patients more closely for signs of postprocedural sepsis and infectious complications. Prophylactic antibiotics prior to biopsy should also be considered.

References

[1] S. M. Sivaraj, V. Vimalraj, P. Saravanaboopathy et al., "Is bactibilia a predictor of poor outcome of pancreaticoduodenectomy?" *Hepatobiliary and Pancreatic Diseases International*, vol. 9, no. 1, pp. 65–68, 2010.

[2] M. C. De Jong, M. B. Farnell, G. Sclabas et al., "Liver-directed therapy for hepatic metastases in patients undergoing pancreaticoduodenectomy: a dual-center analysis," *Annals of Surgery*, vol. 252, no. 1, pp. 142–148, 2010.

[3] C. Gorg, R. Weide, W. B. Schwerk, H. Koppler, and K. Havemann, "Ultrasound evaluation of hepatic and splenic microabscesses in the immunocompromised patient: sonographic patterns, differential diagnosis, and follow-up," *Journal of Clinical Ultrasound*, vol. 22, no. 9, pp. 525–529, 1994.

[4] T. A. Baker, J. M. Aaron, M. Borge, K. Pierce, M. Shoup, and G. V. Aranha, "Role of interventional radiology in the management of complications after pancreaticoduodenectomy," *American Journal of Surgery*, vol. 195, no. 3, pp. 386–390, 2008.

[5] N. K. Lee, S. Kim, J. W. Lee et al., "CT differentiation of pyogenic liver abscesses caused by *Klebsiella pneumoniae* vs non-*Klebsiella pneumoniae*," *British Journal of Radiology*, vol. 84, no. 1002, pp. 518–525, 2011.

[6] D. Mathieu, N. Vasile, and P. L. Fagniez, "Dynamic CT features of hepatic abscesses," *Radiology*, vol. 154, no. 3, pp. 749–752, 1985.

[7] D. A. Gervais, C. Fernandez-Del Castillo, M. J. O'Neill, P. F. Hahn, and P. R. Mueller, "Complications after pancreatoduodenectomy: imaging and imaging-guided interventional procedures," *Radiographics*, vol. 21, no. 3, pp. 673–690, 2001.

[8] L. Lepanto, D. Gianfelice, R. Déry, M. Dagenais, R. Lapointe, and A. Roy, "Postoperative changes, complications, and recurrent disease after Whipple's operation: CT features," *American Journal of Roentgenology*, vol. 163, no. 4, pp. 841–846, 1994.

[9] Y. P. Chou, C. S. Changchien, K. W. Chiu, C. M. Kuo, F. Y. Kuo, and C. H. Kuo, "Salmonellosis with liver abscess mimicking hepatocellular carcinoma in a diabetic and cirrhotic patient: a case report and review of the literature," *Liver International*, vol. 26, no. 4, pp. 498–501, 2006.

[10] R. J. Méndez, M. L. Schiebler, E. K. Outwater, and H. Y. Kressel, "Hepatic abscesses: MR imaging findings," *Radiology*, vol. 190, no. 2, pp. 431–436, 1994.

[11] J. J. Mezhir, Y. Fong, L. M. Jacks et al., "Current management of pyogenic liver abscess: surgery is now second-line treatment,"

Journal of the American College of Surgeons, vol. 210, no. 6, pp. 975–983, 2010.

[12] M. Cheung, L. Temple, and M. Khan, "An unexpected cause of deranged liver function: pyogenic liver abscess," *Journal of the Royal Society of Medicine*, vol. 2, article 4, 2011.

[13] K. T. Brown, R. T. Gandhi, A. M. Covey, L. A. Brody, and G. I. Getrajdman, "Pylephlebitis and liver abscess mimicking hepatocellular carcinoma," *Hepatobiliary and Pancreatic Diseases International*, vol. 2, no. 2, pp. 221–225, 2003.

[14] G. Jackson, M. Kathuria, B. Abraham, and V. J. Schnadig, "Fine needle aspiration diagnosis of necrotizing eosinophilic abscess clinically mimicking hepatic neoplasia: a case report," *Acta Cytologica*, vol. 54, no. 1, pp. 60–62, 2010.

[15] A. Cortes, A. Sauvanet, F. Bert et al., "Effect of bile contamination on immediate outcomes after pancreaticoduodenectomy for tumor," *Journal of the American College of Surgeons*, vol. 202, no. 1, pp. 93–99, 2006.

9

Acute Liver Failure due to Disseminated Varicella Zoster Infection

Elizabeth Caitlin Brewer ⓘ **and Leigh Hunter**

Methodist Hospitals of Dallas, 1441 N Beckley Ave Dallas, TX 75203, USA

Correspondence should be addressed to Elizabeth Caitlin Brewer; drelizabethbrewer@gmail.com

Academic Editor: Melanie Deutsch

Acute liver failure (ALF) can be due to numerous causes and result in fatality or necessitate liver transplantation if left untreated. Possible etiologies of ALF include ischemia, venous obstruction, medications, toxins, autoimmune hepatitis, metabolic and infectious causes including hepatitis A-E, varicella-zoster virus (VZV), cytomegalovirus (CMV), herpes simplex virus (HSV), Epstein-Barr virus (EBV), and adenovirus with VZV being the most rarely reported. Pathognomonic skin lesions facilitate diagnosis of VZV hepatitis, but definitive diagnosis is secured with liver biopsy, tissue histopathology, culture, and specific VZV polymerase chain reaction (PCR). Antiviral treatment with intravenous acyclovir can be effective if initiated in a timely manner; however, comorbidities and complications frequently result in high mortality, especially in immunocompromised hosts as exemplified in this case presentation.

1. Introduction

Varicella zoster virus can cause two clinical syndromes, primary (chickenpox) and secondary (herpes zoster). Primary infection presents mainly in children with a generalized vesicular rash. The virus then establishes latency in the dorsal root ganglia and can later reactivate as "shingles" or herpes zoster, a localized dermatomal vesicular eruption. Cutaneous and extracutaneous dissemination can occur, most commonly in immunocompromised patients [1]. Fulminant hepatic failure due to VZV hepatitis is even more rare and deadly. In review of the literature, only 8 adult cases of acute liver failure from VZV were found, of which only 2 survived [2–9].

2. Case Presentation

A 66-year-old Caucasian woman with past medical history of dermatomyositis, dysphagia, gastro-esophageal reflux, and hypertension presented to the emergency department (ED) with several days of mid-epigastric, constant, moderate intensity, nonradiating abdominal pain. Additionally, she reported 4-5 days of erythematous rash that began on her

face and chest that then spread to her arms and abdomen (Figures 1-2). She also reported white "spots" in her mouth. At that time, CBC, CRP, ESR, CK, and UA were within normal limits. Lipase was 675 U/L and CMP was remarkable for sodium 129 mEq/L, amino alanine transferase (ALT) 158 U/L, and aspartate aminotransferase (AST) 111 U/L; the rest of the CMP including alkaline phosphatase (ALP) was normal. CXR was normal and abdominal radiograph showed evidence of constipation. An abdominal ultrasound was ordered due to elevated lipase and LFTs and showed no evidence of gallbladder dysfunction or liver lesions. She was diagnosed with pancreatitis, thrush, and folliculitis and was discharged home with clear liquid diet orders and prescriptions for nystatin oral solution and oral doxycycline for possible secondary skin infection. Two days later, she returned to the ED with persistent symptoms and decreased urine output. She reported nausea, constipation, and worsened dysphagia, but denied vomiting, weight change, night sweats, fever, chills, chest pain, cough, and shortness of breath. She also denied pertinent past surgeries, family history, recent travel, sexual activity, drug use, and alcohol and tobacco use. She reported allergy to penicillin. Her medication list included prednisone, mycophenolate mofetil

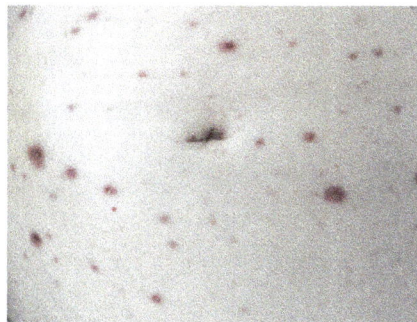

FIGURE 1: Maculopapular rash.

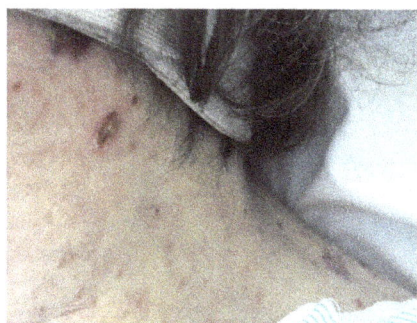

FIGURE 2: Crusted vesicle.

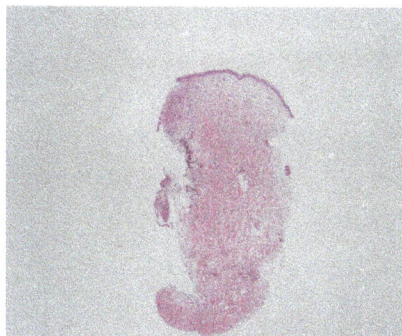

FIGURE 3: Skin biopsy.

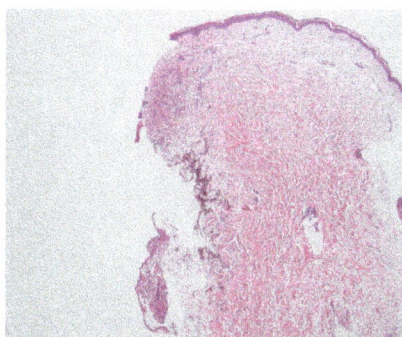

FIGURE 4: Skin biopsy: intact epidermis on one side and lesion on the other.

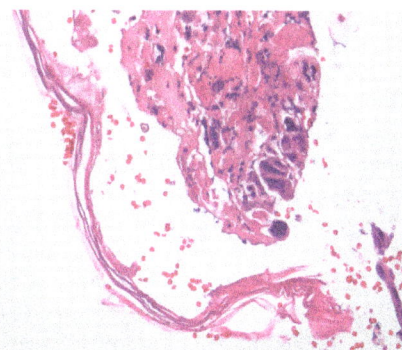

FIGURE 5: Skin biopsy: viral cytoplasmic effect including multinucleated cells and marginalization of chromatin.

(which she held since previous ED visit per doctor recommendations), trimethoprim/sulfamethoxazole (T/S), nystatin oral suspension, carvedilol, ranitidine, estradiol, calcium, and vitamin D. She was told by her dermatologist not to fill the doxycycline prescription from the ED and increase the dose of T/S.

On physical examination, the patient was alert and oriented with normal vital signs. The exam was significant for oral thrush, but normal heart, lung, and abdominal exams. Skin exam showed a diffuse maculopapular eruption with a few vesicles on face, trunk, and extremities. Significant laboratory data was as follows: AST 1389 U/L, ALT 1570 U/L, ALP 68 U/L, international normalized ratio (INR) 1.6, and prothrombin time (PT) 18 seconds. Complete abdominal ultrasound demonstrated normal gallbladder without stones, no biliary ductal dilation, no focal liver lesions, and no ascites or abnormal fluid collections. The patient's dermatologist had performed skin biopsies 2 days prior to admission that showed multinucleated giant cells with viral inclusions suggestive of some type of herpes virus infection (Figures 3–5). The patient was initiated on intravenous (IV) acyclovir, micafungin, vancomycin, aztreonam, and stress dose steroids for presumed disseminated herpes simplex with possible secondary bacterial infection and sepsis. Over the subsequent 48-72 hours, AST and ALT increased to the 4000s, INR increased to 1.8 and PT to 20.6. Due to worsening acute liver failure, she was transferred to our facility for liver transplant evaluation.

On arrival to our hospital, her skin lesions were thought to be most consistent with VZV and skin biopsy cultures

from the outpatient dermatologist later confirmed VZV. IV acyclovir and antibiotics for secondary bacterial sepsis were continued. As part of her liver transplant evaluation, extensive serologic investigation ensued. Acute hepatitis A-E serologies, ANA, IgG4, smooth muscle antibody (Ab), LKM-1 Ab, ceruloplasmin, a-1 antitrypsin, mitochondrial M2 Ab, AFP, HIV, HSV and EBV PCRs, blood cultures, galactomannan, and cryptococcal antigen were submitted and later found to be negative. She was also found to be pANCA MPO positive and PR3 negative. Liver biopsy was performed which revealed multiple areas of necrotic hepatocytes (up to 35% of liver parenchyma) (Figures 6-7) in zones 2 and 3 of the liver. This was associated with some bile

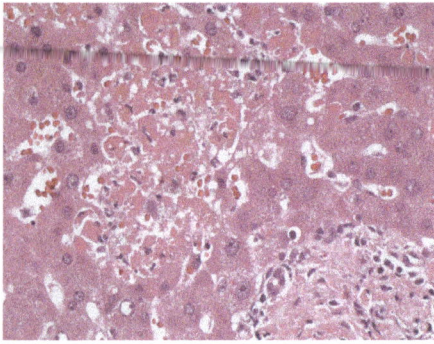

FIGURE 6: Hepatocytes with frank necrosis.

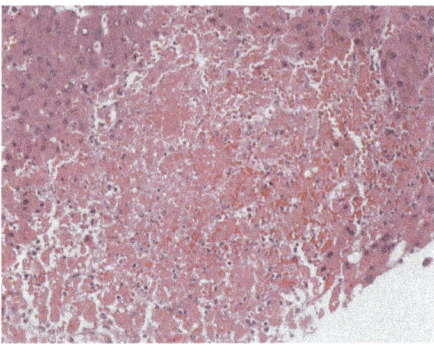

FIGURE 7: Larger foci of hepatocytes with frank necrosis.

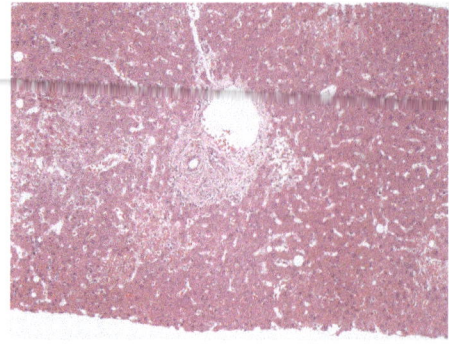

FIGURE 8: Areas of necrosis abutting portal triad with chronic minimal inflammation; no significant steatosis seen and no periportal fibrosis or vasculitis appreciated.

prevented liver transplantation. The patient's code status was eventually changed to "do not resuscitate" and she expired.

3. Discussion

Reactivation of VZV as "shingles" is a common occurrence, but acute liver failure (ALF) due to VZV is exceedingly rare with high mortality [2–9]. The differential diagnosis of ALF includes multiple etiologies including ischemia, venous obstruction, medications, toxins, autoimmune hepatitis, and metabolic and infectious etiologies (predominantly viruses including hepatitis A-E, VZV, CMV, HSV, EBV, and adenovirus) with VZV being the one most rarely reported. By imaging and history, the patient was less likely to have venous obstruction or ischemia from an unrecognized hypotensive event that triggered her hepatitis. She denied exposure to toxins, but had been on prophylactic trimethoprim/sulfamethoxazole for long duration; this was a consideration for drug induced liver injury, but was refuted by biopsy, PCR, and culture results. There was no history of ingestion of other toxins known to cause acute hepatitis before onset of illness. Likewise, the AST to ALT ratio was not in the classic pattern (2:1) for alcoholic hepatitis.

In the setting of VZV hepatitis, definitive diagnosis is made by liver biopsy, histopathology, culture, and VZV PCR. Of note, some cases have been shown to be pANCA positive as well. Thus it is important to utilize physical examination clues to prompt ordering of proper tests along with early empirical antiviral therapy.

Disseminated varicella zoster is most common in immunocompromised patients [1]. Resultant fulminant liver failure from VZV is even more rare and deadly. In review of the literature, only 8 adult cases of acute liver failure from this organism were found, of which only 2 survived. These cases are summarized in Tables 1 and 2. One case report from France involved a 35-year-old woman from the Ivory Coast with past medical history (PMH) of HIV, HBV, and recent neurotoxoplasmosis [2]. A second case report from Spain was a 43-year-old male heart transplant recipient 9 months prior to the time of ALF from a VZV episode [3]. In these cases, IV acyclovir was the staple

extravasation and acute inflammation. No signs of bridging or confluent necrosis were seen. A trichrome stain outlined regions of immature deposition of collagen near necrotic areas. This stain also showed increased perivenular fibrosis around the central veins but no evidence of periportal fibrosis. The portal triads showed nominal chronic inflammation with small lymphocytes, rare large lymphocytes, and a few scattered neutrophils. There was no bile duct injury, paucity, or vasculitis. The hepatocytes did not demonstrate significant steatosis, but there was bile stasis in a few canalicular spaces and hepatocytes. Viral inclusions were not seen. An iron stain showed no accumulation of hemosiderin within the hepatocytes. PCR was negative for HSV, EBV, and CMV and positive for VZV. The necrosis also abutted portal triads seen in the specimens (Figure 8). A Periodic acid-Schiff stain with diastase did not show cytoplasmic globules. Blood PCRs were positive with high levels of VZV and low levels of CMV. The CMV viremia was attributed to secondary reactivation due to her severely immunosuppressed state. VZV immune globulin was considered as therapy, but IVIG was administered instead due to her severe coagulopathy and thrombocytopenia. Outpatient skin biopsy cultures later confirmed VZV; PCR was positive for VZV and negative for HSV.

Her hospital stay was complicated by multidrug-resistant Enterobacter cloacae hospital acquired pneumonia and bacteremia, respiratory failure requiring prolonged intubation, and multiple organ failure. VZV PCR copies decreased with treatment, but her severity of illness and active infection

TABLE 1: Case reports: survivors [2, 3].

Pt Info	PMH	Symptoms	Treatment	Diagnosis	Liver Biopsy
35 y/o African F from Ivory Coast	HIV, HBV and recent neurotoxoplasmosis	Chest pain	IV acyclovir	Vesicle swab VZV + by direct IF and culture; liver bx	>50% hepatic necrosis and inclusion bodies
43 y/o M	S/p heart transplant 9 months earlier	N/V, epigastric pain	IV acyclovir, VZV immune globulin, emergent liver transplant	Skin lesion biopsy: HSV – VZV + liver biopsy	Transjugular liver bx: signs of herpetic hepatitis; histology of hepatectomy: hepatic necrosis consistent with VZV infection

TABLE 2: Case reports: nonsurvivors [4–9].

Pt Info	PMH	Symptoms	Treatment	Diagnosis	Liver Biopsy
49 y/o M	ETOH and tobacco abuse, 15 days post radical dissection neck and laryngectomy for SCC larynx	Abdominal pain, fever, restlessness	"Intensive supportive care"	Post mortem via liver analysis	Post mortem: liver VZV DNA +, hepatic necrosis with intranuclear inclusion bodies
47 y/o Japanese M	MM s/p chemo, steroids, 2 stem cell transplants, moderate GVHD and relapse of MM with more chemo and steroids	Generalized fatigue	FFP, platelets	Retrospective VZV PCR + blood and liver analysis	Autopsy: + anti-VZV IgG stain of liver with hepatic necrosis seen
49 y/o M	No PMH except treatment for pharyngotonsillitis 15 days prior with abx and prednisone	Acute retrosternal pain	IV acyclovir, VZV immune globulin, total hepatectomy	Skin cytology c/w herpes family virus & immuno-cytochemistry stain VZV +; blood VZV DNA +	Liver bx: necrosis only; Post mortem liver VZV DNA +
15 y/o M	None	Fever, abdominal pain, myalgia, skin vesicles	IV acyclovir, MARs	Post mortem liver analysis	Post mortem liver analysis: hepatic necrosis, multinucleation and intranuclear inclusions of Cowdry A bodies; liver VZV PCR +
26 y/o CF	Diagnosed with MS 3 months prior and treated with steroids	Abd pain and vomiting	PO acyclovir ⟶ IV acyclovir	Blood and urine VZV PCR +; post mortem liver analysis	Post mortem liver: hemorrhagic necrosis and VZV PCR +
64 y/o CF	14 months post-op esophago-gastrectomy & splenectomy	Fever, malaise, HA	Vit K	VZV titers D4: 1-64 ⟶ D7: 1-256; liver autopsy analysis	Autopsy liver: hemorrhagic necrosis and signs herpes family virus including Cowdry A intranuclear bodies; EM: intracellular virions consistent with herpes family virus

of treatment [2, 3]. The heart transplant patient also was treated with VZV immune globulin and emergent liver transplant [3]. Other reported cases that did not survive included a 49-year-old German man with PMH of alcohol and tobacco abuse 15 days post radical neck dissection and laryngectomy for laryngeal squamous cell carcinoma who presented for abdominal pain. He received supportive care and was diagnosed post mortem [4]. A Japanese 47-year-old man with multiple myeloma status post chemotherapy, corticosteroids, 2 stem cell transplants, moderate graft versus host disease, and relapse of the myeloma necessitating additional chemotherapy and corticosteroids presented with generalized fatigue. He was treated with fresh frozen plasma, platelet transfusions and was also diagnosed post mortem [5]. Another case reported from Italy was a 49-year-old man with no PMH except treatment for pharyngotonsillitis with steroids and antibiotics 15 days before presentation with retrosternal chest pain and truncal rash. He was treated with IV acyclovir, VZV immune globulin, and total hepatectomy, but was unable to receive a donor liver in time [6]. The next case was of a 15-year-old Roman male with no PMH who was treated with IV acyclovir, MARS (molecular adsorbent re-circulating system), and blood product transfusions. Diagnosis was confirmed with a post mortem liver analysis [7]. An additional case was of a 26-year-old Czech female with diagnosis of multiple sclerosis 3 months prior to admission followed by treatment with steroids who presented with abdominal pain and vomiting and later developed a generalized rash. She was originally treated with oral acyclovir, but because of progressive worsening was changed to IV acyclovir. Despite aggressive treatment, she also expired [8]. The final reported case involved a 64-year-old Caucasian woman in Vermont who was 14 months post esophagogastrectomy/splenectomy and came to the hospital with headache, malaise, and fever. She was diagnosed post mortem with VZV by acute and convalescent antibody titers and liver analysis. She was treated supportively with vitamin K but subsequently died as well [9].

As shown, early IV acyclovir is key to treatment of VZV acute liver failure. Other considered therapies include VZV immune globulin, liver transplant, IVIG, and supportive care [2–9]. Since this cause of liver failure has such high mortality rates and early treatment is critical to survival, VZV hepatitis should be considered in the differential diagnosis of all patients with liver failure who present with a rash.

Additional Points

Learning Points/Take-Home Messages. (1) VZV should be considered as a cause of acute liver failure in the proper clinical setting. (2) Diagnosis of VZV is dependent on liver biopsy, histopathology, culture of tissue, and PCR. (3) Early antiviral medication is essential to decrease morbidity and mortality from disseminated VZV infection. (4) Disseminated VZV with ALF has a very high mortality rate.

References

[1] R. J. Whitley, "Herpesviruses," in *Medical Microbiology*, S. Baron, Ed., University of Texas Medical Branch, Galveston, Tex,

USA, 4th edition, 1996, https://www.ncbi.nlm.nih.govbooks/NBK8157/.

[2] C. Lechiche, V. Le Moing, P. François Perrigault, and J. Reynes, "Fulminant varicella hepatitis in a human immunodeficiency virus infected patient: Case report and review of the literature," *Infectious Diseases*, vol. 38, no. 10, pp. 929–931, 2006.

[3] M. Alvite-Canosa, M. J. Paniagua-Martín, J. Quintela-Fandiño, A. Otero, and M. G. Crespo-Leiro, "Fulminant Hepatic Failure due to Varicella Zoster in a Heart Transplant Patient: Successful Liver Transplant," *The Journal of Heart and Lung Transplantation*, vol. 28, no. 11, pp. 1215-1216, 2009.

[4] U. Drebber, S. F. Preuss, H. U. Kasper, U. Wieland, and H. P. Dienes, "Postoperative fulminant varicella zoster virus hepatitis with fatal outcome: A case report," *Zeitschrift für Gastroenterologie*, vol. 46, no. 1, pp. 45–47, 2008.

[5] H. Saitoh, N. Takahashi, H. Nanjo, Y. Kawabata, M. Hirokawa, and K. Sawada, "Varicella-zoster virus-associated fulminant hepatitis following allogeneic hematopoietic stem cell transplantation for multiple myeloma," *Internal Medicine*, vol. 52, no. 15, pp. 1727–1730, 2013.

[6] U. Maggi, R. Russo, G. Conte et al., "Fulminant multiorgan failure due to varicella zoster virus and HHV6 in an immunocompetent adult patient, and anhepatia," *Transplantation Proceedings*, vol. 43, no. 4, pp. 1184–1186, 2011.

[7] S. Natoli, M. Ciotti, P. Paba et al., "A novel mutation of varicella-zoster virus associated to fatal hepatitis," *Journal of Clinical Virology*, vol. 37, no. 1, pp. 72–74, 2006.

[8] S. Plisek, L. Pliskova, V. Bostik et al., "Fulminant hepatitis and death associated with disseminated varicella in an immunocompromised adult from the Czech Republic caused by a wild-type clade 4 varicella-zoster virus strain," *Journal of Clinical Virology*, vol. 50, no. 1, pp. 72–75, 2011.

[9] J. S. Ross, W. L. Fanning, W. Beautyman, and J. E. Craighead, "Fatal massive hepatic necrosis from varicella-zoster hepatitis," *The American journal of gastroenterology. U.S. National Library of Medicine*, 2017.

10

Hepatic Myelopathy in a Patient with Decompensated Alcoholic Cirrhosis and Portal Colopathy

Madhumita Premkumar, Avishek Bagchi, Neha Kapoor, Ankit Gupta, Gaurav Maurya, Shubham Vatsya, Siddharth Kapahtia, and Premashish Kar

Department of Medicine, B. L. Taneja Block, Maulana Azad Medical College and Associated Hospitals, Bahadur Shah Zafar Marg, New Delhi 110002, India

Correspondence should be addressed to Madhumita Premkumar, drmadhumitap@gmail.com

Academic Editors: G. H. Koek, H. H. Lin, D. Lorenzin, C. Miyabayashi, and H. Uchiyama

Cirrhotic or hepatic myelopathy is a rare neurological complication of chronic liver disease usually seen in adults and presents as a progressive pure motor spastic paraparesis which is usually associated with overt liver failure and a surgical or spontaneous systemic portocaval shunt. We describe the development of progressive spastic paraparesis, in a patient with alcoholic cirrhosis with portal hypertension and portal colopathy who presented with the first episode of hepatic encephalopathy. The patient had not undergone any shunt procedure.

1. Introduction

Hepatic myelopathy (HM) is an insidious onset pure motor spastic paraparesis without sensory or bladder or bowel involvement in patients with liver disease in which the neurological dysfunction cannot be attributed to another disorder. A progressive spastic paraparesis in patients with hepatic failure was first described by Leigh and Card [1], followed by a detailed description of HM by other authors who observed this rare neurological complication of cirrhosis, especially in patients with portosystemic shunts [2–4]. In India, HM was reported for the first time by Pant et al. who described two cases of spastic paraparesis in patients with liver cirrhosis, one with a spontaneous portocaval shunt and the other with a surgical portocaval anastamosis [5]. The typical clinical presentation of this disorder is of a patient with underlying chronic liver disease, developing progressive pure motor spastic paraparesis with minimal or no sensory deficit and without bowel and bladder involvement. Most patients report prior episodes of hepatic encephalopathy, and in many cases, the development of myelopathy follows the creation of surgical shunts [6–8]. Early and accurate diagnosis of HM is important because

patients with early stages of the disease can recover following liver transplantation [9]. Neuropathological studies show demyelination in the lateral corticospinal tracts, with varying degrees of axonal loss [2]. Motor-evoked potential studies may be suitable for the early diagnosis of hepatic myelopathy, even in patients with preclinical stages of the disease [10].

2. Case Presentation

A 45-year-old male farmer, hailing from Uttar Pradesh, north India, presented to us with complaints of difficulty in walking due to stiffness of lower limbs for 2 years, associated with weakness. Initially, the weakness was only present on activities like standing from the squatting position or climbing stairs which over a period of a couple of months progressed to noticing slippage of footwear and dragging of feet while walking. He developed a limping gait, with both legs affected symmetrically. To offset this weakness, he reported the use of a walking stick over the last 6 months. There was no history of fasciculations or wasting. Two weeks ago, he noted fever, which rapidly caused prostration. His family reported altered behavior, forgetfulness, lack of attention with disturbed sleep wake cycle. There was no history of bowel and bladder involvement, ocular or vision abnormalities, seizures, diabetes mellitus, hypertension, tuberculosis, trauma, exposure to industrial toxins or radiation, blood or blood component therapy, bleeding disorders, promiscuity, or similar complaints in the family or neighbourhood. His history was significant for one other factor, occasional intake of *Lathyrus sativus* (khesari dal), but not in a quantity or frequency enough to cause lathyrism. He had significant alcohol intake of about 20–30 grams of alcohol at least 3 times a week since the last 15 years. He did not smoke or consume tobacco. General examination revealed normal vitals, average nutrition, pallor, clubbing, and multiple sebaceous cysts involving the back and mild hepatomegaly along with splenomegaly. Other physical markers of liver disease such as icterus, spider angioma, and palmar erythema, were not present. The patient presented with hepatic encephalopathy, with impaired attention and flapping tremors. Spastic paraparesis (Grade III by Medical Research Council scale) was present along with hyperreflexia and bilateral extensor plantar response. He had ankle and patellar clonus. There were no lower motor neuron signs. There were no features of meningeal irritation or cerebellar involvement. Cranial nerve examination and sensory system was normal.

Investigations revealed mild anemia, mild hyperbilirubinemia, and raised liver enzymes (see Table 1). Cerebrospinal fluid (CSF) examination showed 3 lymphocytes/dL, protein—24 mg%, sugar—67 mg% and was negative for gram's stain, acid fast bacilli, and India ink staining. Ultrasound of the abdomen showed mildly nodular liver with coarsened echotexture with span 13 cm, splenomegaly, a dilated portal vein, and mild ascites. Upper gastrointestinal endoscopy (UGIE) was normal. Electroencephalography revealed background slowing without any spikes suggestive of metabolic encephalopathy. Magnetic resonance imaging (MRI) of the spine and brain showed non specific ischemic changes (see Figures 1, 2, and 3). Patient's serum was nonreactive to hepatitis A, B, C, and E viral markers as well as to HIV I and II. Hb A1c level was within normal limits, which excluded diabetes mellitus.

He developed massive lower gastrointestinal bleed on day 4 and a colonoscopy revealed diffuse portal colopathy with multiple superficial erosions up to the proximal colon. The patient was transfused with fresh frozen plasma but succumbed to the bleed. Postmortem liver biopsy revealed micronodular cirrhosis without steatosis and normal iron stores. 24-hour urinary copper estimation and serum ceruloplasmin were within normal limits. In view of a normal serology, the patient's diagnosis was alcohol-related cirrhosis with portal hypertension with portal colopathy with massive lower GI bleed.

3. Discussion

Hepatic myelopathy or porto-systemic myelopathy is a rare neurological complication of chronic liver disease with portal

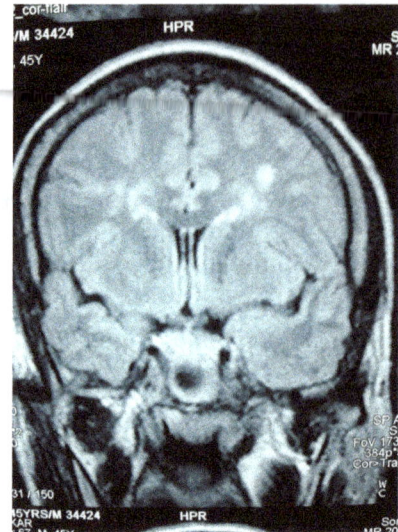

FIGURE 1: Magnetic resonance image of the brain showing nonspecific white matter changes.

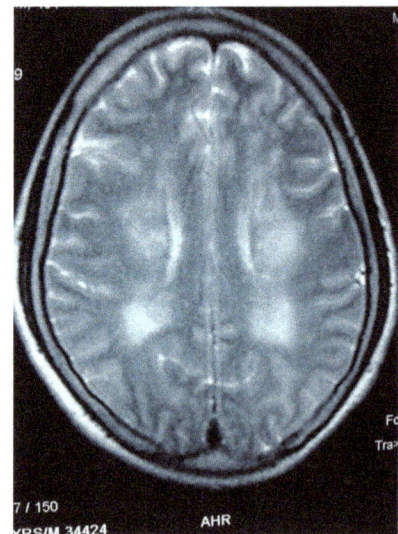

FIGURE 2: MRI Brain showed nonspecific ischemic changes.

hypertension, usually associated with porto-systemic shunting, and presents as pure motor spastic paraparesis without sensory or sphincter involvement. This is thus a diagnosis of exclusion. The exact pathogenesis of HM is still unclear. Most reported cases are of patients with decompensated liver disease, postliver transplant, or postshunt surgery including TIPSS (transjugular intrahepatic portal systemic shunting) [11]. Other rare reported associations of HM are cases of congenital hepatic fibrosis [12], childhood portal vein thrombosis [8], and acute hepatitis E [13].

Our case is interesting for several reasons. Firstly, this patient presented with a long history of progressive spastic paraparesis with no prior episode of hepatic decompensation. The myelopathy was already advanced before his first episode of encephalopathy. He did not

TABLE 1: Hematological and biochemical profile of the patient.

Investigations	Day 1	Day 2	Day 4
Hb (g/dL)	11.0	10.5	11.3
Total leukocyte count (cells/dL)	7560	6700	7200
Differential count	P60/L36/M2/E2	P66/L32/E1/M1	P56/L40/E2/M2
Platelet count (cells/μL)	130,000	133,000	140,000
ESR (mm/1st hour)	54		
Urea (mg/dL)	51	36	55
Creatinine (mg/dL)	0.7	0.7	0.8
Na^+/K^+ (meq/L)	133/4.1	134/3.5	144/4.6
Total bilirubin/direct bilirubin (mg/dL)	1.8/0.5		1.9/0.9
ALT/AST/ALP (IU/L)	99/243/137		93/143/140
Total protein/albumin (g/dL)	8.0/2.2		
Prothrombin time (test/control (seconds))	15/14		>60/14
Hb A1c (g/dL)		5.1	

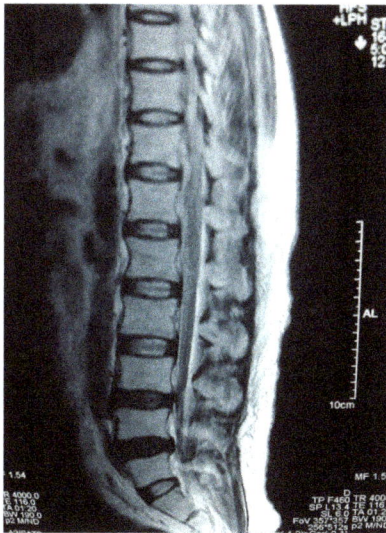

FIGURE 3: MR imaging of dorsolumbar spine did not reveal any abnormalities, with no evidence of compressive myelopathy.

have any prior episodes of gastrointestinal bleeding and the terminal episode of lower gastrointestinal bleeding due to diffuse portal colopathy did not have any antecedent event. Secondly, he had confounding exposure to grass pea, known colloquially as khesari dal (*Lathyrus sativus*). Neurolathyrism is still reported from several states in India, despite extensive awareness programmes about its debilitating neurological effects [14]. The toxin beta oxalyl amino alanine (BOAA) causes lower limb weakness with gluteal atrophy. However, our patient reported infrequent intake of the legume, the weakness was symmetrical, without bladder involvement, and there was no loss of reflexes. The reported toxic dose is about 300 gm of the legume per day for a period of three months [15]. While we were able to exclude certain diagnoses in this case, in view of the long duration of neurological symptoms, the possibility of concomitant predisposing factors like chronic alcoholism and nutrient deficiency cannot be completely ruled out.

It has been hypothesized that the hepatocerebral dysfunction is due to recurrent episodes of hepatic encephalopathy, and prolonged exposure to bypassed nitrogenous waste products such as ammonia, fatty acids, indoles, and mercaptans. These metabolites cause myelin damage resulting in the pathological white matter demyelination in the brain and the spinal cord. The selective predisposition for the motor system has been demonstrated by involvement of the lateral corticospinal tracts in autopsy studies. Other causative factors include nutrient deficiency and deranged liver metabolism. In our patient, the exact cause of myelopathy cannot be explained by the mechanism of recurrent encephalopathy [16].

Conditions which must be excluded include amyotrophic lateral sclerosis, demyelination syndromes like multiple sclerosis and neuromyelitis optica, toxic myelopathy, paraneoplastic syndromes, radiation myelopathy, HTLV-I associated myelopathy, and vascular spinal cord disease. The treatment of HM is difficult and the progression of spastic weakness is relentless. Nonetheless, recent reports have suggested that early detection and liver transplantation may improve prognosis in some cases if not all cases [17–20].

4. Conclusion

Hepatic myelopathy is a rare and debilitating neurological complication of liver failure. Early identification of this disorder and exclusion of other treatable causes is important. The therapeutic potential of liver transplantation for preventing progression and allowing recovery needs to be evaluated further.

Ethical Approval

Written informed consent has been taken from the patient's family. The presentation has been cleared by the department's ethics committee.

References

[1] A. D. Leigh and W. I. Card, "Hepato-lenticular degeneration. A case associated with postero-lateral column degeneration," *Journal of Neuropathology & Experimental Neurology*, vol. 8, pp. 318–346, 1949.

[2] L. Zieve, D. F. Mendelson, and M. Goepfert, "Shunt encephalomyelopathy. II. Occurrence of permanent myelopathy," *Annals of Internal Medicine*, vol. 53, pp. 53–63, 1960.

[3] I. A. Brown, *Liver-Brain Relationships*, Thomas Y Crowell, Springfield, 1957.

[4] S. M. Gospe Jr., R. D. Caruso, M. S. Clegg et al., "Paraparesis, hypermanganesaemia, and polycythaemia: a novel presentation of cirrhosis," *Archives of Disease in Childhood*, vol. 83, no. 5, pp. 439–442, 2000.

[5] S. S. Pant, A. N. Bhargava, M. M. Singh et al., "Myelopathy in hepatic cirrhosis," *British Medical Journal*, vol. 1, pp. 1064–1065, 1963.

[6] G. Mendoza, J. Marti-Fabregas, J. Kulisevsky, and A. Escartin, "Hepatic myelopathy: a rare complication of portacaval shunt," *European Neurology*, vol. 34, no. 4, pp. 209–212, 1994.

[7] J. Panicker, S. Sinha, A. B. Taly, S. Ravishankar, and G. R. Arunodaya, "Hepatic myelopathy: a rare complication following extrahepatic portal vein occlusion and lienorenal shunt," *Neurology India*, vol. 54, no. 3, pp. 298–300, 2006.

[8] J. V. Campellone, D. Lacomis, M. J. Giuliani, and F. J. Kroboth, "Hepatic myelopathy. Case report with review of the literature," *Clinical Neurology and Neurosurgery*, vol. 98, no. 3, pp. 242–246, 1996.

[9] K. Weissenborn, U. J. F. Tietge, M. Bokemeyer et al., "Liver transplantation improves hepatic myelopathy: evidence by three cases," *Gastroenterology*, vol. 124, no. 2, pp. 346–351, 2003.

[10] R. Nardone, T. Buratti, A. Oliviero, A. Lochmann, and F. Tezzon, "Corticospinal involvement in patients with a portosystemic shunt due to liver cirrhosis: a MEP study," *Journal of Neurology*, vol. 253, no. 1, pp. 81–85, 2006.

[11] L. G. Lefer and F. S. Vogel, "Encephalomyelopathy with hepatic cirrhosis following portosystemic venous shunts," *Archives of Pathology*, vol. 93, no. 2, pp. 91–97, 1972.

[12] M. Demirci, E. Tan, B. Elibol, G. Gedikoglu, and O. Saribas, "Spastic paraparesis associated with portal-systemic venous shunting due to congenital hepatic fibrosis," *Neurology*, vol. 42, no. 5, pp. 983–985, 1992.

[13] K. Mandal and N. Chopra, "Acute transverse myelitis following hepatitis E virus infection," *Indian Pediatrics*, vol. 43, no. 4, pp. 365–366, 2006.

[14] K. Sriram, S. K. Shankar, M. R. Boyd, and V. Ravindranath, "Thiol oxidation and loss of mitochondrial complex I precede excitatory amino acid-mediated neurodegeneration," *Journal of Neuroscience*, vol. 18, no. 24, pp. 10287–10296, 1998.

[15] V. Ravindranath, "Neurolathyrism: mitochondrial dysfunction in excitotoxicity mediated by L-β-oxalyl aminoalanine," *Neurochemistry International*, vol. 40, no. 6, pp. 505–509, 2002.

[16] J. C. Kincaid, "Myelitis and myelopathy," in *Clinical Neurology*, R. J. Joynt, Ed., vol. 3, pp. 1–36, JB Lippincott Company, Philadelphia, Pa, USA, 1992.

[17] C. Counsell and C. Warlow, "Failure of presumed hepatic myelopathy to improve after liver transplantation," *Journal of Neurology Neurosurgery and Psychiatry*, vol. 60, no. 5, p. 590, 1996.

[18] R. Troisi, J. Debruyne, and B. De Hemptinne, "Improvement of hepatic myelopathy after liver transplantation," *The New England Journal of Medicine*, vol. 340, no. 2, p. 151, 1999.

[19] C. Caldwell, N. Werdinger, S. Jakab et al., "Use of model for end-stage liver disease exception points for early liver transplantation and successful reversal of hepatic myelopathy with a review of the literature," *Liver Transplantation*, vol. 16, no. 7, pp. 818–826, 2010.

[20] H. S. Malhotra, V. K. Paliwal, M. K. Singh, and A. Agarwal, "Hepatic myelopathy: an unusual complication of advanced hepatic disease," *Annals of Neurosciences*, vol. 14, no. 1, 2007.

11

Acute Liver Failure among Patients on Efavirenz-Based Antiretroviral Therapy

Innocent Lule Segamwenge ⓘ **and Miriam Kaunanele Bernard**

Department of Internal Medicine, Intermediate Hospital Oshakati, Oshakati, Namibia

Correspondence should be addressed to Innocent Lule Segamwenge; sslule@yahoo.com

Academic Editor: Melanie Deutsch

Objectives. To describe the clinical characteristics of patients presenting with fulminant liver failure after varying periods of exposure to Efavirenz containing antiretroviral medications. *Methods.* We report a series of 4 patients with human immunodeficiency virus (HIV) infection who were admitted with acute liver failure (ALF) over a 6-month period. All these patients had been treated with a range of Efavirenz containing antiretroviral regimens and were negative for hepatitis A, B, and C infections as well as other opportunistic infections, all were negative for autoimmune hepatitis, and none had evidence of chronic liver disease or use of alcohol or herbal medications. Information on patient clinical characteristics, current antiretroviral regimen, CD4 count, HIV-1 RNA levels, and clinical chemistry parameters was collected. Informed consent was provided. *Results.* During a 6-month period, four patients without other known risk factors for acute hepatitis presented with symptomatic drug-induced liver injury with varying symptoms and outcomes. The pattern of liver injury was hepatocellular for all the 4 cases. Liver biopsies were done for all the four cases and the results showed a heavy mixed inflammatory cell infiltrate with eosinophils. For three patients withdrawal of Efavirenz from their antiretroviral regimen was sufficient to restore transaminase levels to normal and led to improvement of clinical symptoms. For one patient his clinical course was characterized by fulminant liver failure and fluctuating episodes of hepatic encephalopathy which ultimately resulted in his death. *Conclusion.* Hepatotoxicity of Efavirenz is not as rare as previously described in the literature and does actually present with fatal outcomes. The key message to note is that frequent monitoring of liver enzymes should be done at initiation of antiretroviral therapy and should continue throughout the treatment period.

1. Introduction

Antiretroviral therapy (ART) has dramatically changed the life expectancy and natural course of HIV infection [1, 2]. These drugs however are lifelong and are not without side-effects. Long-term side-effects of highly active antiretroviral therapy now contribute significantly to the morbidity and mortality among HIV patients with good immune reconstitution.

There are several long-term and short-term toxicities of the different antiretroviral drugs affecting many organs in the body [3, 4]. Hepatotoxicity of antiretroviral drugs is one of the more serious and life-threatening complications of antiretroviral drugs.

Non-nucleoside reverse transcriptase inhibitors (NNRTIs) are the drugs most commonly implicated in hepatotoxicity. The two most commonly used NNRTIs Nevirapine and Efavirenz are frequently used as part of the triple combination first-line ART regimen [5]. Nevirapine use has been associated with significant hepatic injury compared to Efavirenz [6]. The toxicity of NNRTIs has also been found to be more common in the first 12 weeks of starting ART and also in patients coinfected with hepatitis B and C [6].

We describe a series of cases presenting with severe Efavirenz associated hepatocellular injury following long-term use of the drug, who were also negative for hepatitis B and C.

TABLE 1: Patient characteristics and laboratory test results.

	Case 1	Case 2	Case 3	Case 4
Age (years)	45	40	40	41
Sex	F	F	M	F
Duration of EFV ART	12 months	4 months	5 months	2 weeks
CD4 count	734	402	667	550
Bilirubin total	208	291	471	273
Direct bilirubin	178	156	257	204
AST (NR: 10–40 U/L)	1288	377	913	913
ALT (NR: 13–40 U/L)	776	249	942	942
ALP (NR: 40–120 U/L)	229	143	139	338
GGT (NR: 9–50 U/L)	1101	145	337	735
R ratio	10.17	5.22	20.33	8.36
Hepatic damage type	Hepatocellular	Hepatocellular	Hepatocellular	Hepatocellular
RUCAM score	6	6	3	8

ALP: alkaline phosphatase; ALT: alanine aminotransferase; AST: aspartate aminotransferase; GGT: gamma-glutamyl transferase; NR: normal range; R ratio: (ALT/upper limit of normal range)/(ALP/upper limit of normal range); RUCAM: Roussel Uclaf Causality Assessment Method, ART: antiretroviral therapy, EFV: Efavirenz.

2. Case Presentation

2.1. Case 1.
A 45-year-old female presented with fatigue and yellow discoloration of eyes and passing yellow urine for over 2 weeks. Her medical history was notable for a history on concurrent HIV infection diagnosed over 3 years previously and she had been on antiretroviral drugs for 1 year. Her antiretroviral regimen is comprised of Tenofovir Disoproxil Fumarate 300 mg (TDF), Lamivudine 300 mg, and Efavirenz 600 mg in a single pill combination tablet (TELURA®, Mylan).

Her CD4 count was 734 cells per mm^3 and her viral load was below the level of detection at less than 40 copies of HIV per milliliter of blood (<40 copies/mL). She had no history of alcohol use nor any other drug use or chronic disease.

Her physical examination was notable for jaundice and tender right hypochondrium. She had no hepatic flap and no other features of hepatic encephalopathy or coagulopathy. The rest of her examination was normal.

Her liver function test showed a hepatocellular pattern of injury (Table 1). She was negative for hepatitis B and C. Her serology for autoimmune hepatitis which included antinuclear antibody (ANA), soluble liver antigen, anti-smooth muscle antibody, and liver kidney microsomal-1 antibodies was all negative. Her antiretroviral drugs were changed to Truvada (Tenofovir and Emtricitabine) and Raltegravir. A liver biopsy was done which showed acute hepatitis with interface activity and hydropic cytoplasmic changes with intermixed chronic inflammation with prominent eosinophil's and scanty neutrophils; these are findings which were more consistent with a drug-induced hepatic injury.

The antiretroviral drugs were all stopped and she was advised not to take any other potentially hepatotoxic drugs. During follow-up 2 months later, she was prescribed Tenofovir and Emtricitabine (Truvada) 300/600 mg once a day and Raltegravir (Isentress) 400 mg twice a day. Her ALT

was 118 U/L (normal range 13–40 U/L), and gamma-glutamyl transferase (GGT) was 943 U/L (normal range 9–50 U/L). Her follow-up at 8 months, GGT was 227 U/L (normal range 9–50 U/L), and ALT and aspartate aminotransferase (AST) were within normal.

2.2. Case 2.
A 40-year-old female presented with yellow discoloration of eyes, urine, and fluctuating level of consciousness over 1 week. Her medical history is noted for HIV infection diagnosed 4 months ago. She has since been on antiretroviral therapy consisting of Tenofovir Disoproxil Fumarate 300 mg (TDF), Lamivudine 300 mg (3TC), and Efavirenz 600 mg a single pill combination tablet (TELURA, Mylan). Her CD4 count was 402 cells per mm^3 and her viral load was below level of detection at less than 40 copies per milliliter of blood (<40 copies/mL). She developed these symptoms 4 months after starting antiretroviral therapy.

She had no history of alcohol use or use of herbal remedies and supplements.

Her physical examination was notable for jaundice and presence hepatic flap; she had no bleeding diathesis and had grade 3 hepatic encephalopathy. Hepatitis screen A, B, and C and her serology for autoimmune hepatitis which included antinuclear antibody (ANA), soluble liver antigen, anti-smooth muscle antibody, and liver kidney microsomal-1 antibodies were all negative.

Her liver function showed hepatocellular pattern of injury shown in Table 1. Following the onset of the symptoms and signs above, her antiretroviral drugs were stopped at the time of presentation to hospital. A liver biopsy was also done which showed prominent inflammation of the portal tracts with infiltrates composed of neutrophils, lymphocytes, and several eosinophils; these are features consistent with medication induced liver injury. Her ALT at 1-month and 2-month follow-up were 42 and 37 U/L (normal range 13–40 U/L), respectively. The ALP was 161 and 105 U/L (normal range

40–120 U/L) at 1 and 2 months. All other blood tests were within normal limits. During her follow-up at 1 month, she was started on Abacavir, Lamivudine (Kivexa) 300/600 mg daily, and Dolutegravir (Tivicay) 50 mg daily. She has since recovered well.

2.3. Case 3. A 46-year-old male presented with yellow discoloration of his eyes and urine over for one month; his medical history was notable for HIV infection that was diagnosed 8 years ago. At the time of admission, he had been on antiretroviral therapy treatment for 8 years. The ART regimen consisted of Zidovudine (AZT), Lamivudine (3TC), and Nevirapine (NVP) (Cipla) a single tablet combination; however, 5 months prior to this presentation, his regimen was changed to Tenofovir Disoproxil Fumarate 300 mg (TDF), Lamivudine 300 mg, and Efavirenz 600 mg in a single pill combination tablet (TELURA, Mylan) (TDF, 3TC, and EFV) in May 2016. The CD4 count was 667 cells per mm^3 and his viral load was below level of detection at less than 40 copies per millimeter of blood (<40 copies/ml). He had no history of drinking alcohol or use traditional herbal remedies.

The physical examination was notable for presence of jaundice, confusion, and excessive somnolence with presence of a hepatic flap. Tests for HBsAg, anti-HCV, anti-HAV IgM, CMV IgM, and EBV, antinuclear antibody (ANA), antimitochondrial antibody (AMA), and anti-smooth muscle antibody (ASMA) were negative. Abdominal ultrasound examination of the liver was normal. His liver function showed marked transaminitis as shown in Table 1. Liver biopsy was done which showed portal tracts with moderately heavy mixed inflammatory cell infiltrates of neutrophils, eosinophils, and lymphocytes. There were no plasma cells. The histological picture was in favor of drug-induced hepatitis.

His ART medications were stopped; however, his clinical course was characterized by recurrent episodes of hepatic encephalopathy without much improvement despite treatment with lactulose, metronidazole, and mannitol. His ALT was 339 U/L (normal range 13–40 U/L) at 1 month. He succumbed to fulminant liver failure after 1-month duration of hospitalization.

2.4. Case 4. A 41-year-old female presented with yellow discoloration of her eyes and urine over 3 weeks; she was diagnosed with HIV infection 9 years ago. She had been on ART treatment since her diagnosis. Her antiretroviral regimen consisted of Zidovudine (AZT) Lamivudine (3TC) and Nevirapine (NVP) (Cipla) a single tablet combination. Her CD4 count is 550 cells per mm^3 and her viral load is below level of detection at less than 40 copies per millimeter of blood (<40 copies/ml). Her ART regimen was changed 2 weeks prior to presentation to Tenofovir Disoproxil Fumarate 300 mg (TDF), Lamivudine 300 mg, and Efavirenz 600 mg in a single pill combination tablet (TELURA, Mylan).

She had no history of alcohol or any other drug use. Her physical examination was notable for jaundice; there was no

evidence of bleeding, no confusion, or other clinical signs of hepatic encephalopathy.

Tests for HBsAg, anti-HCV, anti-HAV IgM, CMV IgM, and EBV, antinuclear antibody (ANA), antimitochondrial antibody (AMA), and anti-smooth muscle antibody (ASMA) were negative. Her ALT above 942 U/L (normal range 13–40 U/L) and AST was above 913 U/L (normal range 10–40 U/L). Abdominal ultrasound examination of the liver was normal. Liver biopsy was done which showed normal hepatocytes with portal tracts having heavy mixed inflammatory cell infiltrates with numerous polymorphs and eosinophils. Cholestasis was evident with no granulomas, neoplasm, no fibrosis, or nodular formation.

Her ART was stopped and serial liver function testing was done to monitor her response to treatment. The ALT at weeks 2 and 4 of follow-up was 128 U/L and 114 U/l (normal range 13–40 U/L), respectively; the ALP was 153 and 185 U/L and GGT 250 and 310, respectively at weeks 2 and 4 of follow-up. She recovered well and at week two she was switched to a regimen consisting of Abacavir 300 mg twice daily, Lamivudine 150 mg twice daily, and Lopinavir boosted with ritonavir 400 m/100 mg twice daily. She recovered well.

3. Discussion

Hepatotoxicity of antiretroviral drugs is one of the more serious and life-threatening complications of antiretroviral drugs. Non-nucleoside reverse transcriptase inhibitors (NNRTIs) are the drugs most commonly implicated in hepatotoxicity yet these drugs are frequently used as part of the triple combination first-line ART regimen [5]. The greatest risk of NNRTI-associated severe hepatotoxicity are observed in patients taking Nevirapine, those with hepatitis B or C coinfection, and those coadministered protease inhibitors [6]. In particular Nevirapine use has been associated with severe hepatotoxicity in other studies, which, in some cases, was associated with an early (12 weeks) hypersensitivity reaction. Likewise, Efavirenz has also been associated with significant hepatotoxicity; however severe hepatotoxicity is relatively uncommon among nonhepatitis C infected individuals and those not receiving protease inhibitor therapy [6].

Our patients presented with severe liver toxicity defined as grade 3-4 elevations (>5 × upper limit of normal) of aminotransferases AST or ALT but were negative for Hepatitis A, B, and C and were not on protease inhibitor therapy, and none was taking Nevirapine. Interestingly, cases 3 and 4 developed severe hepatotoxicity after switching from Nevirapine to Efavirenz. Case 3 developed drug-induced hepatitis after 5 months of changing to Efavirenz-based therapy while case 4 developed the same after only 2 weeks of switching therapy. Sulkowski et al. described the development of de novo severe hepatotoxicity among 7 of 85 (9%) Efavirenz users after changing from Nevirapine [6]. The mechanism underlying the development of this severe toxicity is not known; it is possible that patients may be susceptible to toxicity of a particular drug, rather than NNRTI class, specifically.

The average age was 43 years and all had high CD4 counts with the lowest being 402 and the highest 734 cells per mm^3. High CD4 cell recovery has been associated with severe hepatotoxicity; it is not clear whether this represents immune-mediated liver injury in the hepatotoxicity or medication adherence and drug exposure [7]. The liver biopsies of our patients showed inflammatory cell infiltrates that are comprised predominantly of eosinophils and neutrophils with some biopsies showing lymphocyte infiltrates; these findings suggest that hepatic injury may be immune-mediated in our patients.

All our patients presented with symptomatic liver failure with case 3 having fulminant liver failure with a fatal outcome. Studies looking at grade 3-4 [8] hepatotoxicity of ART reported that most patients were asymptomatic and no deaths were due to liver-related events [7, 9, 10]. Fulminant hepatic failure due to Efavirenz leading to death is rare. Only one death due to fulminant liver failure after starting Efavirenz-based ART has been reported in the literature and two case reports of Efavirenz induced liver failure which required liver transplantation with good outcomes have been reported [11–13].

The timing of hepatotoxicity varied a lot among our patients ranging from two weeks of exposure to Efavirenz for case four to one year for case one. Hepatotoxicity due to Efavirenz has been described to occur between 100 days and 168 days (14 to 24 weeks) [6, 14]. Early and late onset types of antiretroviral-associated hepatotoxicity have been described. The early occurring form (less than 12 weeks after initiation of therapy) frequently goes along with rash, eosinophilia, fever, and arthralgia and seems to be based on an immune-mediated mechanism. The late onset form (after more than 12 weeks of therapy) is supposed to rely on an intrinsic toxic of the drug [14]. Our patient (case 4) who presented with early onset type of hepatotoxicity had no rash, fever, arthralgia, or eosinophilia. However, all our patients had eosinophil inflammatory infiltrate on liver biopsy. It is possible that both immune-mediated mechanisms and intrinsic toxic effects of the Efavirenz all had a role in the mechanism of hepatotoxicity in our patients.

4. Conclusion

Hepatotoxicity of Efavirenz is not as rare as previously described in the literature and does actually present with fatal outcomes. The key message to note is that frequent monitoring of liver enzymes should be done at initiation of antiretroviral therapy and should continue throughout the treatment period.

Authors' Contributions

Innocent Lule Segamwenge conceived the idea and wrote the manuscript. Miriam Kaunanele Bernard investigated and treated the patients. The final manuscript was read and approved by all authors.

Acknowledgments

The authors are grateful to our patients for accepting to have these cases published. They are also grateful to the administration and staff of Intermediate Hospital Oshakati, the Ministry of Health and Social Services of Namibia, and the Namibian Institute of Pathology for the assistance offered in managing the patients.

References

[1] R. Detels, A. Muñoz, G. McFarlane et al., "Effectiveness of potent antiretroviral therapy on time to AIDS and death in men with known HIV infection duration," *Journal of the American Medical Association*, vol. 280, no. 17, pp. 1497–1503, 1998.

[2] F. J. Palella Jr., K. M. Delaney, A. C. Moorman et al., "Declining morbidity and mortality among patients with advanced human immunodeficiency virus infection," *The New England Journal of Medicine*, vol. 338, no. 13, pp. 853–860, 1998.

[3] D. C. Rudorf and S. A. Krikorian, "Adverse effects associated with antiretroviral therapy and potential management strategies," *Journal of Pharmacy Practice*, vol. 18, no. 4, pp. 258–277, 2005.

[4] V. Montessori, N. Press, M. Harris, L. Akagi, and J. S. G. Montaner, "Adverse effects of antiretroviral therapy for HIV infection," *Canadian Medical Association Journal*, vol. 170, no. 2, pp. 229–238, 2004.

[5] L. Mbuagbaw, S. Mursleen, J. H. Irlam, A. B. Spaulding, G. W. Rutherford, and N. Siegfried, "Efavirenz or nevirapine in three-drug combination therapy with two nucleoside or nucleotide-reverse transcriptase inhibitors for initial treatment of HIV infection in antiretroviral-naïve individuals," *Cochrane Database of Systematic Reviews*, vol. 2016, no. 12, Article ID CD004246, 2016.

[6] M. S. Sulkowski, D. L. Thomas, S. H. Mehta, R. E. Chaisson, and R. D. Moore, "Hepatotoxicity associated with nevirapine or efavirenz-containing antiretroviral therapy: role of hepatitis C and B infections," *Hepatology*, vol. 35, no. 1, pp. 182–189, 2002.

[7] M. S. Sulkowski, D. L. Thomas, R. E. Chaisson, and R. D. Moore, "Hepatotoxicity associated with antiretroviral therapy in adults infected with human immunodeficiency virus and the role of hepatitis C or B virus infection," *Journal of the American Medical Association*, vol. 283, no. 1, pp. 74–80, 2000.

[8] U.S. Department of Health and Human Services, National Institutes of Health, National Institute of Allergy and Infectious Diseases, and Division of AIDS, "Division of AIDS (DAIDS) table for grading the severity of adult and pediatric adverse events, corrected version 2.1," 2017, https://rsc.tech-res.com/docs/default-source/safety/daidsgradingcorrectedv21.pdf.

[9] F. W. N. M. Wit, G. J. Weverling, J. Weel, S. Jurriaans, and J. M. A. Lange, "Incidence of and risk factors for severe hepatotoxicity associated with antiretroviral combination therapy," *The Journal of Infectious Diseases*, vol. 186, no. 1, pp. 23–31, 2002.

[10] G. Yimer, W. Amogne, A. Habtewold et al., "High plasma efavirenz level and CYP2B66 are associated with efavirenz-based HAART-induced liver injury in the treatment of naïve HIV patients from Ethiopia: a prospective cohort study," *The Pharmacogenomics Journal*, vol. 12, no. 6, pp. 499–506, 2012.

[11] N. Abrescia, M. D'Abbraccio, M. Figoni et al., "Fulminant hepatic failure after the start of an efavirenz-based HAART regimen in a treatment-naive female AIDS patient without hepatitis virus co-infection," *Journal of Antimicrobial Chemotherapy*, vol. 50, no. 5, pp. 763–765, 2002.

[12] D. L. Fink and E. Bloch, "Liver transplantation for acute liver failure due to efavirenz hepatotoxicity: the importance of routine monitoring," *International Journal of STD & AIDS*, vol. 24, no. 10, pp. 831–833, 2013.

[13] A. Turkova, C. Ball, S. Gilmour-White, M. Rela, and G. Mieli-Vergani, "A paediatric case of acute liver failure associated with efavirenz-based highly active antiretroviral therapy and effective use of raltegravir in combination antiretroviral treatment after liver transplantation," *Journal of Antimicrobial Chemotherapy*, vol. 63, no. 3, pp. 623–625, 2009.

[14] S. Brück, S. Witte, J. Brust et al., "Hepatotoxicity in patients prescribed efavirenz or nevirapine," *European Journal of Medical Research*, vol. 13, no. 7, pp. 343–348, 2008.

12

Transjugular Retrograde Obliteration prior to Liver Resection for Hepatocellular Carcinoma Associated with Hyperammonemia due to Spontaneous Portosystemic Shunt

Fumio Chikamori[1] and Nobutoshi Kuniyoshi[2]

[1] Department of Surgery, Kuniyoshi Hospital, 1-3-4 Kamimachi, Kochi City, Kochi 780-0901, Japan
[2] Department of Internal Medicine, Kuniyoshi Hospital, 1-3-4 Kamimachi, Kochi City, Kochi 780-0901, Japan

Correspondence should be addressed to Fumio Chikamori; chikamo2300@gmail.com

Academic Editors: S. Kapoor, Z.-Y. Lin, and R. T. Marinho

A 67-year-old woman had hepatocellular carcinoma (HCC) measuring 3.7 cm at S8 of the liver with hyperammonemia due to a spontaneous giant mesocaval shunt. Admission laboratory data revealed albumin, 2.9 g/dL; total bilirubin, 1.3 mg/dL; plasma ammonia level (NH_3), 152 g/dL; total bile acid (TBA) 108.5 μmoL/L; indocyanine green retention rate at 15 min (ICG15), 63%. Superior mesenteric arterial portography revealed a hepatofugal giant mesocaval shunt, and the portal vein was not visualized. Before surgery, transjugular retrograde obliteration (TJO) for the mesocaval shunt was attempted to normalize the portal blood flow. Via the right internal jugular vein, a 6 F occlusive balloon catheter was inserted superselectively into the mesocaval shunt. The mesocaval shunt was successfully embolized using absolute ethanol and a 50% glucose solution. Eleven days after TJO, NH_3, TBA, and ICG15 decreased to 56, 44, and 33, respectively. Superior mesenteric arterial portography after TJO revealed a hepatopetal portal flow. Partial hepatectomy of S8 was performed 25 days after TJO. The subsequent clinical course showed no complications, and the woman was discharged on postoperative day 14. We conclude that the combined therapy of surgery and TJO is an effective means of treating HCC with hyperammonemia due to a spontaneous portosystemic shunt.

1. Introduction

Hepatocellular carcinoma (HCC) with hyperammonemia due to a spontaneous portosystemic shunt (PSS) is not common, and the guidelines for such a condition have not been established yet [1]. Liver function is an important factor to determine the treatment strategy for HCC.

To lower morbidity after hepatic resection, the Makuuchi criteria, including the presence or absence of ascites, serum total bilirubin level, and the plasma indocyanine green retention rate at 15 min (ICG15), are widely used [2, 3]. However, the existence of PSS often increases the level of ICG15 and the plasma ammonia level (NH_3) and reduces the hepatopetal portal blood flow. We previously reported that transjugular retrograde obliteration (TJO) for PSS reduced ICG15 and NH_3 [4]. A mesocaval shunt is one of the PSSs. Here, we describe a case of HCC associated with hyperammonemia due to a spontaneous mesocaval shunt treated by the combined therapy of surgery and TJO.

2. Case Report

A 67-year-old woman suffered from HCC with hyperammonemia due to a spontaneous giant mesocaval shunt. Six months before that, she had undergone interferon therapy for hepatitis C. However, follow-up CT examination revealed HCC, so she was referred to our department for further evaluation and treatment.

On admission, her vital signs were stable. The patient was conscious and alert. Her palpebral conjunctivae were pale. Admission laboratory data were as follows: white blood cell count, 4300/μL; hemoglobin, 10.6 g/dL; platelets, 187000/μL; albumin, 2.9 g/dL; total bilirubin, 1.3 mg/dL;

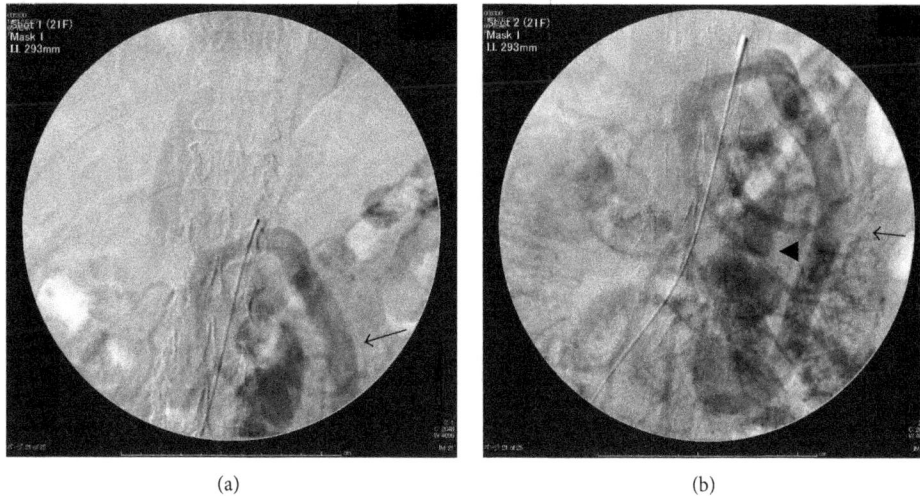

(a)   (b)

FIGURE 1: (a) Superior mesenteric arterial portogram shows hepatofugal giant mesocaval shunt (arrow). Portal vein was not visualized. (b) Superior mesenteric arterial portogram: mesenteric venous blood was drained into the inferior vena cava via dilated inferior mesenteric vein (arrow), left ovarian vein (arrowhead) and left renal vein.

aspartate aminotransferase, 46 IU/L; alanine aminotransferase, 14 IU/L; cholinesterase, 132 U/L; prothrombin time, 62%; hepaplastin test, 62%: NH_3, 152 g/dL; total bile acid (TBA), 108.5 μmol/L: ICG15, 63%. Tumor marker levels were as follows: alpha-fetoprotein (AFP), 88.5 nG/mL; protein induced by vitamin K absence or antagonist II (PIVKA-II), 5130 mAU/mL. Hepatic function was classified as Child-Pugh class A (score 6). Hepatitis B surface antigen was negative. Hepatitis C virus (HCV) antibody was positive, but HCV-RNA was not detected. Ultrasonography and contrast enhanced computed tomography revealed HCC measuring 3.7 cm in diameter at S8 of the liver and a markedly tortuous mesocaval shunt. An endoscopic examination revealed no esophagogastric varices. Superior mesenteric arterial portography revealed a hepatofugal giant mesocaval shunt, and the portal vein was not visualized (Figures 1(a) and 1(b)).

Before surgery, TJO for the mesocaval shunt was attempted to normalize the portal blood flow, NH_3, and ICG15. Via the right internal jugular vein, an 8 F cobra shaped sheath was inserted into the left renal vein. Then, a 6 F occlusive balloon catheter was inserted superselectively into the mesocaval shunt (Figure 2(a)). On the 1st day of TJO, 8 mL of absolute ethanol and 100 mL of a 50% glucose solution were injected into the mesocaval shunt intermittently.

On the 2nd day, the marginal vein which communicated with the portal vein and the superior rectal vein which communicated with the bilateral internal iliac veins were revealed, so 1 mL of absolute ethanol and 20 mL of a 50% glucose solution were injected again (Figures 2(b), 2(c), and 2(d)). On the 3rd day, the marginal vein was not visualized. After confirming the thrombus formation in the mesocaval shunt, the catheter was removed (Figure 2(e)).

Eleven days after TJO, NH_3, TBA, and ICG15 decreased to 56, 44, and 33, respectively. Superior mesenteric arterial portography after TJO revealed a hepatopetal portal blood

flow (Figure 3). Partial hepatectomy of S8 was performed 25 days after TJO. The subsequent clinical course showed no complications, and the woman was discharged on postoperative day 14. AFP/PIVKA-II levels 2 and 14 weeks after surgery decreased to 21.2/79 and 3.7/24, respectively. Follow-up examinations for 6 months after the combined therapy have not indicated any recurrence of HCC or hyperammonemia.

3. Discussion

We successfully treated HCC with hyperammonemia due to a spontaneous PSS by the combined therapy of surgery and TJO. HCC with hyperammonemia is an uncommon condition. Hepatic failure is the most lethal complication of hepatectomy. Insufficient portal blood flow is one of the causes of hepatic failure [5]. The treatment for such a condition has not yet been established. Hepatectomy with simultaneous ligation of spontaneous PSS has been reported [6–8]. However, hepatectomy for patients with poor liver function is invasive, so we have to evaluate preoperative liver function precisely. If liver function is modified by abnormal portal blood flow, we have to reevaluate it after normalization of portal blood flow.

We applied the interventional radiology technique (IVR) to normalize the portal blood flow. Vascular anatomy is important for treating PSS by IVR. A mesocaval shunt is one of the PSSs, and it is supplied by the inferior mesenteric vein and drained by the gonadal or renal vein. In addition, we have to recognize that the shunt communicates with superior rectal and sigmoid veins. There are three IVR approaches for mesocaval shunt obliteration. Percutaneous transhepatic obliteration (PTO) [9, 10] and transileocolic vein obliteration (TIO) [11] are embolization techniques via the blood supply route. Retrograde transvenous obliteration (RTO) is an embolization technique via the blood drainage route. PTO

(a)

(b)

(c)

(d)

(e)

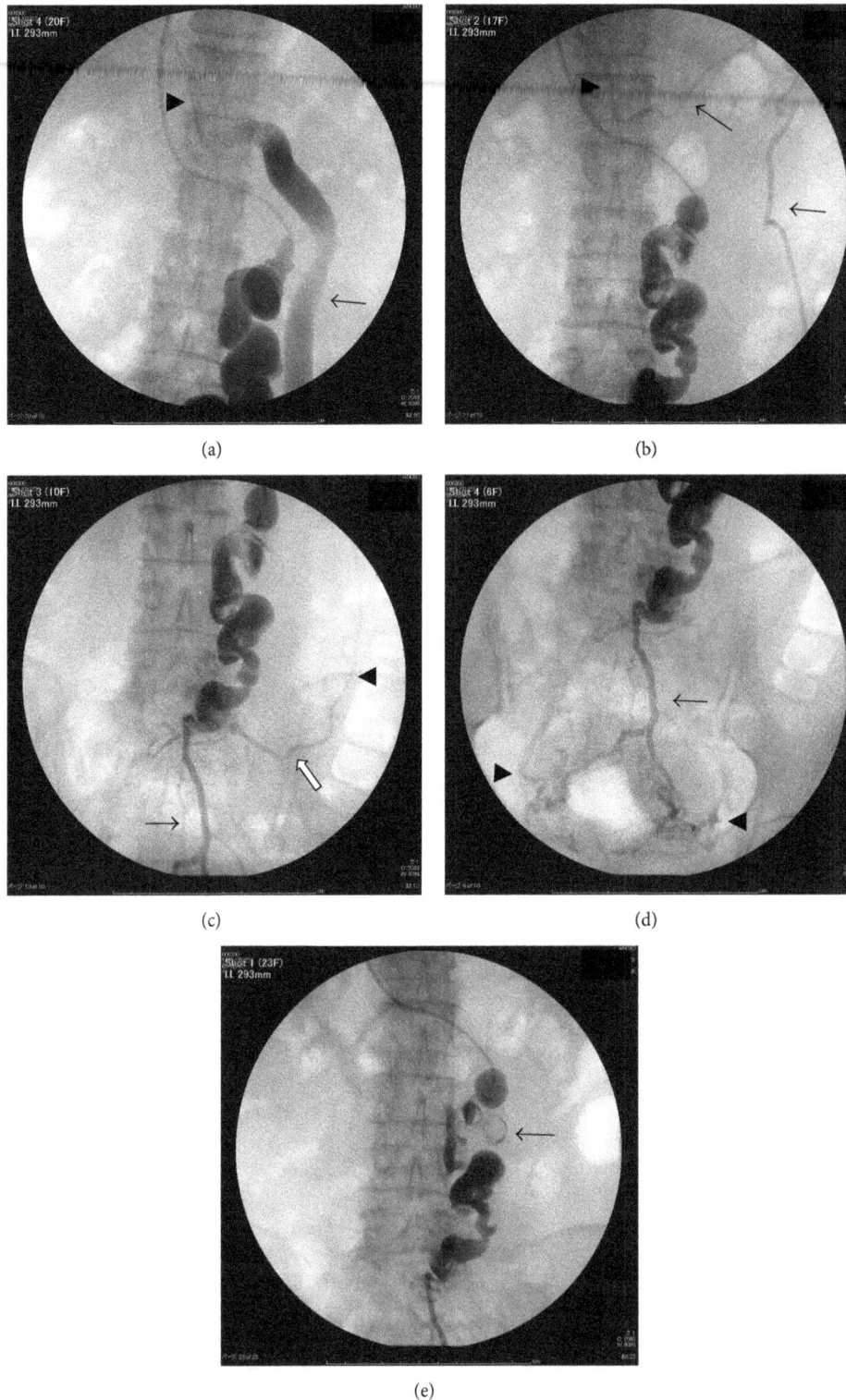

FIGURE 2: (a) Transjugular retrograde obliteration (TJO) on the 1st day: retrograde shunt venogram shows left ovarian vein and dilated inferior mesenteric vein (arrow) and portal vein (arrowhead). (b) Retrograde shunt venogram on the 2nd day shows marginal vein (arrow) communicated with portal vein (arrowhead). (c) Retrograde shunt venogram on the 2nd day shows superior rectal (arrow), sigmoid (white arrow), and marginal veins (arrowhead). (d) Retrograde shunt venogram on the 2nd day shows superior rectal vein (arrow) communicated with bilateral internal iliac veins (arrowhead). (e) Retrograde shunt venogram on the 3rd day shows thrombus formation (arrowhead) in the mesocaval shunt. The marginal vein communicated with portal vein was not visualized.

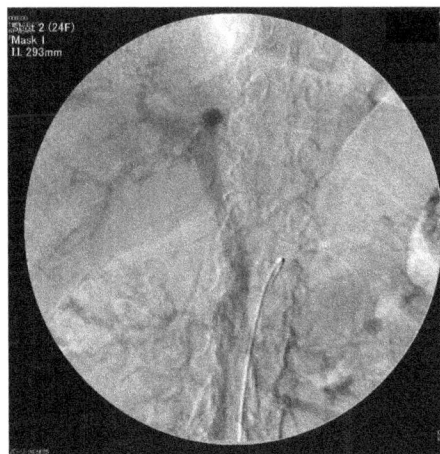

FIGURE 3: Superior mesenteric arterial portogram after TJO shows hepatopetal portal blood flow.

for varices is occasionally used for acute variceal hemorrhage; however, it has the risk of intraperitoneal bleeding and is invasive. Minilaparotomy is necessary for TIO. Therefore, we chose RTO in the present case.

There are only a few reports of combined therapy using surgery and RTO for HCC with PSS [12, 13]. RTO such as TJO [14] or balloon-occluded transvenous obliteration (B-RTO) [15] is popular in Japan for gastric variceal treatment. TJO was reported as a transjugular approach, which maintains the balloon catheter for 24 hours, and B-RTO was reported as a transfemoral approach, which maintains the catheter for 30 minutes originally [14, 15]. TJO has an advantage over the femoral approach in being able to obliterate the shunt superselectively. Superselective obliteration can reduce the volume of sclerosant required for shunt obliteration.

We already confirmed that TJO for chronic portosystemic encephalopathy reduced NH_3 and ICG15 [3]. In the present case, we applied TJO for the mesocaval shunt before hepatectomy to normalize the portal blood flow during which we should pay attention to the communicating routes of the mesocaval shunt, which seem to be a giant solitary line on a superior mesenteric arterial portogram. Actually, it is not solitary and communicates with the superior rectal and sigmoid veins. A retrograde shunt venogram on the 2nd day revealed these communicating routes. The superior rectal vein communicates with the bilateral iliac veins, which lead to systemic circulation, but the sigmoid vein communicates with the marginal vein which leads to portal circulation. The most important issue is how to disconnect the mesocaval shunt from the portal circulation completely. Therefore, we had to reinject the sclerosant on the 2nd day. We could confirm that the marginal vein was not visualized by retrograde shunt venography on the 3rd day. TJO contributed to the protecting portal blood steal after hepatectomy, and the patient's postoperative course was uneventful. We conclude that the combined therapy of surgery and TJO is an effective means of treating HCC with hyperammonemia due to a spontaneous PSS.

References

[1] N. Watanabe, A. Toyonaga, S. Kojima et al., "Current status of ectopic varices in Japan: results of a survey by the Japan Society for Portal Hypertension," *Hepatology Research*, vol. 40, no. 8, pp. 763–776, 2010.

[2] Y. Seyama and N. Kokudo, "Assessment of liver function for safe hepatic resection," *Hepatology Research*, vol. 39, no. 2, pp. 107–116, 2009.

[3] S. Miyagawa, M. Makuuchi, S. Kawasaki, and T. Kakazu, "Criteria for safe hepatic resection," *American Journal of Surgery*, vol. 169, no. 6, pp. 589–594, 1995.

[4] F. Chikamori, N. Kuniyoshi, S. Shibuya, and Y. Takase, "Transjugular retrograde obliteration for chronic portosystemic encephalopathy," *Abdominal Imaging*, vol. 25, no. 6, pp. 567–571, 2000.

[5] M. Kajikawa, A. Harada, H. Kobayashi et al., "Transient hepatofugal portal blood flow after hepatectomy in a patient with cirrhosis: report of a case," *Surgery Today*, vol. 26, no. 9, pp. 719–722, 1996.

[6] T. Hayashi, H. Kohno, A. Yamanoi, H. Kubota, M. Tachibana, and N. Nagasue, "Surgical treatment of hepatocellular carcinoma associated with spontaneous portosystemic shunts," *European Journal of Surgery*, vol. 165, no. 6, pp. 543–549, 1999.

[7] Q. Wang, K. Sun, X. H. Li, B. G. Peng, and L. J. Liang, "Surgical treatment for hepatocellular carcinoma and secondary hypersplenism," *Hepatobiliary and Pancreatic Diseases International*, vol. 5, no. 3, pp. 396–400, 2006.

[8] H. Li, Y. L. Hu, Y. Wang, D. S. Zhang, and F. X. Jiang, "Simultaneous operative treatment of patients with primary liver cancer associated with portal hypertension," *Hepatobiliary and Pancreatic Diseases International*, vol. 1, no. 1, pp. 92–93, 2002.

[9] A. Lunderquist and J. Vang, "Transhepatic catheterization and obliteration of the coronary vein in patients with portal hypertension and esophageal varices," *The New England Journal of Medicine*, vol. 291, no. 13, pp. 646–649, 1974.

[10] F. Chikamori, N. Kuniyoshi, S. Kagiyama, T. Kawashima, S. Shibuya, and Y. Takase, "Role of percutaneous transhepatic obliteration for special types of varices with portal hypertension," *Abdominal Imaging*, vol. 32, no. 1, pp. 92–95, 2007.

[11] K. Ota, M. Okazaki, H. Higashihara et al., "Combination of transileocolic vein obliteration and balloon-occluded retrograde transvenous obliteration is effective for ruptured duodenal varices," *Journal of Gastroenterology*, vol. 34, no. 6, pp. 694–699, 1999.

[12] K. Morita, A. Taketomi, Y. Yamashita et al., "A case of hepatocellular carcinoma resected after improvement of liver function by balloon-occluded retrograde transvenous obliteration," *Japanese Journal of Gastroenterological Surgery*, vol. 41, no. 4, pp. 418–423, 2008.

[13] N. Hashimoto, T. Akahoshi, T. Shoji et al., "Successful treatment for hepatic encephalopathy aggravated by portal vein thrombosis with balloon-occluded retrograde transvenous obliteration," *Case Reports in Gastroenterology*, vol. 5, no. 2, pp. 366–371, 2011.

[14] F. Chikamori, S. Shibuya, Y. Takase, A. Ozaki, and K. Fukao, "Transjugular retrograde obliteration for gastric varices," *Abdominal Imaging*, vol. 21, no. 4, pp. 299–303, 1996.

[15] H. Kanagawa, S. Mima, H. Kouyama et al., "A successfully treated case of fundic varices by retrograde transvenous obliteration with balloon," *Nihon Shokakibyo Gakkai Zasshi*, vol. 88, no. 7, pp. 1459–1462, 1991.

13

Nonalcoholic Steatohepatitis in a Patient with Ataxia-Telangiectasia

Trinidad Caballero,[1,2] Mercedes Caba-Molina,[1] Javier Salmerón,[2] and Mercedes Gómez-Morales[1]

[1] *Pathology Department, San Cecilio University Hospital and School of Medicine, University of Granada, Avenida de Madrid 11, 18012 Granada, Spain*
[2] *Networked Biomedical Research Center for Hepatic and Digestive Diseases (CIBERehd), Carlos III Institute of Health, Spain*

Correspondence should be addressed to Trinidad Caballero; trinidad@ugr.es

Academic Editors: H. Miura and T. Tanwandee

Ataxia-telangiectasia (A-T) is a rare disease characterized by neurodegenerative alterations, telangiectasia, primary immunodeficiency, extreme sensitivity to radiation, and susceptibility to neoplasms. A-T patients have inactivation of ataxia-telangiectasia-mutated (ATM) protein, which controls DNA double-strand break repair and is involved in oxidative stress response, among other functions; dysfunctional control of reactive oxygen species may be responsible for many of the clinical manifestations of this disease. To the best of our knowledge, hepatic lesions of steatohepatitis have not previously been reported in A-T patients. The present study reports the case of a 22-year-old man diagnosed with A-T at the age of 6 years who was referred to our Digestive Disease Unit with a three-year history of hyperlipidemia and liver test alterations. Core liver biopsy showed similar lesions to those observed in nonalcoholic steatohepatitis. Immunohistochemical staining disclosed the absence of ATM protein in hepatocyte nuclei. We suggest that the liver injury may be mainly attributable to the oxidative stress associated with ATM protein deficiency, although other factors may have made a contribution. We propose the inclusion of A-T among the causes of nonalcoholic steatohepatitis, which may respond to antioxidant therapy.

1. Introduction

Ataxia-telangiectasia (A-T) is a rare autosomal recessive hereditary neurodegenerative and progressive disease caused by mutations in the ataxia-telangiectasia-mutated (ATM) gene that produce the absence or inactivation of ATM protein kinase. Clinical manifestations of A-T include early-onset neurological alterations (cerebellar ataxia caused by Purkinje and granule cell degeneration), late-onset oculocutaneous telangiectasias, early aging, sterility, hypersensitivity to ionizing radiation, immunodeficiency, and susceptibility to neoplasms [1, 2], especially leukemia, lymphomas, and breast cancer [3, 4]. Patients with A-T can also have impaired cellular and humoral immunity (IgA, IgE, or IgG2 immunodeficiency) and elevated serum alpha-fetoprotein (AFP), which can be useful for the diagnosis [4, 5].

ATM protein participates in double-strand-break repair mechanisms and can be activated by exogenous and endogen oxidative stress; ATM activation increases antioxidant levels and induces DNA oxidative damage repair [6]. Along with p53, ATM plays an important role in maintaining genomic integrity [5]. Many of the clinical alterations observed in A-T patients may be related to the dysfunctional control of reactive oxygen species (ROS) observed when ATM is deficient [1].

Nonalcoholic steatohepatitis (NASH) is a progressive form of nonalcoholic fatty liver disease histologically characterized by hepatocyte steatosis, ballooning (with or without Mallory-Denk body [MDB] formation), and lobular necroinflammatory lesions, which tend to be associated with pericellular and perisinusoidal fibrosis; many of these changes are localized in the acinar zone 3 [7, 8]. Although various factors

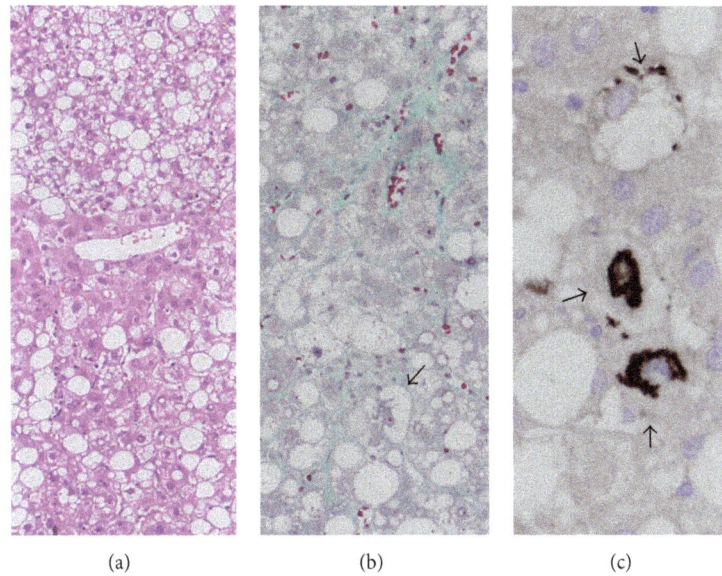

(a) (b) (c)

FIGURE 1: Histological changes in liver biopsy from patient with ataxia-telangiectasia. Hepatic lobule showing hepatocytes with macrovesicular and multivesicular steatosis (hematoxylin-eosin (a)) and perisinusoidal and pericellular fibrosis around ballooning hepatocytes, some containing Mallory-Denk bodies (arrow) (Gomori trichrome (b)), which are more evident with immunohistochemical staining for p62 protein, arrows (c) (original magnification: ×10, ×20, and ×40, resp.).

may contribute to the development of these alterations, ROS-mediated oxidative stress is known to play a major role in their genesis [9, 10].

We present the first report of NASH lesions in an A-T patient who had shown alterations in liver tests over the previous two years. We discuss the pathogenic mechanisms that may be implicated in the genesis of liver damage in this disease.

2. Case Report and Results

A 22-year-old male, with a height of 160 cm and body mass index of 17.5, was referred to the Department of Digestive Diseases for elevated serum transaminases. The family history was not relevant. He was diagnosed with A-T in infancy, and cerebellar atrophy was revealed by magnetic resonance imaging at the age of six years. At the time of his referral, his progressive motor alteration had left him wheelchair bound. His history also included agammaglobulinemia (IgA) since childhood, requiring immunoglobulin substitution therapy; H1N1 influenza A virus infection; repeated respiratory infections; and recurrent herpetic keratitis, treated with valacyclovir for the previous 10 years.

Tests over the two years before his referral to the Digestive Disease Unit evidenced elevated serum AST, ALT, and GGT values and dyslipidemia; in the biopsy taken at his referral, the serum values were 204 U/L (N ≤ 37), 376 U/L (N ≤ 40), and 442 U/L (N ≤ 50), respectively. Serum TG (167 mg/dL, N ≤ 150) and LDL (139 mg/dL, N ≤ 130) levels were mildly elevated, HDL was normal, and he evidenced thrombocytosis ($502 \times 10^3 \mu$L) and a very high AFP level (1202 ng/mL; N ≤ 10). Blood pressure, basal glucose, thyroid hormones, and alfa-1 antitrypsin values were normal; viral serology (HAV, HBV, HCV, HEV, CMV, HSV, EBV, VZV) and autoantibody (ANA, AMA, AML, LKM1, ATA) screening results were negative, and no iron or copper metabolism anomalies were detected. Ultrasound scan detected liver steatosis. A percutaneous liver biopsy was taken.

Liver biopsy was fixed in 10% neutral formalin and embedded in paraffin; 4μm sections were obtained and stained with hematoxylin-eosin, PAS-diastase, Gomori trichrome, Gordon-Sweet reticulin, and Prussian blue (Perls). Immunohistochemical techniques were also applied with an automated system (Lab Vision Autostainer 720) using primary antibodies against p62 protein (monoclonal antibody 3P62LCK, 1/500 dilution, BD transduction), which binds to MDBs, and against ATM protein (monoclonal antibody Y170, prediluted, Master Diagnóstica, Granada, Spain).

Histological examination of the liver biopsy revealed the characteristic features of steatohepatitis, that is, moderate macrovesicular and multivesicular steatosis (Figure 1(a)) and ballooning hepatocytes, some containing MDBs, in perivenular areas, along with pericellular and perisinusoidal fibrosis (Figure 1(b)). Some foci of lobular inflammation were also observed, but no fibrosis or inflammatory infiltration of portal tracts was detected; therefore, the lesions were classified as stage 1A. Immunohistochemical study with the anti-p62 antibody revealed the presence of MDBs in the cytoplasm of several ballooning hepatocytes localized in acinar zone 3 of numerous lobules (Figure 1(c)). Staining for ATM protein showed that expression of this protein was absent in the hepatocyte nuclei (Figure 2(a)), whereas it was found in normal liver and in liver specimens from patients with steatohepatitis of different etiologies (Figures 2(b) and 2(c)) (unpublished observation).

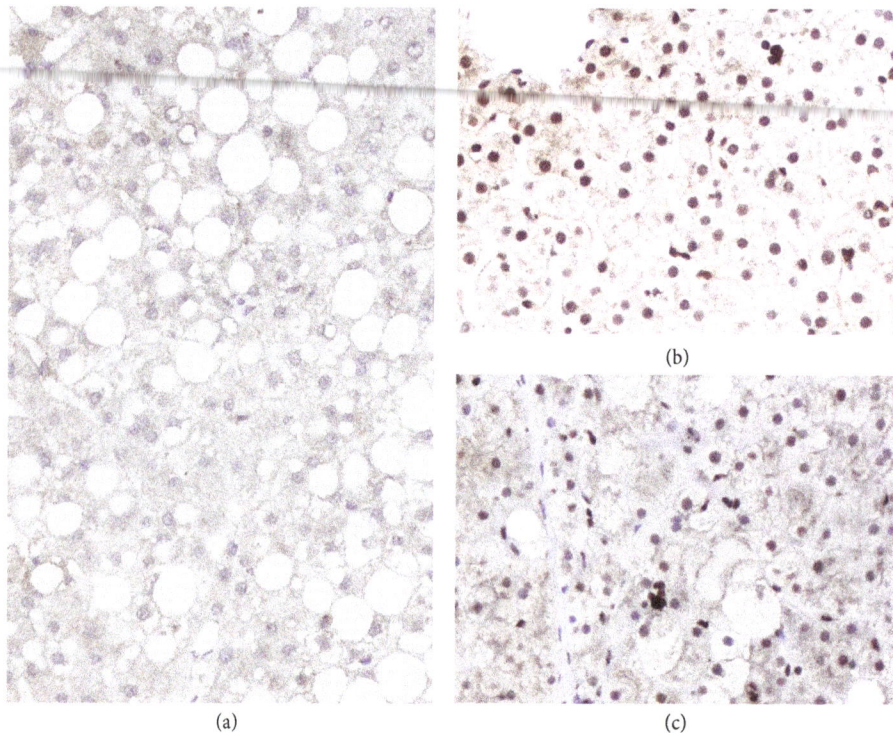

FIGURE 2: Immunohistochemical staining of liver biopsies with anti-ATM antibody. Absence of hepatocyte nuclear staining in the A-T patient (a). Nuclear immunostaining is observed in a normal liver (b) and in a liver biopsy specimen from an obese patient with nonalcoholic steatohepatitis (c) (immunoperoxidase, original magnification: ×20).

3. Discussion

A-T is a rare hereditary and recessive disease whose clinical manifestations are related to the presence of a defective or nonfunctional ATM protein due to ATM gene mutation [1, 5]. A-T is a clinically heterogeneous disease, and there are milder forms with a slower or later neurological progression [2] that may produce various neuropathological alterations [11].

ATM protein is a serine/threonine protein kinase, chief activator of the DNA damage response induced by DNA double-strand breaks after ionizing radiation and other insults, and it may be activated by oxidative stress [1, 5, 6]. ATM protein is involved in several cellular biological processes such as neural and immune system homeostasis, cell cycle checkpoints, genomic stability and insulin signaling, among others, which are controlled by signaling pathways triggered after ATM activation [11–13]. ATM protein is distributed in the cytoplasm and, mainly, in the nucleus of the various types of cells in which it is abundant [13].

Many of the alterations observed in A-T patients may be related to the dysfunctional control of ROS, given that cells lacking ATM exhibit high ROS concentrations and hypersensitivity to oxidative stress-inducing agents [1, 6]. Chronic activation of stress response pathways has been observed in tissues with pathological changes, such as the cerebellum, and other areas of the central nervous system may become affected if the life of the patient is prolonged [1, 10].

Serum AFP level was elevated in our patient, as also reported in more than 95% of A-T patients [5], and this elevation may be of value in the differential diagnosis between A-T and other A-T-like diseases. The increased serum AFP in A-T is not related to hepatic injury and is of uncertain origin, although a relationship with cerebellar Purkinje cell degeneration has been proposed, based on the elevated AFP levels observed in various diseases characterized by neural tube defects [4]. High AFP levels have also been described in diseases produced by AFP gene mutation, including hereditary persistence of alpha-fetoprotein [14]; inflammatory liver diseases, usually associated with malignant transformation; and germinal cell neoplasms.

NASH, a potentially aggressive and progressive form of nonalcoholic fatty liver disease, displays similar histological lesions to those in alcoholic hepatitis, with a distribution in the acinar zone 3 of hepatic lobules and a variable severity [7], although MDBs and fibrosis are less pronounced in NASH, as in the present case. The origin of these lesions is multifactorial, although an important role is played by ROS-induced oxidative damage [9], which produces injury in several cell components, including protein and DNA damage and membrane lipid peroxidation. The characteristic histologic lesions of NASH (ballooning, MDBs, necrosis/apoptosis of hepatocytes, inflammation, and fibrosis) represent the morphological expression of oxidative stress [8, 15].

Steatosis is the first event ("hit") in the development of steatohepatitis [16]. Macrovesicular steatosis can be induced if mild and prolonged alteration of mitochondrial

β-oxidation occurs [17], which may explain the onset of liver injury in this patient, along with other factors (e.g., dyslipidemia).

Although the most common cause of nonalcoholic fatty liver disease is the metabolic syndrome, it has also been related to other causes, including nutritional and metabolic status, drugs, genetic factors, and infectious agents, among others [8]. However, A-T has never been cited as a possible etiology.

Patients with A-T are reported to be at increased risk of diabetes mellitus type 2 (DM-2), although their short life expectancy and the typically late onset of DM-2 means that its associated complications are not usually observed in these patients [12]. DM-2 may be associated with metabolic syndrome and nonalcoholic fatty liver disease. Basal glucose levels were normal in the patient in all determinations carried out during the followup; although the patient showed elevated TG and HDL when the biopsy was taken, these values are normal at present after dietetic modification and statin treatment. No other parameters of metabolic syndrome were altered.

NASH and A-T share the same pathogenic mechanism of ROS generation. ROS may contribute to the mitochondrial dysfunction that plays a role in the development of lesions in NASH, which has been considered a mitochondrial disease [15]. In turn, excessive ROS production has been attributed to mitochondrial dysfunction in other diseases, including neurodegenerative conditions [13], and may be induced by the morphofunctional mitochondrial changes in A-T patients.

The development of steatohepatitis in our patient may be the result of oxidative stress due to inactive ATM protein, although other possible contributory factors include dyslipidemia, physical inactivity, and pharmacological treatments, which can induce further ROS generation and/or antioxidant depletion of hepatocytes.

The relatively long survival of the patient, probably attributable to his less severe form of A-T, may be responsible for the development of the hepatic lesions. We propose A-T as a candidate for inclusion among the causes of NASH. Further studies of larger series of patients with A-T are required to confirm our observations, although this is a challenging task given the low incidence of this disease (1 per 40,000–100,000 newborns [5]).

In summary, A-T patients with a relatively long survival may develop hepatic lesions similar to those in nonalcoholic steatohepatitis, and A-T should therefore be considered as a possible cause of NASH. Oxidative stress due to the functional deficiency of ATM protein is involved in the pathogenesis of hepatic lesions in this patient, which may therefore be susceptible to antioxidant therapy. We propose that NASH may be considered as a late phenotypic manifestation of A-T.

Abbreviations

A-T: Ataxia-telangiectasia
ATM: Ataxia telangiectasia mutated
AFP: Alpha-fetoprotein
ROS: Reactive oxygen species
NASH: Nonalcoholic steatohepatitis
MDB: Mallory-Denk body
ALT: Alanine aminotransferase
AST: Aspartate aminotransferase
GGT: Gamma-glutamyltransferase
N: Normal
TG: Triglycerides
LDL: Low-density lipoproteins
HDL: High-density lipoproteins
HAV: Hepatitis A virus
HBV: Hepatitis B virus
HCV: Hepatitis C virus
HEV: Hepatitis E virus
Ab: Antibody
CMV: Cytomegalovirus
EBV: Epstein-Barr virus
HSV: Herpes simplex virus
VZV: Varicella zoster virus
ANA: Anti-nuclear Abs
AMA: Anti-mitochondrial Abs
SML: Smooth-muscle Abs
LKM1: Liver/kidney microsomal Abs
ATA: Anti-transglutaminase Abs
DM-2: Diabetes mellitus-type 2.

Acknowledgment

The authors are grateful to Máster Diagnóstica (Granada, Spain) for the immunohistochemical ATM protein detection.

References

[1] A. Barzilai, G. Rotman, and Y. Shiloh, "ATM deficiency and oxidative stress: a new dimension of defective response to DNA damage," *DNA Repair*, vol. 1, no. 1, pp. 3–25, 2002.

[2] A. M. R. Taylor and P. J. Byrd, "Molecular pathology of ataxia telangiectasia," *Journal of Clinical Pathology*, vol. 58, no. 10, pp. 1009–1015, 2005.

[3] J. Boultwood, "Ataxia telangiectasia gene mutations in leukaemia and lymphoma," *Journal of Clinical Pathology*, vol. 54, no. 7, pp. 512–516, 2001.

[4] L. G. Ball and W. Xiao, "Molecular basis of ataxia telangiectasia and related diseases," *Acta Pharmacologica Sinica*, vol. 26, no. 8, pp. 897–907, 2005.

[5] A. Mavrou, G. T. Tsangaris, E. Roma, and A. Kolialexi, "The ATM gene and ataxia telangiectasia," *Anticancer Research*, vol. 28, no. 1, pp. 401–405, 2008.

[6] Z. Guo, R. Deshpande, and T. T. Paull, "ATM activation in the presence of oxidative stress," *Cell Cycle*, vol. 9, no. 24, pp. 4805–4811, 2010.

[7] E. M. Brunt, "Nonalcoholic steatohepatitis: definition and pathology," *Seminars in Liver Disease*, vol. 21, no. 1, pp. 3–16, 2001.

[8] P. Angulo, "Medical progress: nonalcoholic fatty liver disease," *New England Journal of Medicine*, vol. 346, no. 16, pp. 1221–1231, 2002.

[9] M. Parola and G. Robino, "Oxidative stress-related molecules and liver fibrosis," *Journal of Hepatology*, vol. 35, no. 2, pp. 297–306, 2001.

[10] M. M. M. Verhagen, J.-J. Martin, M. van Deuren et al., "Neuropathology in classical and variant ataxia-telangiectasia," *Neuropathology*, vol. 32, pp. 234–244, 2012.

[11] P. J. McKinnon, "ATM and the molecular pathogenesis of ataxia telangiectasia," *Annual Review of Pathology: Mechanisms of Disease*, vol. 7, pp. 303–321, 2012.

[12] S. Ditch and T. T. Paull, "The ATM protein kinase and cellular redox signaling: beyond the DNA damage response," *Trends in Biochemical Sciences*, vol. 37, no. 1, pp. 15–22, 2012.

[13] M. Ambrose and R. A. Gatti, "Pathogenesis of ataxia-telangiectasia: the next generation of ATM functions," *Blood*, vol. 121, pp. 4036–4045, 2013.

[14] J. R. Blesa, R. Giner-Durán, J. Vidal et al., "Report of hereditary persistence of α-fetoprotein in a Spanish family: molecular basis and clinical concerns," *Journal of Hepatology*, vol. 38, no. 4, pp. 541–544, 2003.

[15] D. Pessayre and B. Fromenty, "NASH: a mitochondrial disease," *Journal of Hepatology*, vol. 42, no. 6, pp. 928–940, 2005.

[16] C. P. Day and O. F. W. James, "Steatohepatitis: a tale of two "Hits"?" *Gastroenterology*, vol. 114, no. 4, pp. 842–845, 1998.

[17] G. Labbe, D. Pessayre, and B. Fromenty, "Drug-induced liver injury through mitochondrial dysfunction: mechanisms and detection during preclinical safety studies," *Fundamental and Clinical Pharmacology*, vol. 22, no. 4, pp. 335–353, 2008.

14

Sorafenib-Induced Liver Failure: A Case Report and Review of the Literature

Anneleen Van Hootegem, Chris Verslype, and Werner Van Steenbergen

Liver Unit, Department of Pathophysiology, University Hospital Gasthuisberg, Catholic University of Leuven, 3000 Leuven, Belgium

Correspondence should be addressed to Werner Van Steenbergen, werner.vansteenbergen@uzleuven.be

Academic Editors: I. Gentile, B. Mauro, and F. Pérez Roldán

In patients with hepatocellular carcinoma characterized by vascular invasion and/or extrahepatic disease, Sorafenib is considered treatment of choice. Although mild liver test abnormalities were reported in less than 1% of the patients in the two large randomized, controlled phase III trials, four cases of severe acute Sorafenib-induced hepatitis have been described. One of these four cases died from liver failure. In this paper, a patient with HCC with lung metastases developed high fever and a severe hepatitis that rapidly evolved into liver coma and death, two weeks after the initiation of Sorafenib. Biochemical parameters pointed to a hepatocellular type of injury. Clinical and biochemical presentations were compatible with a drug-induced hypersensitivity syndrome such as it has mainly been described for aromatic anticonvulsants, sulphonamides, and allopurinol. We hypothesize that an underlying cytochrome P450 dysfunction with the presence of reactive drug metabolites might lead to this potentially fatal Sorafenib-induced severe liver dysfunction.

1. Introduction

Hepatocellular carcinoma (HCC) is a highly prevalent malignancy with liver cirrhosis as the major predisposing factor. Choice of the treatment should be based on an individualised evaluation of each patient. It depends on multiple variables such as the size and number of tumoral nodules, degree of liver function, general health of the patient, the presence of portal invasion and of metastatic disease and requires a multidisciplinary approach [1–3]. In patients with advanced disease marked by vascular invasion and/or extrahepatic disease and presenting with an acceptable Child-Pugh score A or B and performance status not higher than 2, targeted therapy with the multikinase inhibitor Sorafenib is now considered the treatment of choice. This drug has been shown to lead to clinical relevant improvements in time to progression and in survival, with a magnitude of improvement in survival comparing with molecular-targeted therapies for other advanced cancers [1, 3, 4]. Sorafenib is considered to have an easily manageable associated toxicity without a treatment-related mortality [1, 4, 5].

As most patients who present with HCC have an underlying liver disease, an important issue related to this therapy is its potential liver toxicity. Liver dysfunction was reported in less than 1% of the Sorafenib-treated patients in the two randomized, double-blind, placebo-controlled multicentre, phase III trials (the SHARP trial and the Asia-Pacific trial) [6, 7]. Only four cases of Sorafenib-induced severe hepatitis have been described [8–11]. Liver toxicity occurred in two patients with underlying liver disease [8, 9] as well as in two cases with a previously normal liver function [10, 11]. One of the patients with a preexisting normal liver died of liver failure [10].

In this paper, we describe a patient with metastatic hepatocellular carcinoma who developed an acute fulminant hepatitis with fatal outcome two weeks after the start of treatment with Sorafenib. It is the purpose of the authors to bring this potential complication to the attention of hepatologists and oncologists involved in the treatment of HCC.

2. Case Report

A 76-year-old male Caucasian patient with a previous history of repeated episodes of acute alcoholic hepatitis was referred to our Liver Unit in June, 2007, because of the incidental finding on CT scan of a tumoral mass in segment IV of the liver. He was also known with arterial hypertension and with recurrent stomach ulcers for which he was treated since many years with perindopril and with omeprazole, respectively. On admission, the clinical examination was normal except for palmar erythema. Laboratory evaluation showed an alpha-foetoprotein (AFP) concentration of $525 \mu g/L$ (nl < 14); haemoglobin was $14,7 g/dL$, alkaline phosphatase $110 U/l$ (nl < 270), AST $46 U/l$ (nl < 38), ALT $39 U/l$ (nl < 41), and gamma-GT $54 U/l$ (nl < 53). Oesophageal varices were excluded, and a tumorectomy was performed. The resection specimen showed an undifferentiated hepatocellular carcinoma with vascular invasion; the nontumoral liver parenchyma was characterized by the presence of Mallory bodies and a septal stage of fibrosis. In October, 2008, and in February, 2009, radiofrequency ablation (RFA) was performed for recurrent HCC in segment IV. In February, 2009, previous to the second ablation therapy, AFP was $14 \mu g/l$, alkaline phosphatase $147 U/l$, AST $63 U/l$, ALT $45 U/l$, and gamma-GT $104 U/l$. There was no further use of alcohol since the diagnosis of cirrhosis, and HCC had been made.

In November, 2009, a repeated CT scan of thorax and liver was performed because of a rise in AFP up to $75 \mu g/l$; several small lung metastases were observed. In March, 2010, AFP had risen up to $743 \mu g/l$, and an increase in size of the lung metastases as well as a single, 17 mm large HCC-nodule in segment VII of the liver were visualized. At that time, alkaline phosphatase was $154 U/l$, AST $125 U/l$, ALT $60 U/l$, and gamma-GT $304 U/l$. Serum albumin was $46,9 g/dL$, and the prothrombin time was $1,1 INR$, indicative of a well-preserved liver function. The Child-Pugh status was A5. Sorafenib was started the first week of May, 2010, at a dosage of 400 mg per day during the first week and with an increase up to 800 mg daily from the second week of treatment onward. One week after the start of the 800 mg regime, the patient developed a flu-like syndrome with high spiking fever up to $40°C$, tinnitus, nausea and severe vomiting, severe muscle cramps, anorexia, and watery diarrhea with a frequency of more than 10 stools per day. He was seen as an outpatient the first week of June, 2010. Clinical examination at that time revealed the presence of scleral jaundice and of a marked hepatomegaly, findings that had never been observed during previous examinations. Total bilirubin was $3,6 mg/dL$ with a direct fraction of $2 mg/dL$; alkaline phosphatase was $135 U/l$, AST $525 U/l$, ALT $343 U/l$, gamma-GT $215 U/l$, ferritin $2099 \mu g/l$, albumin $3,2 g/l$, and the prothrombin time was now $1,5 INR$. The total white blood cell count was $7.4 \times 10^9/l$ with a neutrophil count of $5.7 \times 10^9/l$; blood eosinophils were normal. Serology for hepatitis A, B, and C, as well as antinuclear antibodies were negative. Sonography showed a large liver without focal liver lesions or dilated bile ducts and with only a minimal amount of ascites so that a diagnostic paracentesis was not considered to be useful. As the diarrhea had already improved at the time of the consultation, stool cultures have not been performed. Sorafenib was stopped but the patient went rapidly into a severe jaundice and a deep liver coma and died on June 16, 2010. As his family refused any further hospitalisation, we were not able to perform a liver biopsy.

3. Discussion

In patients with advanced hepatocellular carcinoma characterized by vascular invasion and/or extrahepatic disease and presenting with an acceptable Child-Pugh score A or B, Sorafenib is considered the treatment of choice. Sorafenib is an oral multikinase inhibitor that blocks tumor cell proliferation by targeting Raf/MEK/ERK signalling pathway and that has an antiangiogenic effect by targeting vascular endothelial growth factor receptor [5, 6]. Overall, oral Sorafenib is a well-tolerated treatment option with an acceptable safety profile with hand-foot skin reaction and diarrhea as the most frequent side effects [6, 7]. Liver dysfunction was reported in less than 1% of the Sorafenib-treated patients in the SHARP trial and the Asia-Pacific trial [6, 7]. Outside the mild liver dysfunction reported in both these randomized, placebo-controlled multicentre, phase III trials, four cases of Sorafenib-induced severe hepatitis have been described [8–11]. Liver toxicity occurred in two patients with underlying liver disease [8, 9] as well as in two cases with a previously normal liver function, already suggesting an idiosyncratic drug reaction [10, 11]. One of the patients with a preexisting normal liver died of liver failure [10]. Here, we report a second patient with an apparent Sorafenib-induced liver failure resulting in death shortly after the start of Sorafenib therapy.

Our patient presented with a clinical-biochemical picture of an acute hepatitis with severe general symptoms consisting of high fever, anorexia and vomiting, watery diarrea, and severe muscle cramps, and with a marked rise in aminotransferases about ten times above the upper limit of normal. These symptoms occurred two weeks after the start of Sorafenib and one week after increasing the dosage from 400 to 800 mg daily. In three other cases reported, Sorafenib-induced hepatitis also presented with flu-like symptoms with fever [8] or high fever up to $39°C$ [11], with skin rash and diarrhea [8], nausea [11], with a hepatocellular type of injury with high transaminases [9, 11], and with a histological picture of hepatocellular centrolobular necrosis [8, 11]. In our patient, the hepatocellular type of injury was also evident from a high R ratio of 16,8, as calculated from the ratio (ALT/ULN)/(alkaline phosphatase/ULN), with a ratio >5 indicating hepatocellular injury and <2 cholestatic injury [12]. Besides the symptoms such as fever and rash and the early onset within one to eight weeks after Sorafenib-introduction reported in our and in other cases, the presence of eosinophilic infiltration in the portal tracts and a positive lymphocyte transformation test that was subsequently performed in the patient reported by Herden et al. [11] suggests an allergic, drug-induced hypersensitivity syndrome (DHIS) as the pathogenetic mechanism of the Sorafenib-induced hepatitis [12–16]. Interestingly, in the patient with severe Sorafenib-induced hepatitis reported by Schramm et al. [8], prednisolone was given as a treatment for the acute hepatitis and transaminases returned to baseline levels within 10 days. The management of DHIS involves discontinuation of the offending drug as well as the administration of moderate to high doses of systemic glucocorticosteroids, especially in cases with extensive involvement of the internal organs such as myocarditis [13, 14]. In our case, Sorafenib was stopped but the patient rapidly went into a deep liver coma and the family refused any further hospitalisation, so that steroid treatment could not be given. Because of this refusal for hospitalisation, it was also not possible to perform a liver biopsy. In our opinion, however, the clinical evolution as well as the biochemical findings occurring shortly after the start of Sorafenib treatment were sufficient to make a diagnosis of a severe drug-induced liver damage obvious.

A severe drug reaction with systemic symptoms can also be part of the so-called DRESS syndrome or drug reaction with eosinophilia and systemic symptoms; this syndrome is not always characterized by eosinophilia, and its main features are skin rash with a diversity of cutaneous eruptions, high fever, and organ involvement with, amongst others, hepatomegaly and hepatitis with potential evolution towards liver failure and death. Other noteworthy features are a delayed onset, usually 2–6 weeks after initiation of the drug, and the possible persistence or aggravation of symptoms despite discontinuation of the culprit drug [15, 16]. Although our patient did not show any skin eruption, the high fever with hepatomegaly and death from liver failure might be compatible with DRESS syndrome. Moreover, one patient that was previously reported with Sorafenib hepatitis did show a cutaneous rash [8], whereas an eosinophilic infiltration in portal tracts was found in another case [11]. Also for the DRESS syndrome with internal organ involvement, treatment with systemic corticosteroids is proposed [15, 16].

The drug-induced hypersensitivity syndrome and the DRESS syndrome are most frequently related to the use of antiepileptic agents such as carbamazepine, phenobarbital, and phenytoin; antibiotics such as sulphonamides; dapsone, sulfasalazine, and allopurinol [14, 15]. Biologically reactive metabolites are thought to be responsible for a delayed immunologically mediated reaction with macrophage and T-lymphocyte activation and cytokine release [13, 14]. Defects in detoxification enzymes for aromatic anticonvulsants, slow acetylator phenotype, and an increased susceptibility of lymphocytes to toxic metabolites in the case of sulphonamides have been implicated in the pathogenesis of these clinical conditions [15, 16]. The oxidative metabolism of Sorafenib occurs primarily in the liver and is mediated by the cytochrome P450 (CYP)3A4. Eight Sorafenib metabolites have been identified with pyridine N-oxide being the main circulating metabolite in plasma [5]. It could be hypothesized that an underlying cytochrome P450 dysfunction and the presence of biologically reactive drug metabolites might lead to this Sorafenib-induced severe liver dysfunction. DHIS and DRESS have also been associated with human herpesvirus 6 (HHV-6) reactivation [17, 18], and, according to Shiohara et al. [17], HHV-6 reactivation is even one of their 6 diagnostic criteria for DIHS/DRESS. In this regard, the clinical symptoms with high fever observed during the course of DIHS/DRESS could be mediated by antiviral T cells, which could explain amongst others a further deterioration of liver function after withdrawal of the offending drug [17]. HHV-6 serology and PCR-DNA have therefore been applied in the diagnosis of patients with these conditions [17, 18]. Serologic

examination for HHV-6 has not been performed in our patient.

In conclusion, it could be suggested to add Sorafenib to the list of drugs that may lead to the drug-induced hypersensitivity syndrome and possibly also to the DRESS syndrome. The appearance of high fever and liver test abnormalities after initiation of Sorafenib should lead to an immediate discontinuation of the drug and to the initiation of therapy with corticosteroids in case of severe hepatitis. In case of detection of further cases of severe Sorafenib-induced hepatitis in patients with HCC, a study of HHV-6 antibodies and DNA could be useful to study the possible role of HHV-6 reactivation in the pathogenesis of this potentially lethal liver disease.

References

[1] J. Bruix and M. Sherman, "Management of hepatocellular carcinoma: an update," *Hepatology*, vol. 53, no. 3, pp. 1020–1022, 2011.

[2] S Tremosini, M Reig, C Rodriguez de Lope, A Forner, and J. Bruix, "Treatment of early hepatocellular carcinoma: towards personalised therapy," *Digestive and Liver Disease*, vol. 42S, pp. S242–S248, 2010.

[3] R. Cabrera and D. R. Nelson, "Review article: the management of hepatocellular carcinoma," *Alimentary Pharmacology and Therapeutics*, vol. 31, no. 4, pp. 461–476, 2010.

[4] A. Villanueva and J. M. Llovet, "Targeted therapies for hepatocellular carcinoma," *Gastroenterology*, vol. 140, pp. 1410–1426, 2011.

[5] G. M. Keating and A. Santoro, "Sorafenib: A review of its use in advanced hepatocellular carcinoma," *Drugs*, vol. 69, no. 2, pp. 223–240, 2009.

[6] J. M. Llovet, S. Ricci, V. Mazzaferro et al., "Sorafenib in advanced hepatocellular carcinoma," *New England Journal of Medicine*, vol. 359, no. 4, pp. 378–390, 2008.

[7] A. L. Cheng, Y. K. Kang, Z. Chen et al., "Efficacy and safety of sorafenib in patients in the Asia-Pacific region with advanced hepatocellular carcinoma: a phase III randomised, double-blind, placebo-controlled trial," *The Lancet Oncology*, vol. 10, no. 1, pp. 25–34, 2009.

[8] C. Schramm, G. Schuch, and A. W. Lohse, "Sorafenib-induced liver failure," *American Journal of Gastroenterology*, vol. 103, no. 8, pp. 2162–2163, 2008.

[9] L. Llanos, P. Bellot, P. Zapater, M. Pérez-Mateo, and J. Such, "Acute hepatitis in a patient with cirrhosis and hepatocellular carcinoma treated with sorafenib," *American Journal of Gastroenterology*, vol. 104, no. 1, pp. 257–258, 2009.

[10] V. Gupta-Abramson, A. B. Troxel, A. Nellore et al., "Phase II trial of sorafenib in advanced thyroid cancer," *Journal of Clinical Oncology*, vol. 26, no. 29, pp. 4714–4719, 2008.

[11] U. Herden, L. Fischer, H. Schäfer, B. Nashan, V. Von Baehr, and M. Sterneck, "Sorafenib-induced severe acute hepatitis in a stable liver transplant recipient," *Transplantation*, vol. 90, no. 1, pp. 98–99, 2010.

[12] R. J. Fontana, L. B. Seeff, R. J. Andrade et al., "Standardization of nomenclature and causality assessment in drug-induced liver injury: summary of a clinical research workshop," *Hepatology*, vol. 52, no. 2, pp. 730–742, 2010.

[13] M. Ben M'Rad, S. Leclerc-Mercier, P. Blanche et al., "Drug-induced hypersensitivity syndrome: clinical and biologic disease atterns In 24 patients," *Medicine*, vol. 88, no. 3, pp. 131–140, 2009.

[14] K. Gomułka, D. Kuliczkowska, M. Cisło, Z. Woźniak, and B. Panaszek, "Drug-induced hypersensitivity syndrome—a literature review and the case report," *Pneumonologia i Alergologia Polska*, vol. 79, no. 1, pp. 52–56, 2011.

[15] H. Bocquet, M. Bagot, and J. C. Roujeau, "Drug-induced pseudolymphoma and drug hypersensitivity syndrome (Drug Rash with Eosinophilia and Systemic Symptoms: DRESS)," *Seminars in Cutaneous Medicine and Surgery*, vol. 15, no. 4, pp. 250–257, 1996.

[16] P. Cacoub, P. Musette, V. Descamps et al., "The DRESS syndrome: a literature review," *American Journal of Medicine*, vol. 124, no. 7, pp. 588–597, 2011.

[17] T. Shiohara, M. Inaoka, and Y. Kano, "Drug-induced hypersensitivity syndrome(DIHS): a reaction induced by a complex interplay among herpesviruses and antiviral and antidrug immune responses," *Allergology International*, vol. 55, no. 1, pp. 1–8, 2006.

[18] I. Gentile, M. Talamo, and G. Borgia, "Is the drug-induced hypersensitivity syndrome (DIHS) due to human herpesvirus 6 infection or to allergy-mediated viral reactivation? Report of a case and literature review," *BMC Infectious Diseases*, vol. 10, article 49, 2010.

15

Onset of Celiac Disease after Treatment of Chronic Hepatitis C with Interferon Based Triple Therapy

Amandeep Singh,[1,2] Nayere Zaeri,[1] and Immanuel K. Ho[1,3]

[1]*Crozer Chester Medical Center, One Medical Center Boulevard, Upland, PA 19018, USA*
[2]*Cleveland Clinic Foundation, 9500 Euclid Avenue, Cleveland, OH 44195, USA*
[3]*Division of Gastroenterology, Pennsylvania Hospital, 230 W. Washington Square, 4th Floor, Philadelphia, PA 19106, USA*

Correspondence should be addressed to Amandeep Singh; bansraoaman@yahoo.com

Academic Editor: Ivan Gentile

Background. Patients treated with interferon (IFN) based therapies may develop exacerbation of autoimmune disease. We herein present the case of a 53-year-old female patient who developed celiac disease (CD) as a result of triple therapy (interferon, ribavirin, and boceprevir) for chronic HCV. *Case.* 53-year-old Caucasian female with past medical history of IV drug abuse was referred for abnormal LFTs. Laboratory data showed HCV RNA of 4,515,392 IU/mL, HCV genotype 1a, with normal LFTs. She was treated with 4 weeks of pegylated interferon alfa-2a plus ribavirin, followed by triple therapy using boceprevir for a total of 28 weeks. Approximately 4 weeks after initiation of triple therapy patient developed loose nonbloody bowel movements and was also found to have anemia. Biopsies from first and second portions of the duodenum were consistent with CD. The patient was treated with a gluten-free diet. Her intestinal symptoms improved and the hemoglobin returned to normal. *Conclusion.* Chronic HCV patients being treated with interferon alfa can develop celiac disease during or after therapy. For patients with positive autoantibodies, all-oral-IFN-free regimens should be considered. Celiac disease should be considered in patients who develop CD-like symptoms while on and shortly after cessation of interferon alfa therapy.

1. Introduction

Chronic hepatitis C (HCV) is one of the most common causes for liver transplantation. There are at least 5.2 million persons living with chronic HCV in the United States today [1]. The standard of care for treatment of chronic HCV genotype 1 infection before the approval of newer interferon-free regimens was a triple combination regimen therapy involving pegylated interferon alfa, ribavirin, and a NS3/4A protease inhibitor (boceprevir, telaprevir, and simeprevir) or a nucleotide analogue NS5B polymerase inhibitor (sofosbuvir) or peginterferon and ribavirin alone. Some patients may develop autoimmune side effects related to underlying disorders while on interferon treatment [2]. We herein present a case of a 53-year-old female who was started on triple therapy (interferon, ribavirin, and boceprevir) for HCV and subsequently developed celiac disease (CD) as a result of therapy.

2. Case Description

C. K., a 53-year-old Caucasian female, was referred by her primary care physician for abnormal liver function tests. She was first diagnosed with HCV exposure in 2005 with genotype 3a and had undergone pegylated interferon monotherapy weekly for six months. She achieved end of treatment response. Subsequently, she continued to use intravenous drugs. On presentation to our clinic on 05/04/2011, patient was found to have reinfection with genotype 1a with an HCV viral load of 29,000 IU/mL. She had no nausea, vomiting, heartburn, abdominal pain, or dysphagia. She had lost some weight but she was dieting. She denied any intravenous drug and alcohol use in last 3 years.

Her past medical history was notable for methicillin resistant staphylococcus aureus (MRSA) endocarditis, vertebral osteomyelitis, hyperlipidemia, diverticulosis, and *Helicobacter pylori* gastritis. There was no family history of celiac

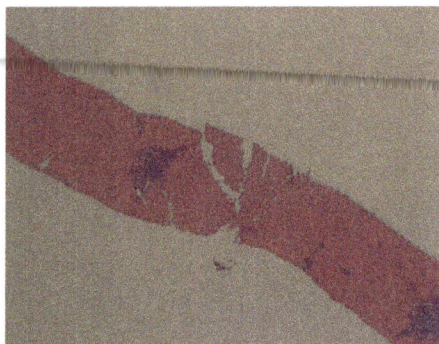

FIGURE 1: Liver biopsy showing grade 2 inflammation activity and stage 1 fibrosis.

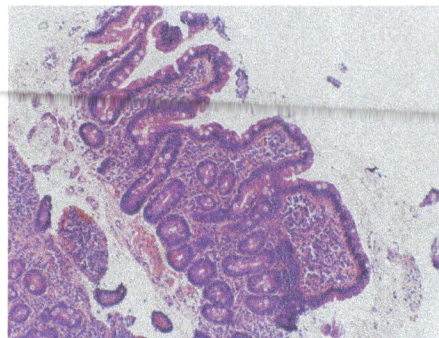

FIGURE 2: Duodenal biopsy showing mild villous blunting, crypt hyperplasia, and intraepithelial lymphocytes characteristic of celiac disease.

disease, type 1 diabetes or any other autoimmune diseases. She is a former smoker. Her medications included butalbital/acetaminophen/caffeine, simvastatin, and esomeprazole.

Initial physical examination showed temperature of 98.2°F, pulse of 72 beats/minute, BP of 116/70 mm/Hg, and weight of 146 pounds. Physical examination was normal "without stigmata of liver disease or malnutrition and so forth."

Laboratory data on initial visit showed normal complete blood count (CBC), complete metabolic profile (CMP), and iron studies. Pt was found to have HCV viral load of 4,515,392 IU/ml and genotype 1a. Other causes of liver disease including hepatitis B, autoimmune hepatitis, Wilson disease, and HIV were ruled out. The patient underwent a liver biopsy which showed Metavir grade 2 inflammatory activity and stage 1 fibrosis (Figure 1).

Colonoscopy was also done on 6/25/2008 at different facility, which did not show any polyps but showed diverticular disease of descending colon and sigmoid colon. The patient underwent upper gastrointestinal endoscopy (EGD) done on 10/7/2009 which was unremarkable.

Treatment was initiated on dual therapy with pegylated interferon alfa-2a at 180 μg subcutaneous weekly plus ribavirin 600 mg orally twice per day for a 4-week lead-in phase, followed by triple therapy using boceprevir (BOC) 800 mg orally three times per day for total of 28 weeks. HCV viral loads which were collected at weeks 4, 8, 12, 21, and 24 were undetectable by polymerase chain reaction. During treatment, the patient developed neutropenia and anemia, which were treated with pegfilgrastim and darbepoetin alfa.

Approximately 4 weeks after initiation of triple therapy the patient developed loose nonbloody bowel movements, which was not reported at the time. She experienced nausea and decreased appetite but no vomiting or abdominal pain. Occasionally she felt bloated. There was no fever, chills, or skin rash.

Three months following cessation of treatment the patient complained of ongoing weakness and dyspnea on exertion which had begun after the initiation of therapy but which had not resolved completely. She had ten-pound weight loss during treatment which persisted, but she also now

admitted to having 5-6 watery loose bowel movements for the preceding five months. Repeat CBC showed low hemoglobin of 10.7 g/dL (baseline 14 g/dL). The patient failed to give stool samples for analysis. She underwent an EGD and colonoscopy. During EGD, mucosa in the stomach and second and third part of duodenum appeared normal but biopsies from second portion of the duodenum revealed mild villous blunting, mild crypt hyperplasia, and minimal intraepithelial lymphocytes consistent with CD (Figure 2). The tissue transglutaminase IgA was 85 U/mL. The patient was started on gluten-free diet. Her intestinal symptoms improved and the hemoglobin returned to normal.

3. Discussion

Development of CD has been reported in patients with chronic hepatitis C [3, 4] and CD activation after the initiation of interferon alfa has also been described [5–8]. There are studies which deny any clear association or increased prevalence of CD in patients with HCV [9–11] but, on the contrary there are studies to support the increased prevalence of celiac autoantibodies in patients with chronic hepatitis C and risk of activation of silent CD during interferon treatment [7, 8].

Autoimmune side effects including hyperthyroidism, hypothyroidism, diabetes mellitus, interstitial pneumonitis, autoimmune thrombocytopenic purpura, hemolytic anemia, rheumatoid arthritis, and systemic lupus erythematosus have all been reported to exacerbate or develop during interferon therapy [2].

CD is an autoimmune disease prevalent in Caucasians of European descent (1 : 200–300) and is mediated by CD4 lymphocytes in response to ingested gluten in genetically predisposed individuals. Gama interferon production, stimulated by gluten, activates CD4 lymphocytes in lamina propria of small intestine mucosa resulting in intestinal mucosa damage with villous atrophy, crypts hyperplasia; with mucosa infiltration with CD3[+] lymphocytes [6]. CD may present in various clinical modes such as potential, latent, silent, atypical, and classical modes.

Interferon alfa and ribavirin treatment for chronic HCV may unmask the symptoms of celiac disease [5–8]. However, diarrhea, the hallmark symptom of celiac disease, may also occur as a result of IFN-alpha therapy [12]. Interferon use has the potential to exacerbate autoimmune disease either by direct effects on tissues or through its effect on the immune system by altering lymphocyte population and the profile of cytokine production. While interferon alfa acts in differentiation of T helper (Th) 2 cells to Th1 cells and improve T-cell and natural killer cell cytotoxicity [6], ribavirin promotes a Th1 cytokine-mediated immune response, suppressing Th2 response [13]. Similarly, gluten induced activation of lamina propria Th1 cells followed by secretion of IFN gamma is an important pathogenic mechanism in CD [14]. Thus one might speculate that Th1/Th2 imbalance may play a role in the activation of CD in some patients. Our patient was on boceprevir (BOC), along with IFN and ribavirin.

This is a case of patient manifesting celiac disease on and after treatment with interferon based triple regimen. Whether BOC has additive effects on IFN-ribavirin is unknown. Our experience with this case raises again the important question of whether CD screening should be performed prior to initiation of interferon based therapy for chronic hepatitis C [15]. Although screening for celiac disease before initiation of interferon therapy has been suggested [16, 17], current screening recommendations for celiac disease are targeted towards pediatric and adult patients already diagnosed with certain autoimmune diseases (including autoimmune thyroid disease, autoimmune liver disease, primary biliary cirrhosis, and type 1 diabetes mellitus) [18, 19]. Screening for CD in the setting of HCV treatment with interferon has not yet been recommended. Patients with positive autoantibodies require careful consideration of IFN-free regimens. If IFN-free regimens are not available there should be a low threshold for obtaining tissue transglutaminase IgA from patients if diarrhea, weight loss, or anemia developed while on or after the use the interferon therapy and if the suspicion of CD is high, intestinal biopsy should be pursued even if serologies are negative and a gluten-free diet must be started preemptively.

4. Conclusion

Chronic HCV patients being treated with interferon alfa can develop celiac disease during or after therapy. For patients with positive autoantibodies, all-oral-IFN-free regimens should be considered. Celiac disease should be considered in patients who develop CD-like symptoms while on and shortly after cessation of interferon alfa therapy.

Authors' Contribution

Amandeep Singh, primary author/guarantor, was responsible for data collection, literature search, and writing of case report.

References

[1] E. Chak, A. H. Talal, K. E. Sherman, E. R. Schiff, and S. Saab, "Hepatitis C virus infection in USA: an estimate of true prevalence," *Liver International*, vol. 31, no. 8, pp. 1090–1101, 2011.

[2] F. L. Dumoulin, L. Leifeld, T. Sauerbruch, and U. Spengler, "Autoimmunity induced by interferon-α therapy for chronic viral hepatitis," *Biomedicine and Pharmacotherapy*, vol. 53, no. 5-6, pp. 242–254, 1999.

[3] K. D. Fine, F. Ogunji, Y. Saloum, S. Beharry, J. Crippin, and J. Weinstein, "Celiac sprue: another autoimmune syndrome associated with hepatitis C," *The American Journal of Gastroenterology*, vol. 96, no. 1, pp. 138–145, 2001.

[4] A. Teml and H. Vogelsang, "Re: celiac sprue: another autoimmune syndrome associated with hepatitis C," *American Journal of Gastroenterology*, vol. 96, no. 8, pp. 2522–2523, 2001.

[5] E. V. Martins Jr. and A. K. Gaburri, "Celiac disease onset after pegylated interferon and ribavirin treatment of chronic hepatitis C," *Arquivos de Gastroenterologia*, vol. 41, no. 2, pp. 132–133, 2004.

[6] L. E. Adinolfi, E. D. Mangoni, and A. Andreana, "Interferon and ribavirin treatment for chronic hepatitis C may activate celiac disease," *American Journal of Gastroenterology*, vol. 96, no. 2, pp. 607–608, 2001.

[7] E. Durante-Mangoni, P. Iardino, M. Resse et al., "Silent celiac disease in chronic hepatitis C: impact of interferon treatment on the disease onset and clinical outcome," *Journal of Clinical Gastroenterology*, vol. 38, no. 10, pp. 901–905, 2004.

[8] J. L. Narciso-Schiavon and L. D. L. Schiavon, "Autoantibodies in chronic hepatitis C: a clinical perspective," *World Journal of Hepatology*, vol. 7, no. 8, pp. 1074–1085, 2015.

[9] L. Hernandez, T. C. Johnson, A. J. Naiyer et al., "Chronic hepatitis C virus and celiac disease, is there an association?" *Digestive Diseases and Sciences*, vol. 53, no. 1, pp. 256–261, 2008.

[10] T. Thevenot, J. Denis, V. Jouannaud et al., "Coeliac disease in chronic hepatitis C: a French multicentre prospective study," *Alimentary Pharmacology and Therapeutics*, vol. 26, no. 9, pp. 1209–1216, 2007.

[11] T. Thevenot, A. Boruchowicz, J. Henrion, B. Nalet, and H. Moindrot, "Celiac disease is not associated with chronic hepatitis C," *Digestive Diseases and Sciences*, vol. 52, no. 5, pp. 1310–1312, 2007.

[12] G. Dusheiko, "Side effects of alpha interferon in chronic hepatitis C," *Hepatology*, vol. 26, no. 3, pp. 112S–121S, 1997.

[13] R. C. Tam, B. Pai, J. Bard et al., "Ribavirin polarizes human T cell responses towards a Type 1 cytokine profile," *Journal of Hepatology*, vol. 30, no. 3, pp. 376–382, 1999.

[14] D. Schuppan, "Current concepts of celiac disease pathogenesis," *Gastroenterology*, vol. 119, no. 1, pp. 234–242, 2000.

[15] M. P. Manns, J. Mccone, M. N. Davis et al., "Overall safety profile of boceprevir plus peginterferon alfa-2b and ribavirin in patients with chronic hepatitis C genotype 1: a combined analysis of 3 phase 2/3 clinical trials," *Liver International*, vol. 34, no. 5, pp. 707–719, 2014.

[16] M. R. Nejad and S. M. Alavian, "Should routine screening for celiac disease be considered before starting interferon/ribavirin treatment in patients affected by chronic hepatitis C or not?" *Bratislavské lekárske listy*, vol. 113, no. 4, article 251, 2012.

[17] G. Casella, M. T. Bardella, D. Perego, and V. Baldini, "Should routine screening for coeliac disease be considered before starting interferon/ribavirin treatment in patients affected by chronic hepatitis C?" *European Journal of Gastroenterology & Hepatology*, vol. 16, no. 4, p. 429, 2004.

[18] S. Aggarwal, B. Lebwohl, and P. H. R. Green, "Screening for celiac disease in average-risk and high-risk populations," *Therapeutic Advances in Gastroenterology*, vol. 5, no. 1, pp. 37–47, 2012.

[19] A. Rubio-Tapia, I. D. Hill, C. P. Kelly, A. H. Calderwood, and J. A. Murray, "ACG clinical guidelines: diagnosis and management of celiac disease," *The American Journal of Gastroenterology*, vol. 108, no. 5, pp. 656–676, 2013.

16

Severe Aplastic Anemia following Parvovirus B19-Associated Acute Hepatitis

Masanori Furukawa,[1] Kosuke Kaji,[1] Hiroyuki Masuda,[1] Kuniaki Ozaki,[1] Shohei Asada,[1] Aritoshi Koizumi,[1] Takuya Kubo,[1] Norihisa Nishimura,[1] Yasuhiko Sawada,[1] Kosuke Takeda,[1] Tsuyoshi Mashitani,[1] Masayuki Kubo,[2] Itsuto Amano,[2] Tomoyuki Ootani,[3] Chiho Ohbayashi,[3] Koji Murata,[4] Tatsuichi Ann,[4] Akira Mitoro,[1] and Hitoshi Yoshiji[1]

[1]Third Department of Internal Medicine, Nara Medical University, Kashihara, Nara, Japan
[2]Second Department of Internal Medicine, Nara Medical University, Kashihara, Nara, Japan
[3]Department of Diagnostic Pathology, Nara Medical University, Kashihara, Nara, Japan
[4]Division of Gastroenterology, Bell Land General Hospital, Sakai, Osaka, Japan

Correspondence should be addressed to Kosuke Kaji; kajik@naramed-u.ac.jp

Academic Editor: Melanie Deutsch

Human parvovirus (HPV) B19 is linked to a variety of clinical manifestations, such as erythema infectiosum, nonimmune hydrops fetalis, and transient aplastic anemia. Although a few cases have shown HPVB19 infection as a possible causative agent for hepatitis-associated aplastic anemia (HAAA) in immunocompetent patients, most reported cases of HAAA following transient hepatitis did not have delayed remission. Here we report a rare case of severe aplastic anemia following acute hepatitis with prolonged jaundice due to HPVB19 infection in a previously healthy young male. Clinical laboratory examination assessed marked liver injury and jaundice as well as peripheral pancytopenia, and bone marrow biopsy revealed severe hypoplasia and fatty replacement. HPVB19 infection was diagnosed by enzyme immunoassay with high titer of anti-HPVB19 immunoglobulin M antibodies. Immunosuppressive therapy was initiated 2 months after the onset of acute hepatitis when liver injury and jaundice were improved. Cyclosporine provided partial remission after 2 months of medication without bone marrow transplantation. Our case suggests that HPVB19 should be considered as a hepatotropic virus and a cause of acquired aplastic anemia, including HAAA.

1. Introduction

Acute hepatitis is mainly caused by hepatitis A–E viruses (HAV–HEV), and it is rarely thought to be caused by infection of other viruses, including herpes simplex virus, Epstein-Barr virus, cytomegalovirus, coxsackievirus, echovirus, adenovirus, rubella virus, GB virus, and TT virus.

Human parvovirus (HPV) B19 is a very common viral agent that presents worldwide without ethnic or geographical boundaries. Infection with HPVB19 is known to cause several clinical manifestations, such as erythema infectiosum (fifth disease), transient aplastic crisis, pure red cell aplasia, nonimmune hydrops fetalis, glomerulopathy, and anemia in end-stage renal disease [1, 2]. In addition to these typical symptoms, HPVB19 is associated with acute hepatitis [3]. Although HPVB19-related hepatitis often shows complete and spontaneous remission, particularly in adults, it sometimes induces fulminant hepatitis complicated with acquired aplastic anemia, the so-called hepatitis-associated aplastic anemia (HAAA) [4–8].

Here we report a rare case of severe aplastic anemia following acute hepatitis with prolonged jaundice due to HPVB19 infection in a previously healthy young male.

2. Case Report

A 17-year-old male was admitted to Bell Land General Hospital with a 2-week history of nausea and fatigue. He

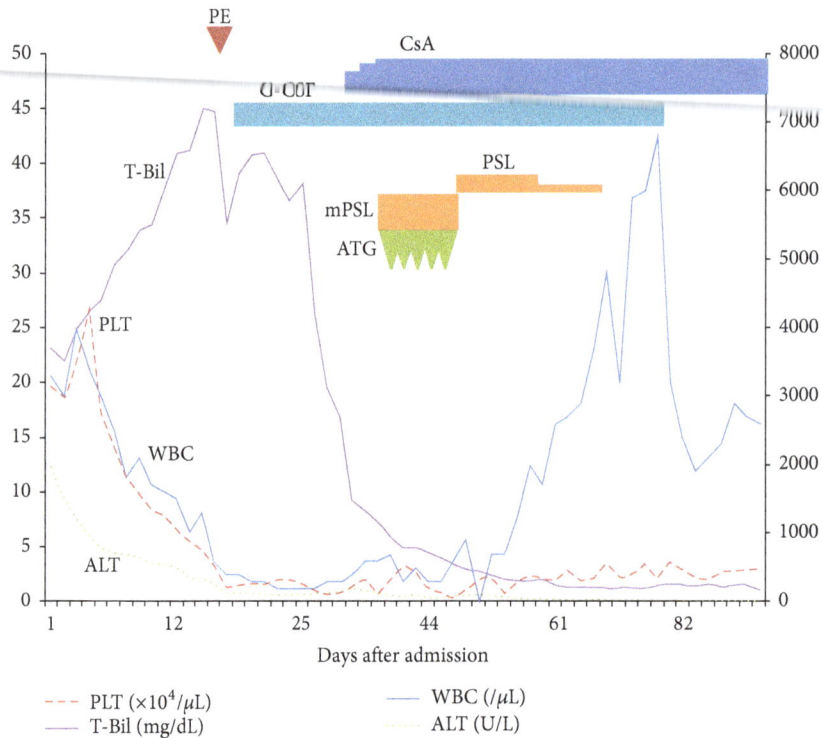

FIGURE 1: The change in laboratory investigation and the course of treatment. PLT, platelet; T-Bil, total bilirubin; WBC, white blood cell count; ALT, alanine aminotransferase; PE, plasmapheresis; G-CSF, granulocyte colony-stimulating factor; CsA, cyclosporine; ATG, anti-thymocyte globulin; mPSL, methylprednisolone; PSL, prednisolone.

had neither significant drug history nor past medical history, including liver dysfunction. All vital signs were normal, and his consciousness was not impaired. He appeared to be systemically icteric, but there was no evidence of erythema. Abdominal palpitation revealed hepatomegaly, but splenomegaly was not observed.

His development after hospital admission is shown in Figure 1. Laboratory investigation on admission (day 1) revealed an extremely elevated aspartate transaminase (AST) level of 2,432 U/L, alanine transaminase (ALT) level of 1,950 U/L, and total bilirubin (T-Bil) level of 23.1 mg/dL. Prothrombin time (PT) activity declined to 30.4% (international normalized ratio, 1.94). Initially, his blood cell count was almost within the normal limits, with white blood cell count (WBC) of $33 \times 10^2/\mu L$, hemoglobin (Hb) level of 14.6 g/dL, and platelet count (PLT) of $19.6 \times 10^4/\mu L$. The serologic test showed negative findings for anti-HAV immunoglobulin M (HAV IgM), HB surface antigen, HB core IgM, HCV IgG, HEV IgA, cytomegalovirus IgM, Epstein-Barr virus IgM, and human immunodeficiency virus IgM/IgG antibodies. Both antinucleic and antimitochondrial antibodies were also negative (Table 1). Ultrasonography demonstrated hepatomegaly without evidence of biliary obstruction, hepatic vein occlusion, ascites, or splenomegaly. During hospitalization, AST and ALT levels gradually decreased, although the decline in PT activity was prolonged and the T-Bil level was markedly increased. Moreover, at day 10, a complete blood count showed WBC of $17 \times 10^2/\mu L$, Hb level of 11.9 g/dL, and PLT of $8.4 \times 10^3/\mu L$, indicating the development of pancytopenia. Because his

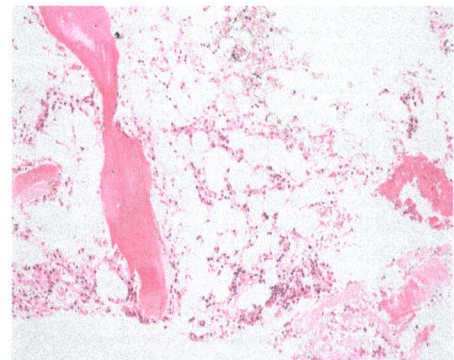

FIGURE 2: Representative picture of H&E stained bone marrow tissue specimen (original magnification, ×100). His bone marrow showed severe marrow hypocellularity.

condition was exacerbated despite plasmapheresis and his pancytopenia was suspected of being myelopathy-derived, he was transferred to Nara Medical University Hospital on day 18.

Initial laboratory examination after transfer demonstrated an improved AST level of 97 U/L, ALT level of 127 U/L, and PT activity of 62%, whereas an elevated T-Bil level at 34.5 mg/dL was still observed, and pancytopenia grossly progressed to WBC of $4 \times 10^2/\mu L$, Hb level of 9.2 g/dL, reticulocyte count of $4.6 \times 10^4/\mu L$, and PLT of $1.3 \times 10^4/\mu L$. Bone marrow examination showed fatty replacement and hypocellularity, a nucleic cell count of 7000/μL, and no aberrant karyotype (Figure 2). Additional tests for herpes simplex

TABLE 1: Initial acute hepatitis workup.

Hepatitis A IgM	Nonreactive
Hepatitis B core IgM	Nonreactive
Hepatitis B surface antigen	Nonreactive
HBV-DNA (real-time PCR)	Negative
Hepatitis C IgG antibody	Nonreactive
HIV 1 & 2 antibody	Nonreactive
HTLV 1 & 2 antibody	Nonreactive
CMV antigenemia (C7-HRP)	Negative
HSV IgG antibody (EIA)	Positive
HSV IgM antibody (EIA)	Negative
VZV IgG antibody (EIA)	Positive
VZV IgM antibody (EIA)	Negative
EBV IgG antibody (FA)	Positive
EBV IgM antibody (FA)	Negative
EB nuclear antigen (EBNA) IgG (FA)	Positive
EBV ultraquantitative	Negative
Echo virus type 3 antibody (FA)	Negative
Parvovirus B19 IgM antibody (EIA)	Positive
Parvovirus B19 DNA PCR	Positive
Antinuclear antibodies	Negative
Antimitochondrial antibodies	Negative
TSH (μIU/ml)	0.48
FT3 (pg/ml)	1.5
FT4 (ng/ml)	1.24
PR3-ANCA (U/ml)	Negative
MPO-ANCA (U/ml)	Negative
Ferritin (ng/ml)	1199.5
Iron (μg/dl)	211
TIBC (μg/dl)	227
Ceruloplasmin (mg/dl)	24.4
IgG (mg/dl)	967
IgA (mg/dl)	182.1
IgM (mg/dl)	90.7
AFP tumor marker (ng/ml)	4835.6
HGF (ng/ml)	3.59

virus IgM, varicella-zoster virus IgM, echovirus type 3 (HI), human T-cell lymphotropic virus 1 IgG, and antineutrophilic cytoplasmic antibodies were all negative. Meanwhile, HPVB19 IgM (EIA) was positive with an optical density value of 3.73 (reference values: <0.8, negative; 0.8–0.99, equivocal; and ≥1.0, positive). HPVB19 DNA was positively detected by quantitative polymerase chain reaction, in agreement with the high titer of HPVB19 IgM antibody (Table 1). Therefore, he was diagnosed with HAAA induced by HPVB19 infection.

When liver injury and jaundice improved with conservative treatment and alimentation, we initiated oral administration of cyclosporine as remission induction therapy for HAAA at 2.5 mg/kg/day on day 32 and gradually increased the dosage to 3.5 mg/kg/day, adjusting trough levels to 150–250 ng/mL. However, there was only slight improvement, and consequently both antithymocyte globulin (ATG) and methylprednisolone were administered in combination with cyclosporine at a dosage of 2.5 mg/kg/day and 2 mg/kg/day, respectively, from day 42 to 46. We continuously administered methylprednisolone until day 70 with gradual tapering of dose, and we treated the patient with granulocyte colony-stimulating factor and transfusion on demand. On day 98

after remission induction with cyclosporine, his pancytopenia improved with WBC of $26 \times 10^2/\mu$L, reticulocyte count of $9.6 \times 10^4/\mu$L, and PLT of $3 \times 10^4/\mu$L without bone marrow transplantation. At present, he is continuously treated with cyclosporine as an outpatient of our hospital.

3. Discussion

HPVB19 is the first known human virus in the Parvoviridae family, genus *Erythroparvovirus*, which is a nonenveloped, icosahedral virus containing a single-stranded linear DNA genome [9]. HPVB19 infection rarely presents any symptoms in most immunocompetent individuals, but it causes several well-known clinical manifestations, including erythema infectiosum, arthropathy, transient aplastic crisis, nonimmune hydrops fetalis, meningitis, encephalitis, and myocarditis, particularly in childhood [10]. Symptoms usually begin 6 days after exposure and last for approximately a week. Recently, it has been reported that HPVB19 infection is considered as one of the causes of acute hepatitis [11]. Yoto et al. reported a case of pediatric acute hepatitis in the course of erythema infectiosum, and a case of cryptogenic acute hepatitis without exanthema was suspected to be induced by HPVB19 [12]. Mihály et al. also reported that HPVB19-related hepatitis may occur in 4.1% of patients infected with this virus [13]. Liver damage associated with HPVB19 shows a wide spectrum of disease severity from transient elevation of transaminase levels to fulminant liver failure. However, liver dysfunction induced by HPVB19 is often improved spontaneously in general cases and less frequently leads to a serious condition.

The pathogenic mechanism of hepatic injury by HPVB19 infection has not been elucidated. There are two theories: one is direct viral invasion and the other is an indirect immunological response, namely, virus-associated hemophagocytic syndrome (VAHS) [11]. HPVB19 can infect cells that possess globosides, which are glycosphingolipids acting as the receptor for HPVB19, such as erythroid precursors, megakaryocytes, endothelial cells, and hepatocytes [14, 15]. HPVB19 directly enters the hepatocytes through globosides and produces nonstructural protein (NS1) without the production of viral progeny [16]. NS1 expression significantly upregulates p21/WAF1 expression, a cyclin-dependent kinase inhibitor that induces G1 arrest leading to apoptosis by activation of caspase-3 and caspase-9 [17, 18]. On the other hand, HPVB19 infection reportedly induces VAHS, which increases circulating CD8$^+$ cytotoxic T cells and IFN-γ and TNF-α secretion, triggering symptoms such as high fever, liver injury, enlarged liver and spleen, coagulation factor abnormalities, pancytopenia, and a build-up of histiocytes in various tissues resulting in the destruction of blood-producing cells [19–21]. In the present case, the bone marrow did not show hemophagocytosis but showed aplastic anemia, indicating that VAHS did not primarily participate in the onset of acute hepatitis.

Our patient progressively developed aplastic anemia following severe hepatitis, which is defined as HAAA. This is a well-known and distinct variant of acquired aplastic anemia, in which acute hepatitis leads to marrow failure and pancytopenia [22–24]. HAAA is associated with immunological abnormalities mediated by CD8$^+$ Kupffer cells [25]. Patients with HAAA show a decreased ratio of CD4/CD8 cells and a high percentage of CD8$^+$ cells, and the residual CD8$^+$ cells in the bone marrow produce large amounts of IFN-γ [26]. HAAA has been reported in 2%–10% of cases of aplastic anemia [27]. Etiological factors have been attributed to pathogenic viruses, autoimmune responses, liver transplantation, bone marrow transplantation, radiation, and drugs administered to regulate the viral replication, whereas it has been reported that the causal virus was unidentified in majority of cases of HAAA in Japan.

A relationship between HAAA and HPVB19 infection is also controversially described. Langnas et al. have shown that HPVB19 is a possible causative agent of fulminant liver failure and HAAA, while Wong et al. advocated that there is no pathophysiological association [8, 28]. In the present case, it was not definitively concluded that HPVB19 infection was involved in the development of HAAA because we were unable to perform liver biopsy because of the patient's hyperbilirubinemia and thrombocytopenia. If we had the opportunity to perform liver biopsy, we could evaluate the existence of HPVB19 by immunohistochemistry or quantitative polymerase chain reaction.

Clinical guidelines for HPVB19 infection treatment have not been established as most of the symptoms, including liver dysfunction, frequently recover without any treatment. However, HAAA progresses rapidly and is usually fatal if untreated; that is, the mean survival rate of progressed severe bone marrow aplasia is 2 months, and the fatality rate ranges from 78% to 88% [29–31]. Therefore, therapeutic intervention is urgently required for the survival of patients developing HAAA. The primary curative option for treatment of severe HAAA is immunosuppressive therapy [32]. The response rate to immunosuppressive therapy is reportedly 70% [22]. Brown et al. have demonstrated that immunosuppressive therapy with cyclosporine and ATG provides a beneficial outcome in patients with HAAA [27]. Successful treatment with immunosuppressive therapy is usually associated with rapid resolution of acute hepatitis in patients. Cyclosporine and ATG may improve hepatitis as well as bone marrow failure via suppression of cytotoxic T lymphocytes [19]. In addition to immunosuppressive therapy, bone marrow transplantation is also a critical option for the treatment of HAAA. Doney et al. reported 85% survival in patients treated with hematopoietic cell transplantation [32]. Safadi et al. also demonstrated that no cases of recurrent hepatitis occurred during the bone marrow transplantation follow-up period, with patients having reasonable survival rates [33].

In conclusion, HAAA is a distinct clinical syndrome characterized by the onset of bone marrow failure following acute hepatic injury through immunologic mechanisms. The causal trigger of HAAA mostly appears to be an undetermined virus, and, in the present case, HPVB19 is strongly considered as a candidate virus. Most unrecognized, and thus untreated, cases show extremely poor prognosis. Immunosuppressive therapy is reportedly effective, but the long-term outcome for patients with HAAA treated with immunosuppressive ther-

apy is still obscure. Our case suggests that HPVB19 should be considered as a hepatotropic virus and a cause of acquired aplastic anemia. With the accumulation of cases in the future, further elucidation of the disease state and establishment of a treatment method for HPVB19-related hepatitis and HAAA are needed.

References

[1] B. J. Cohen and M. M. Buckley, "The prevalence of antibody to human parvovirus B 19 in England and Wales," *Journal of Medical Microbiology*, vol. 25, no. 2, pp. 151–153, 1988.

[2] H. A. Kelly, D. Siebert, R. Hammond, J. Leydon, P. Kiely, and W. Maskill, "The age-specific prevalence of human parvovirus immunity in Victoria, Australia compared with other parts of the world," *Epidemiology and Infection*, vol. 124, no. 3, pp. 449–457, 2000.

[3] S. Arista, S. De Grazia, V. Di Marco, R. Di Stefano, and A. Craxì, "Parvovirus B19 and "cryptogenic" chronic hepatitis," *Journal of Hepatology*, vol. 38, no. 3, pp. 375–376, 2003.

[4] D. S. Krygier, U. P. Steinbrecher, M. Petric et al., "Parvovirus B19 induced hepatic failure in an adult requiring liver transplantation," *World Journal of Gastroenterology*, vol. 15, no. 32, pp. 4067–4069, 2009.

[5] L. Sun and J.-C. Zhang, "Acute fulminant hepatitis with bone marrow failure in an adult due to parvovirus B19 infection," *Hepatology*, vol. 55, no. 1, pp. 329–330, 2012.

[6] R. M. Al-Abdwani, F. A. Khamis, A. Balkhair, M. Sacharia, and Y. A. Wali, "A child with human parvovirus B19 infection induced aplastic anemia and acute hepatitis: Effectiveness of immunosuppressive therapy," *Pediatric Hematology and Oncology*, vol. 25, no. 7, pp. 699–703, 2008.

[7] C. Dame, C. Hasan, U. Bode, and A. M. Eis-Hübinger, "Acute liver disease and aplastic anemia associated with the persistence of B19 dna in liver and bone marrow," *Pediatric Pathology & Molecular Medicine*, vol. 21, no. 1, pp. 25–29, 2002.

[8] A. N. Langnas, R. S. Markin, M. S. Cattral, and S. J. Naides, "Parvovirus B19 as a possible causative agent of fulminant liver failure and associated aplastic anemia," *Hepatology*, vol. 22, no. 6, pp. 1661–1665, 1995.

[9] L. D. Rogo, T. Mokhtari-Azad, M. H. Kabir, and F. Rezaei, "Human parvovirus B19: a review," *Acta Virologica*, vol. 58, no. 3, pp. 199–213, 2014.

[10] N. S. Young and K. E. Brown, "Mechanisms of disease: parvovirus B19," *New England Journal of Medicine*, vol. 350, no. 6, pp. 586–597, 2004.

[11] C. Bihari, A. Rastogi, P. Saxena et al., "Parvovirus B19 associated hepatitis," *Hepatitis Research and Treatment*, vol. 2013, Article ID 472027, 9 pages, 2013.

[12] Y. Yoto, T. Kudoh, K. Haseyama, N. Suzuki, and S. Chiba, "Human parvovirus B19 infection associated with acute hepatitis," *Lancet*, vol. 347, no. 9005, pp. 868–869, 1996.

[13] I. Mihály, A. Trethon, Z. Arányi et al., "Observations on human parvovirus B19 infection diagnosed in 2011," *Orvosi Hetilap*, vol. 153, no. 49, pp. 1948–1957, 2012.

[14] K. E. Brown and N. S. Young, "The simian parvoviruses," *Reviews in Medical Virology*, vol. 7, no. 4, pp. 211–218, 1997.

[15] T. L. Moore, "Parvovirus-associated arthritis," *Current Opinion in Rheumatology*, vol. 12, no. 4, pp. 289–294, 2000.

[16] L. L. W. Cooling, T. A. W. Koerner, and S. J. Naides, "Multiple glycosphingolipids determine the tissue tropism of parvovirus B19," *Journal of Infectious Diseases*, vol. 172, no. 5, pp. 1198–1205, 1995.

[17] E. Morita, A. Nakashima, H. Asao, H. Sato, and K. Sugamura, "Human parvovirus B19 nonstructural protein (NS1) induces cell cycle arrest at G1 phase," *Journal of Virology*, vol. 77, no. 5, pp. 2915–2921, 2003.

[18] B. D. Poole, Y. V. Karetnyi, and S. J. Naides, "Parvovirus B19-induced apoptosis of hepatocytes," *Journal of Virology*, vol. 78, no. 14, pp. 7775–7783, 2004.

[19] B. Rauff, M. Idrees, S. A. R. Shah et al., "Hepatitis associated aplastic anemia: a review," *Virology Journal*, vol. 8, article 87, 2011.

[20] R. Andreesen, W. Brugger, C. Thomssen, A. Rehm, B. Speck, and G. W. Lohr, "Defective monocyte-to-macrophage maturation in patients with aplastic anemia," *Blood*, vol. 74, no. 6, pp. 2150–2156, 1989.

[21] T. Muta, Y. Tanaka, E. Takeshita et al., "Recurrence of hepatitis-associated aplastic anemia after a 10-year interval," *Internal Medicine*, vol. 47, no. 19, pp. 1733–1737, 2008.

[22] R. Gonzalez-Casas, L. Garcia-Buey, E. A. Jones, J. P. Gisbert, and R. Moreno-Otero, "Systematic review: hepatitis-associated aplastic anaemia—a syndrome associated with abnormal immunological function," *Alimentary Pharmacology & Therapeutics*, vol. 30, no. 5, pp. 436–443, 2009.

[23] E. Lorenz and K. Quaiser, "Panmyelophatie nach hepatitis epidemica," *Wiener Medizinische Wochenschrift*, vol. 105, pp. 19–22, 1955 (German).

[24] Y. Osugi, H. Yagasaki, M. Sako et al., "Antithymocyte globulin and cyclosporine for treatment of 44 children with hepatitis associated aplastic anemia," *Haematologica*, vol. 92, no. 12, pp. 1687–1690, 2007.

[25] C. Cengiz, N. Turhan, O. F. Yolcu, and S. Yilmaz, "Hepatitis associated with aplastic anemia: do CD8(+) Kupffer cells have a role in the pathogenesis?" *Digestive Diseases and Sciences*, vol. 52, no. 9, pp. 2438–2443, 2007.

[26] D. G. Bowen, A. Warren, T. Davis et al., "Cytokine-dependent bystander hepatitis due to intrahepatic murine CD8 T-cell activation by bone marrow-derived cells," *Gastroenterology*, vol. 123, no. 4, pp. 1252–1264, 2002.

[27] K. E. Brown, J. Tisdale, A. J. Barrett, C. E. Dunbar, and N. S. Young, "Hepatitis-associated aplastic anemia," *The New England Journal of Medicine*, vol. 336, no. 15, pp. 1059–1064, 1997.

[28] S. Wong, N. S. Young, and K. E. Brown, "Prevalence of parvovirus B19 in liver tissue: no association with fulminant hepatitis or hepatitis-associated aplastic anemia," *Journal of Infectious Diseases*, vol. 187, no. 10, pp. 1581–1586, 2003.

[29] P. Bannister, K. Miloszewski, D. Barnard, and M. S. Losowsky, "Fatal marrow aplasia associated with non-A, non-B hepatitis," *British Medical Journal (Clinical Research Ed.)*, vol. 286, no. 6374, pp. 1314–1315, 1983.

[30] J. K. Davies and E. C. Guinan, "An update on the management of severe idiopathic aplastic anaemia in children," *British Journal of Haematology*, vol. 136, no. 4, pp. 549–564, 2007.

[31] J. M. Valdez, P. Scheinberg, N. S. Young, and T. J. Walsh, "Infections in patients with aplastic anemia," *Seminars in Hematology*, vol. 46, no. 3, pp. 269–276, 2009.

[32] K. Doney, W. Leisenring, R. Storb, and F. R. Appelbaum, "Primary treatment of acquired aplastic anemia: outcomes with bone marrow transplantation and immunosuppressive therapy," *Annals of Internal Medicine*, vol. 126, no. 2, pp. 107–115, 1997.

[33] R. Safadi, R. Or, Y. Ilan et al., "Lack of known hepatitis virus in hepatitis-associated aplastic anemia and outcome after bone marrow transplantation," *Bone Marrow Transplantation*, vol. 27, no. 2, pp. 183–190, 2001.

17

Early Onset of Tenofovir-Related Fanconi Syndrome in a Child with Acute Hepatitis B: A Case Report and Systematic Review of Literature

Renato Pascale,[1] **Viola Guardigni,**[1,2] **Lorenzo Badia,**[1,2] **Francesca Volpato,**[1]
Pierluigi Viale,[1] **and Gabriella Verucchi**[1,2]

[1]*Infectious Diseases Unit, Department of Medical and Surgical Science, S. Orsola-Malpighi Hospital,*
University of Bologna, Bologna, Italy
[2]*Research Centre for the Study of Hepatitis, University of Bologna, Bologna, Italy*

Correspondence should be addressed to Viola Guardigni; v.guardigni@gmail.com

Academic Editor: Mauro Vigano

Tenofovir disoproxil fumarate- (TDF-) related nephropathy is known to be a long-term complication of this drug, more commonly observed in HIV-infected patients, but occurring also in hepatitis B. Cases of Fanconi Syndrome associated with TDF have been reported in adult patients, usually as a long-term complication of chronic hepatitis B treatment. We present here a case of a 12-year-old male developing a severe acute HBV hepatitis treated with TDF. The patient achieved an early virological and biochemical response, but with a subsequent onset of proximal renal tubular damage, consistent with Fanconi Syndrome. After withdrawing this drug and switching to Entecavir, a complete resolution of tubulopathy and, after 6 months, a complete HBsAg seroconversion occurred. To our knowledge, this is the first report of an early renal injury due to TDF-therapy in a pediatric patient treated for acute hepatitis B.

1. Introduction

In 1992, World Health Organization set the inclusion of hepatitis B vaccine into their childhood vaccination programs as a goal for all countries worldwide [1]. Indeed, in the United States, acute hepatitis B cases from the National Notifiable Disease Surveillance System showed an overall low incidence rate of 0.9/100,000 population in 2011 [2]. Similar trend was reported in Italy, with an incidence of 0.85/100,000 population, in 2012 [3]. Severe acute hepatitis B is defined by coagulopathy (INR > 1.5) or a protracted course (i.e., persistent symptoms or marked jaundice for >4 weeks) or signs of acute liver failure, representing a risk for an incipient fulminant hepatitis. European Association For The Study Of The Liver and European Society of Pediatric Gastroenterology suggest that both pediatric and adult patients with this condition might benefit from treatment with Nucleoside Analogue (NA) in order to prevent development of fulminant hepatitis [4, 5].

Reports mainly described lamivudine (LAM) therapy even if, in many experts' opinion, Entecavir (ETV) or Tenofovir disoproxil fumarate (TDF) should be used [5, 6], since these third-generation NAs have higher antiviral potency and are less likely to induce resistance than LAM [4, 7, 8]. Moreover, a case of fulminant hepatitis B in a 4-month-old infant successfully treated with Tenofovir was reported [9].

We present here the first case of an early-onset renal injury, consistent with Fanconi Syndrome, during TDF-therapy in a child treated for acute hepatitis B. Furthermore, we report a systematic review of scientific literature on this topic.

2. Methods

We conducted a literature search using PubMed, PubMed Central, and Medline databases, reviewing all the case reports published in English. Search terms included "Tenofovir",

"Fanconi Syndrome", "Renal injury", "Hepatits B", and "children". The initial search was performed in January 2015 and repeated for new references in May 2017.

3. Case Report

A 12-year-old male affected by an osteosarcoma of femur, diagnosed in August 2012, after several neoadjuvant cycles of chemotherapy with adriamycin, cisplatin, ifosfamide, and methotrexate, underwent a surgical removal of femur in December 2012. After surgery, additional chemotherapy cycles were performed, and, during the last one (in June 2013), an unexpected hypertransaminasemia (ALT: 456 U/L) was detected. Further laboratory tests confirmed ALT and AST alterations progressively worsening (AST: 280 UI/ml and ALT: 620 UI/ml). The serologic panel showed acute HBV infection (HBsAg positive, HBcIgM positive, HBeAg negative, and HBeAb positive, HBV-DNA: >170.000.000 UI/ml), even though it was shown that the child was correctly vaccinated for HBV, as his parents and relatives were. D genotype was identified. Considering that HBsAg was negative at presurgical screening (while HBsAb was not tested), a diagnosis of acute HBV infection in a patient nonresponder to vaccination was formulated, hypothesizing an infection occurred during his surgical or oncological course. Despite moderate elevation in aminotransferases and INR (1.40) we decided to start an off-label treatment with Tenofovir considering a substantial risk for evolution toward a fulminant hepatitis B (which is more likely in childhood than in other age ranges [6]). The dosage assessed by age and body weight was 245 mg once a day. After 30 days of therapy, HBV-DNA had decreased of 4 log(10), HBsAg was declining, and transaminases and coagulation parameters were normalized; no signs of acute encephalopathy developed at any time. Considering patient's oncological history and the planned further chemotherapy cycles, we decided to maintain NA-treatment until HBsAg clearance. Nevertheless, after 5 months of TDF-treatment, normoglycemic glycosuria (glycemia 88 mg/dl, glycosuria 70 mg/dl), phosphaturia with hypophosphatemia (reduced tubular absorption of phosphorus (56%), phosphatemia 1.9 mg/dl, proteinuria (albuminuria 100 mg/dl at dipstick, proteinuria: 0.2 g/24 h), glomerular filtration rate (GFR) 70 ml/min/1.73 m^2, and urine creatinine 0.47 g/day were detected, leading to diagnosis of Fanconi Syndrome associated with TDF-therapy.

Assuming that tubular damage was possibly related to TDF (enhancing a preexisting renal impairment secondary to chemotherapy), the latter was withdrawn and a concomitant switch to ETV was decided. At that time, there were no indications for pediatric use of ETV but, considering reports of safety and efficacy in pediatric population treated for chronic HBV infection, a dosage of 0.015 mg/kg/day was prescribed. ETV therapy was well tolerated and maintained HBV-DNA negativity. Indeed, after 2 months of this treatment a complete resolution of tubulopathy was observed and after 6 months a complete HBs seroconversion (HBsAg negative; HBsAb: 15 UI/ml) occurred (Figure 1). Currently, the oncological disease is in remission and NA therapy has been stopped after 18 months from seroconversion. Persistence of HBs

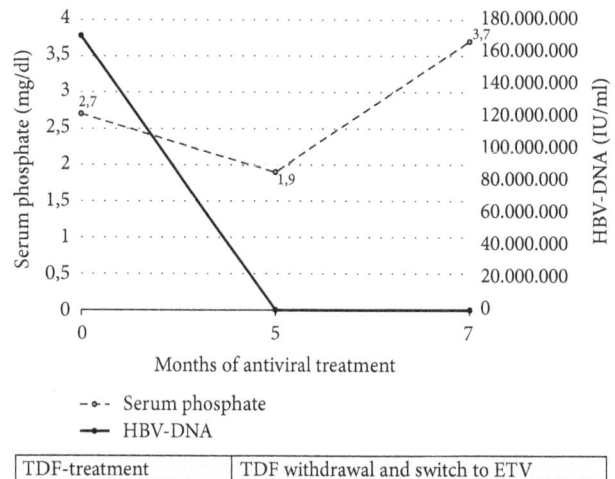

FIGURE 1: Serum phosphate and HBV-DNA levels over Tenofovir treatment and after its withdrawal.

seroconversion has been confirmed after 2 years from the end of treatment.

4. Discussion

Fanconi Syndrome, characterized by normoglycemic glycosuria, hypophosphatemia, aminoaciduria, proteinuria, metabolic acidosis, and hypouricemia, may be caused by NtRTIs (like TDF) [16] and is widely reported in HIV-infected patients, also pediatric. Probably, in this special population, the direct role of HIV damaging kidney and concomitant use of other drugs, such as protease inhibitor, are closely related to renal impairment [17–19].

Renal injury due to TDF monotherapy in hepatitis B infection is less common, although several studies have reported chronic tubular damage and reduction in eGFR in patients treated with this antiviral [4] and Tenofovir alafenamide (TAF) has been now demonstrated to be safer than TDF in registrational trials [4, 6]. To date, there are few published reports of TDF-related Fanconi syndrome (Table 1): all of them have been described in adult patients with CHB. To the best of our knowledge, this is the first report of an early-onset TDF-related renal injury in a child with acute hepatitis B.

Majority of patients described in literature [10–15, 20] developed tubular complications after long-term TDF-administration (after an average of 24 months) for hepatitis B, suggesting that Fanconi Syndrome is a late onset complication of this drug. Our case presents some peculiarities: early onset of the tubulopathy (reported only by Samarkos et al. [14] and Hwang et al. [15]), young age of the patients, and TDF-administration for acute HBV-related hepatitis. In our patient chemotherapy could have played an important role in enhancing kidney damage, since he had been recently treated with ifosfamide and cisplatin, which are drugs with a well-known nephrotoxicity [16]. This relevant predisposing factor, not characterizing the other patients reported in literature, might explain such an early onset of TDF-related toxicity.

TABLE 1: Review of cases of TDF-associated Fanconi Syndrome during Hepatitis B therapy.

	Age	Sex	TDF-treatment duration	Risk factor	Serum creatinine (mg/dl)	eGFR* (ml/min)	Serum phosphate (mg/dl)	Serum bicarbonate (mmol/L)	Uric Acid (mg/dl)	Phosphate fractional excretion (%)	Glycosuria° (mg/dl)	Proteinuria (≤24 h)
Murray et al. [10]	39	M	24 months	Adefovir exposure	1.44	59	1.86	n/a	3.5	n/a	yes	0.6
Murray et al. [10]	54	M	24 months	Hypertension	1.53	51	2.1	n/a	1.34	elevated	n/a	0.2
Magalhães-Costa et al. [11]	82	M	6 months	Adefovir exposure, diabetes	n/a	n/a	1.1	13.9	1.7	65.8%	yes	yes
Gracey et al. [12]	58	M	42 months	Adefovir exposure	1.32	55	2.1	19.3	n/a	n/a	500	0.5
Gracey et al. [12]	62	M	45 months	Hypertension	3.35	18	1.7	19.5	n/a	n/a	400	n/a
Viganò et al. [13]	44	F	3 months	Diabetes	3.22	20	2.6	11	2.5	elevated^	n/a	yes
Samarkos et al. [14]	58	M	12 months	Adefovir exposure, hypertension	1.45	n/a	1.4	17.1	n/a	elevated^^	500	0.96
Hwang et al. [15]	40	M	36 months	No	1.5	58.6	1.3	n/a	1.9	41%	200	0.3
Our case	12	M	5 months	Ifosfamide, Cisplatin	0.47	70	1.9	n/a	n/a	56%	70	0.2

*By MDRD formula; °by dipstick. ^Tubular maximal transport of phosphate reabsorption to the glomerular filtration rate transport (TmP/GFR): 0.008 mg/dl; ^^TmP/GFR: 0.66 mmol/L.

After the switch to Entecavir, tubular function progressively improved and HBV-DNA continued to be undetectable. At the time of decision, ETV was not yet registered for pediatric use, while safety and effectiveness of ETV in treating children with CHB are now proved [8, 10] and the drug is registered for use in this population. Acute HBV symptomatic infection is rare in pediatric age (due to vaccination), and it can vary from a mild to a fulminant hepatitis. Classic symptoms are present in 30–50% of older children and adolescents with acute hepatitis B and include fever, jaundice, nausea and vomiting, abdominal pain, liver tenderness, and fatigue, which last approximately 2-3 months [4, 5]. In our report, the patient had only laboratory tests alteration (increase in transaminases and coagulation parameters), without clinical findings.

HBV vaccination has an excellent record of safety and effectiveness (response in over 90% of the immunecompetent individuals) [21]. However, a substantial rate of nonresponse to vaccination may occur. Almost 1–10% of healthy individuals fail to generate a protective antibody response to hepatitis B vaccine (more frequent in healthy adults compared to neonates) [22]; many factors associated with a nonresponse to HBV vaccination have been described, including incorrect administration of the vaccine, impaired vaccine storage conditions, drug abuse, smoking, genetic factors, obesity, chronic kidney disease, celiac disease, thalassemia, type I diabetes mellitus, and Down's Syndrome [21–23]. We considered our patient as nonresponder to hepatitis B vaccination but we do not know how the child became infected with HBV: it might be speculated that it happened during his many hospitalizations. Indeed, though unexpected, cases of transmission of HBV in health-care setting have been reported also in recent years [24].

We decided to start NA therapy considering the severity of illness, with risk of acute hepatic failure development. The potential need of long-term therapy with risk to develop resistance, induced us to prefer a third-generation NA rather than lamivudine [4, 7, 8]. Our first choice was TDF, which is known to have higher antiviral potency and to induce a lower rate of resistance than lamivudine [7]. At the time of the decision there were already many data supporting the use of TDF in children and adolescents suffering of chronic hepatitis B (CHB), as well as part of antiretroviral therapy in HIV-infected children [10, 19, 25]. Particularly, in the study of Murray et al. TDF was shown to be highly effective and safe for HBV suppression in 52 adolescents with CHB observed for 72 weeks [10]. An anecdotal case of fulminant hepatitis B of a 4-month-old infant successfully treated with Tenofovir was also reported [9].

In conclusion, despite the presence of an effective vaccine, new HBV infections are still possible (also in health-care settings) and testing HBV markers should be mandatory in every patient exposed to immunosuppressive treatment, regardless of vaccination report. Last generation NAs (e.g., TDF, ETV) are effective not only in CHB but also in acute hepatitis B.

Our case highlights the potential risks for TDF-related renal injury and raises some concerns about using this antiviral in frail patients with concomitant risk factors for acute tubular damage, such as chemotherapy. Therefore, a close monitoring of renal and tubular function in patients undergoing TDF-treatment should be performed in any case, and the choice of NA for hepatitis B should be based on patients' characteristics, considering the high virological efficacy of all the available antivirals.

References

[1] R. J. Kim-Farley, "EPI for the 1990s," *Vaccine*, vol. 10, no. 13, pp. 940–948, 1992.

[2] K. Iqbal, R. M. Klevens, M. A. Kainer et al., "Epidemiology of Acute Hepatitis B in the United States from Population-Based Surveillance, 2006-2011," *Clinical Infectious Diseases*, vol. 61, no. 4, pp. 584–592, 2015.

[3] C. Sagnelli, M. Ciccozzi, M. Pisaturo et al., "The impact of viral molecular diversity on the clinical presentation and outcome of acute hepatitis B in Italy," *New Microbiologica*, vol. 38, no. 2, pp. 137–147, 2015.

[4] P. Lampertico, K. Agarwal, T. Berg et al., "EASL 2017 Clinical Practice Guidelines on the management of hepatitis B virus infection," *Journal of Hepatology*, vol. 67, no. 2, pp. 370–398, 2017.

[5] E. M. Sokal, M. Paganelli, S. Wirth et al., "Management of chronic hepatitis B in childhood: ESPGHAN clinical practice guidelines: consensus of an expert panel on behalf of the European Society of Pediatric Gastroenterology, Hepatology and Nutrition," *Journal of Hepatology*, vol. 59, no. 4, pp. 814–829, 2013.

[6] C.-Y. Chen, Y.-H. Ni, H.-L. Chen, F. L. Lu, and M.-H. Chang, "Lamivudine treatment in infantile fulminant hepatitis B," *Pediatrics International*, vol. 52, no. 4, pp. 672–674, 2010.

[7] A. S. Lok, "Drug therapy: Tenofovir," *Hepatology*, vol. 52, no. 2, pp. 743–747, 2010.

[8] T. Miyauchi, T. Kanda, M. Shinozaki et al., "Efficacy of lamivudine or entecavir against virological rebound after achieving HBV DNA negativity in chronic hepatitis B patients," *International Journal of Medical Sciences*, vol. 10, no. 6, pp. 647–652, 2013.

[9] A. Diamanti, M. R. Sartorelli, A. Alterio et al., "Successful Tenofovir Treatment for Fulminant Hepatitis B Infection in an Infant," *The Pediatric Infectious Disease Journal*, vol. 30, no. 10, pp. 912–914, 2011.

[10] K. F. Murray, L. Szenborn, J. Wysocki et al., "Randomized, placebo-controlled trial of tenofovir disoproxil fumarate in adolescents with chronic hepatitis B," *Hepatology*, vol. 56, no. 6, pp. 2018–2026, 2012.

[11] P. Magalhães-Costa, L. Matos, P. Barreiro, and C. Chagas, "Fanconi syndrome and chronic renal failure in a chronic hepatitis B monoinfected patient treated with tenofovir," *Revista Espanola de Enfermedades Digestivas*, vol. 107, no. 8, pp. 512–514, 2015.

[12] D. M. Gracey, P. Snelling, P. McKenzie, and S. I. Strasser, "Tenofovir-associated Fanconi syndrome in patients with chronic hepatitis B monoinfection," *Antiviral Therapy*, vol. 18, no. 7, pp. 945–948, 2013.

[13] M. Viganò, A. Brocchieri, A. Spinetti et al., "Tenofovir-induced Fanconi syndrome in chronic hepatitis B monoinfected patients that reverted after tenofovir withdrawal," *Journal of Clinical Virology*, vol. 61, no. 4, pp. 600–603, 2014.

[14] M. Samarkos, V. Theofanis, I. Eliadi, J. Vlachogiannakos, and A. Polyzos, "Tenofovir-associated Fanconi syndrome in a patient with chronic hepatitis D," *Journal of Gastrointestinal and Liver Diseases*, vol. 23, no. 3, p. 342, 2014, http://www.ncbi.nlm.nih .gov/pubmed/25267967.

[15] H. S. Hwang, C. W. Park, and M. J. Song, "Tenofovir-associated Fanconi syndrome and nephrotic syndrome in a patient with chronic hepatitis B monoinfection," *Hepatology*, vol. 62, no. 4, pp. 1318–1320, 2015.

[16] A. M. Hall, P. Bass, and R. J. Unwin, "Drug-induced renal fanconi syndrome," *QJM: An International Journal of Medicine*, vol. 107, no. 4, pp. 261–269, 2014.

[17] L. Aurpibul and T. Puthanakit, "Review of tenofovir use in HIV-infected children," *Pediatric Infectious Disease Journal*, vol. 34, no. 4, pp. 383–391, 2015.

[18] M. Goicoechea, S. Liu, B. Best et al., "Greater tenofovir-associated renal function decline with protease inhibitor-based versus nonnucleoside reverse-transcriptase inhibitor-based therapy," *The Journal of Infectious Diseases*, vol. 197, no. 1, pp. 102–108, 2008.

[19] M. Purswani, K. Patel, J. B. Kopp et al., "Tenofovir Treatment Duration Predicts Proteinuria in a Multiethnic United States Cohort of Children and Adolescents With Perinatal HIV-1 Infection," *The Pediatric Infectious Disease Journal*, vol. 32, no. 5, pp. 495–500, 2013.

[20] F. Conti, G. Vitale, C. Cursaro, M. Bernardi, and P. Andreone, "Tenofovir-induced Fanconi syndrome in a patient with chronic hepatitis B monoinfection," *Annals of Hepatology*, vol. 15, no. 2, pp. 273–276, 2016.

[21] M. Filippelli, E. Lionetti, A. Gennaro et al., "Hepatitis B vaccine by intradermal route in non responder patients: An update," *World Journal of Gastroenterology*, vol. 20, no. 30, pp. 10383–10394, 2014.

[22] S. Park, J. Markowitz, M. Pettei et al., "Failure to Respond to Hepatitis B Vaccine in Children With Celiac Disease," *Journal of Pediatric Gastroenterology and Nutrition*, vol. 44, no. 4, pp. 431–435, 2007.

[23] J. Chen, Z. Liang, F. Lu et al., "Toll-like receptors and cytokines/cytokine receptors polymorphisms associate with non-response to hepatitis B vaccine," *Vaccine*, vol. 29, no. 4, pp. 706–711, 2011.

[24] J. L. Perry, R. D. Pearson, and J. Jagger, "Infected health care workers and patient safety: A double standard," *American Journal of Infection Control*, vol. 34, no. 5, pp. 313–319, 2006.

[25] P. Rosenthal, "Another drug in the armamentarium to combat hepatitis B virus in adolescents," *Hepatology*, vol. 56, no. 6, pp. 2016-2017, 2012.

18

Severe Acute Hepatitis B in HBV-Vaccinated Partner of a Patient with Multiple Myeloma Treated with Cyclophosphamide, Bortezomib, and Dexamethasone and Autologous Stem Cell Transplant

Majed M. Almaghrabi,[1] Kyle J. Fortinsky,[2] and David Wong[2]

[1]*Division of Internal Medicine, University of Toronto, Toronto, ON, Canada*
[2]*Division of Hepatology, University of Toronto, Toronto, ON, Canada*

Correspondence should be addressed to David Wong; dave.wong@uhn.ca

Academic Editor: Mauro Vigano

Hepatitis B reactivation can occur with various forms of immunosuppression. Cyclophosphamide, Bortezomib, and Dexamethasone (CYBOR-D) chemotherapy is commonly used for the treatment of multiple myeloma and has not been noted in guidelines to be causative in HBV reactivation. Indeed, current guidelines do not recommend providing antiviral prophylaxis to patients with prior HBV infection. We present a case of HBV reactivation as a result of CYBOR-D and autologous stem cell transplant which is complicated by the patient's partner who developed acute hepatitis B. Our case highlights the need to review the role of antiviral prophylaxis for patients undergoing treatment of multiple myeloma and also the role of ensuring immunity for close contacts of these patients who may also be at risk.

1. Introduction

The natural history of chronic hepatitis B virus (HBV) infection is characterized by various stages that are influenced by the host immune response. Resolved HBV infection is defined by undetectable levels of HBV proteins (HBsAg) and viral load (HBV DNA) in a patient with evidence of previous exposure (positive anti-HBc) [1, 2]. HBV reactivation occurs most often in patients with resolved HBV infection who are exposed to profound immunosuppression. Current guidelines describe certain high-risk patients who may benefit from antiviral therapy as prophylaxis against HBV reactivation including those with certain forms of cancer or those on specific chemotherapeutic agents [3, 4]. However, the guideline recommendations are largely based upon expert opinion.

Multiple myeloma (MM) is a cancer resulting in monoclonal expansion of IgG against one epitope potentially at the expense of immunity to other antigens such as HBV. While the precise mechanism within the host immune response is largely unknown, recent studies suggest that T-cells may not be the major players in the natural history of chronic HBV infection [5]. Importantly, since therapies targeted against CD20 can result in HBV reactivation even after HBsAg loss, this suggests that B-lymphocytes and plasma cells likely play a role in immunity against HBV infection [6]. In patients undergoing autologous stem cell transplant (ASCT), host immunity is presumably restored immediately after chemoablation of cancer cells [7]. Moreover, HBV immunity can be adoptively transferred in allogeneic bone marrow transplants. For example, the marrow from a donor who has immunity to HBV can result in HBsAg clearance in a recipient with chronic HBV infection [8]. Conversely, marrow from a donor without immunity to HBV can result in HBsAg recurrence in a recipient who had prior HBV infection that resolved [9].

A few recent studies have reported cases of HBV reactivation in patients with MM being treated with Bortezomib-based chemotherapy [10, 11]. Tsukune et al. reported 9 patients with MM who received Bortezomib-based chemotherapy and developed HBV reactivation [12]. Lee et al. reported 12 patents with MM who all received A3CT (2 of whom were on Bortezomib therapy) and all developed HBV reactivation [13].

The HBV serological status and the type of immunosuppressive therapy are the major determinants in the current guidelines for prevention and treatment of HBV in patients undergoing immunosuppressive therapy. Patients who are HBsAg positive/anti-HBc positive or HBsAg negative/anti-HBc positive undergoing immunosuppressive therapy with B-cell depleting agents, anthracycline derivatives, tyrosine kinase inhibitors, cytokine inhibitors, or integrin inhibitors are recommended to receive antiviral prophylaxis as they are considered to be at moderate to high risk of HBV reactivation [3]. Proteosome inhibitors (e.g., Bortezomib) are not mentioned in the guidelines which suggests they do not require antiviral prophylaxis. Neither the product monograph for Bortezomib nor FDA safety labeling mentions a risk of hepatitis B reactivation. Additionally, current guidelines do not mention screening family members or household contacts for immunity against HBV even when patients themselves are at high risk of HBV reactivation.

The current report describes a case whereby HBV immunity was maintained after the diagnosis of multiple myeloma but was subsequently lost after chemotherapy and autologous stem cell transplant. The current case report adds to the increasing body of literature that suggests Bortezomib-based chemotherapy regimens may lead to HBV reactivation. Importantly, our case is the first report published on acute hepatitis B in a family member of a patient who develops HBV reactivation despite a history of HBV vaccination. Our case highlights important considerations in the management of patients who are undergoing immunosuppressive therapy and their families.

2. Case 1

A 68-year-old Canadian man, originally born in Italy, was referred to our hepatology clinic for management of HBV reactivation after his wife was diagnosed with acute HBV (see Case 2 for details of wife). He was diagnosed with MM and was treated with five cycles of Cyclophosphamide, Bortezomib, and Dexamethasone (CYBOR-D) prior to undergoing an autologous stem cell transplant (ASCT). After the transplant, he was put on Lenalidomide for maintenance therapy. Prophylactic HBV antiviral therapy was not given. His past medical history was remarkable only for resolved HBV infection (HBsAg negative, anti-HBc positive, and anti-HBs positive), which was noted prior to transplantation.

After CYBOR-D chemotherapy, anti-HBs became negative and ALT was elevated. In February 2013 his anti-HBs was positive and in December 2014 his anti-HBs was found to be negative. In February 2016, his family physician provided HBV vaccination presumably because he was unaware of his prior HBV infection. Testing for HBV reactivation was not done until his wife presented with transaminitis, jaundice, and fatigue.

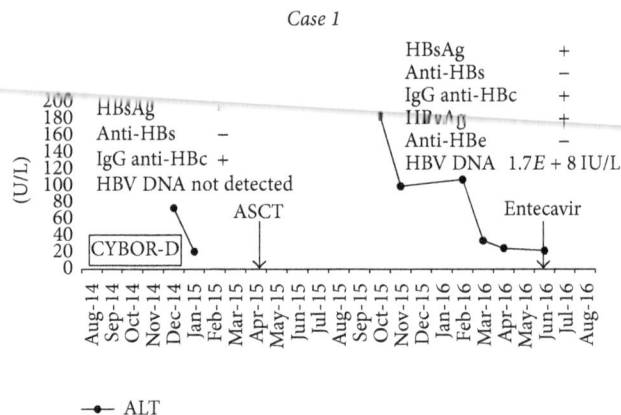

FIGURE 1: Liver enzymes and HBV tests in relation to chemotherapy, autologous stem cell transplant, and entecavir therapy.

Once his wife was diagnosed with acute HBV, he was diagnosed with HBV reactivation: HBsAg positive (titer > 124,925 IU/mL), HBeAg positive, HBV DNA > 1.70E8 IU/mL, and ALT persistently normal. His anti-HCV was negative and he remained immune to hepatitis A. In retrospect, liver enzymes had been abnormal (ALT peak 182) during the HBV vaccination period but were normal when his wife presented with acute hepatitis (see Figure 1). An abdominal ultrasound was unremarkable and a FibroScan was consistent with F1 (minimal) fibrosis. He was started immediately on entecavir for HBV reactivation.

At 4 months' follow-up, he remained asymptomatic from a liver perspective. His liver enzymes and liver function were normal and his HBV viral load was reduced to 4.64E4 IU/mL on entecavir.

3. Case 2

A 68-year-old Canadian woman, originally born in Canada, was admitted to hospital for 2 days after developing jaundice and severe fatigue over the past two weeks. Her past medical history was significant for osteoarthritis, where she was taking daily acetaminophen (<2 grams per day). She denied any sick contacts, recent travel, or symptoms suggestive of an underlying autoimmune disorder. She denied taking any additional medications or herbal supplements. She was a nonsmoker and denied any alcohol or illicit drug use. She had no prior blood transfusions, tattoos, needle stick injuries, incarceration, or recent travel to an HBV endemic country. She reported receiving prior immunization to hepatitis B in 1988 prior to a trip to India but had not been tested for adequate anti-HBs levels.

On examination, she was afebrile and hemodynamically stable. She appeared jaundiced but there were no signs of hepatic encephalopathy. Liver edge was mildly tender and palpable, 4 cm below the costal margin. There was no splenomegaly, ascites, or other stigmata of chronic liver disease. She had no rashes or arthritis. The remainder of her physical examination was unrevealing.

Blood tests showed marked transaminitis (see Figure 2), INR 1.3, and Bilirubin up to 411 umol/L. HBV serology was

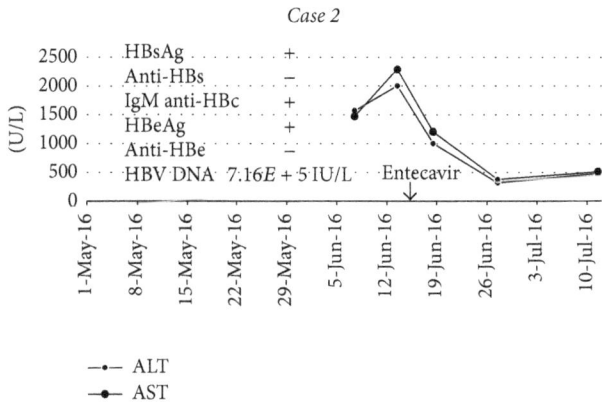

Figure 2: Liver enzymes and HBV tests in relation to entecavir therapy.

consistent with an acute HBV infection as evidenced by a positive IgM anti-HBc, HBsAg, and HBeAg. Abdominal ultrasound revealed an enlarged liver that was 14.8 cm but was otherwise unremarkable. She was treated with entecavir for symptomatic acute HBV infection and her fatigue mostly resolved after a week of therapy.

At 4 months' follow-up, the patient was feeling well, and her liver enzymes and liver function were normal. Her viral load was undetectable and her HBsAg was negative indicating successfully cleared infection; entecavir therapy was stopped.

4. Discussion

Most cases of HBV reactivation in the literature describe HBsAg seroreversion that leads to either low-level viremia without ALT elevation or more significant reactivation with high-level viremia and ongoing immune-mediated liver injury with ALT elevation. Interestingly, our patient in Case 1 developed HBsAg seroreversion with only transient hepatitis before entering what looked like the immune tolerant phase. There have only been 2 previous reported cases of patients with MM who received Bortezomib and had HBV reactivation followed directly by an immunotolerant phase [10, 11].

The precise role of antiviral prophylaxis in patients with resolved HBV who are undergoing ASCT remains controversial [3, 4, 13]. Tsukune et al. recommend serial monitoring of HBsAg or HBV DNA as a strategy to detect reactivation [12]. There do appear to be certain risk factors for HBV. Patients with negative anti-HBs seem to be at higher risk of HBV reactivation when compared to patients with a positive anti-HBs [13].

It is interesting to note that the patient's wife developed acute hepatitis B several months after we suspect the patient developed reactivation. Unfortunately, despite a rise in our patient's liver enzymes after ASCT, he was not recognized to have reactivation until his wife developed acute HBV. The delay between reactivation and his wife's acute HBV infection may be attributable to a rising HBV DNA level during that period as he was becoming more infectious.

There may have been several factors contributing to our patients HBV reactivation including Cyclophosphamide,

Bortezomib, Dexamethasone, ASCT, and Lenalidomide therapy. Lenalidomide is a potent immunomodulator and T-cell stimulator. It has been recommended to be used with caution in patients infected with HBV, though the role of immunomodulators in HBV reactivation is still undetermined [14]. ASCT has also been raised as a risk factor for HBV reactivation [15]. Bortezomib, a proteasome inhibitor, has been previously reported in a few cases of HBV reactivation in MM patients [10, 11]. Given its mechanism of action, Bortezomib may impair intracellular viral antigen processing leading to impaired maintenance of T-cell memory [16]. Recent guidelines, however, do not acknowledge that HBV reactivation might occur in patients exposed to Bortezomib therapy [3, 4]. Lastly, there is evidence that systemic corticosteroids such as Dexamethasone may also increase the risk of reactivation [17].

Interestingly, our patient lost anti-HBs, which prompted his family physician to repeat vaccination instead of testing for HBV reactivation. There are no data to support the strategy of HBV vaccination in those who lose anti-HBs after immunosuppression. Although patients with a negative anti-HBs may be at higher risk for reactivation compared to patients with a positive anti-HBs, current guidelines do not suggest prophylaxis for patients based upon their anti-HBs status alone. In general, prophylaxis with HBV antiviral therapy is initiated at the beginning of chemotherapy until approximately 6 months after completing therapy. Moreover, current guidelines do not recommend routine testing for family members or close contacts of patients at risk for reactivation.

The majority of patients with acute hepatitis B recover spontaneously without need for antiviral treatment. However, those who have symptomatic acute HBV infection may benefit from antiviral therapy to shorten duration and severity of symptoms. Those who remain HBeAg positive with high-level viremia more than 3 months after infection may benefit from antiviral therapy to prevent establishment of chronic infection. In regard to treatment, there are different choices of antiviral therapies including lamivudine, tenofovir, and entecavir [18].

This report highlights a case of HBV reactivation in a patient with MM treated with Bortezomib containing chemotherapy. It is still unclear if antiviral therapy versus careful monitoring is the best strategy for such patients. As the risk of reactivation is low and can take place over many years [12], it may be reasonable to monitor HBsAg every 6 months for 3 to 5 years after therapy rather than treating all with antivirals for 5 years.

Our case described a unique situation where the patient lost anti-HBs and vaccination did not prevent reactivation. Clinicians should consider more careful monitoring of patients undergoing Bortezomib-based chemotherapy and pay especially close attention to patients without anti-HBs. HBV vaccination in those who lose anti-HBs should not be undertaken until HBsAg testing to rule out HBV reactivation has been done. Furthermore, testing to monitor for HBV reactivation should be performed routinely during and immediately after treatment. Lastly, our case describes an unusual complication of a family member developing acute HBV as a result of reactivation in her husband. This occurred despite the wife being vaccinated many years priorly. The authors suggest that clinicians consider screening close household contacts of patients at risk for HBV reactivation in order to identify those without immunity to HBV who could benefit from repeat vaccination. Our cases portray the importance of considering both the patient and family members or close contacts who can also be adversely affected by medical treatments.

References

[1] C. S. Coffin, S. K. Fung, and M. M. Ma, "Management of chronic hepatitis B: Canadian association for the study of the liver consensus guidelines," *Canadian Journal of Gastroenterology*, vol. 26, no. 12, pp. 917–938, 2012.

[2] H. J. Yim and A. S.-F. Lok, "Natural history of chronic hepatitis B virus infection: what we knew in 1981 and what we know in 2005," *Hepatology*, vol. 43, no. 1, pp. S173–S181, 2006.

[3] K. R. Reddy, K. L. Beavers, S. P. Hammond, J. K. Lim, and Y. T. Falck-Ytter, "American Gastroenterological Association Institute guideline on the prevention and treatment of hepatitis B virus reactivation during immunosuppressive drug therapy," *Gastroenterology*, vol. 148, no. 1, pp. 215–219, 2015.

[4] J. P. Hwang, M. R. Somerfield, D. E. Alston-Johnson et al., "Hepatitis B virus screening for patients with cancer before therapy: American Society of Clinical Oncology provisional clinical opinion update," *Journal of Clinical Oncology*, vol. 33, no. 19, pp. 2212–2220, 2015.

[5] J.-J. Park, D. K. Wong, A. S. Wahed et al., "Hepatitis B virus–specific and global T-cell dysfunction in chronic hepatitis B," *Gastroenterology*, vol. 150, no. 3, pp. 684–695.e5, 2016.

[6] L.-T. Hsiao, T.-J. Chiou, J.-P. Gau et al., "Risk of reverse seroconversion of hepatitis B virus surface antigen in rituximab-treated non-Hodgkin lymphoma patients: a large cohort retrospective study," *Medicine*, vol. 94, no. 32, Article ID e1321, 2015.

[7] J. Storek, M. Geddes, F. Khan et al., "Reconstitution of the immune system after hematopoietic stem cell transplantation in humans," *Seminars in Immunopathology*, vol. 30, no. 4, pp. 425–4237, 2008.

[8] S. I. Strasser and G. B. McDonald, "Hepatitis viruses and hematopoietic cell transplantation: a guide to patient and donor management," *Blood*, vol. 93, no. 4, pp. 1127–1136, 1999.

[9] L. Milazzo, M. Corbellino, A. Foschi et al., "Late onset of hepatitis B virus reactivation following hematopoietic stem cell transplantation: successful treatment with combined entecavir plus tenofovir therapy," *Transplant Infectious Disease*, vol. 14, no. 1, pp. 95–98, 2012.

[10] S. Hussain, R. Jhaj, S. Ahsan, M. Ahsan, R. E. Bloom, and S. R. Jafri, "Bortezomib induced hepatitis B reactivation," *Case Reports in Medicine*, vol. 2014, Article ID 964082, 5 pages, 2014.

[11] H. Tanaka, I. Sakuma, S. Hashimoto et al., "Hepatitis B reactivation in a multiple myeloma patient with resolved hepatitis B infection during bortezomib therapy: case report," *Journal of Clinical and Experimental Hematopathology*, vol. 52, no. 1, pp. 67–69, 2012.

[12] Y. Tsukune, M. Sasaki, T. Odajima et al., "Incidence and clinical background of hepatitis B virus reactivation in multiple myeloma in novel agents' era," *Annals of Hematology*, vol. 95, no. 9, pp. 1465–1472, 2016.

[13] J. Y. Lee, S. H. Lim, M.-Y. Lee et al., "Hepatitis B reactivation in multiple myeloma patients with resolved hepatitis B undergoing chemotherapy," *Liver International*, vol. 35, no. 11, pp. 2363–2369, 2015.

[14] D. H. T. Mya, S. T. Han, Y. C. Linn, W. Y. K. Hwang, Y. T. Goh, and D. C. L. Tan, "Risk of hepatitis B reactivation and the role of novel agents and stem-cell transplantation in multiple myeloma patients with hepatitis B virus (HBV) infection," *Annals of Oncology*, vol. 23, no. 2, pp. 421–426, 2012.

[15] K. Matsue, T. Aoki, J. Odawara et al., "High risk of hepatitis B-virus reactivation after hematopoietic cell transplantation in hepatitis B core antibody-positive patients," *European Journal of Haematology*, vol. 83, no. 4, pp. 357–364, 2009.

[16] J. Li, B. Huang, Y. Li, D. Zheng, Z. Zhou, and J. Liu, "Hepatitis B virus reactivation in patients with multiple myeloma receiving bortezomib-containing regimens followed by autologous stem cell transplant," *Leukemia and Lymphoma*, vol. 56, no. 6, pp. 1710–1717, 2015.

[17] W. Yeo, B. Zee, S. Zhong et al., "Comprehensive analysis of risk factors associating with Hepatitis B virus (HBV) reactivation in cancer patients undergoing cytotoxic chemotherapy," *British Journal of Cancer*, vol. 90, no. 7, pp. 1306–1311, 2004.

[18] C. Jochum, R. K. Gieseler, I. Gawlista et al., "Hepatitis B-associated acute liver failure: immediate treatment with entecavir inhibits hepatitis B virus replication and potentially its sequelae," *Digestion*, vol. 80, no. 4, pp. 235–240, 2009.

19

Herpes Simplex Virus Hepatitis: A Presentation of Multi-Institutional Cases to Promote Early Diagnosis and Management of the Disease

Ashwinee Natu,[1] **Guiseppe Iuppa,**[2] **and Clifford D. Packer**[3]

[1]*Department of Internal Medicine, University Hospitals Cleveland Medical Center, 11100 Euclid Ave., Cleveland, OH 44106, USA*
[2]*Department of Transplant Surgery, Cleveland Clinic, 9500 Euclid Ave., Cleveland, OH 44195, USA*
[3]*Department of Internal Medicine, Louis Stokes VA Medical Center, 10701 East Blvd., Cleveland, OH 44106, USA*

Correspondence should be addressed to Ashwinee Natu; ashwinee.natu@gmail.com

Academic Editor: Melanie Deutsch

Objective. To compare three cases of Herpes simplex virus (HSV) hepatitis to increase early diagnosis of the disease. *Case 1.* A 23-year-old man with Crohn's disease and oral HSV. HSV hepatitis was diagnosed clinically and he improved with acyclovir. *Case 2.* An 18-year-old G1P0 woman with transaminitis. Despite early empiric acyclovir therapy, she died due to fulminant liver failure. *Case 3.* A 65-year-old woman who developed transaminitis after liver transplant. Diagnosis was confirmed by biopsy and she had resolution of acute liver failure with acyclovir. *Conclusion.* It is imperative that clinicians be aware of patients at high risk for developing HSV hepatitis to increase timely diagnosis and prevent morbidity and fatality.

1. Introduction

Herpes simplex virus (HSV) hepatitis is a rare diagnosis that can rapidly progress to fulminant liver failure. Timely diagnosis and treatment of this disease are imperative in reducing patient morbidity and mortality. We describe three cases of HSV hepatitis that highlight the commonalities and differences in presentation and discuss keys to early diagnosis.

2. Case 1

A 23-year-old man with severe fistulizing Crohn's disease was admitted to the hospital with abdominal pain. Symptoms included right upper quadrant abdominal pain, fever, tachycardia, and increased nonbloody bowel movements. He had been on a prednisone taper and vedolizumab. Initial lab findings were significant for an elevation in aminotransferases (ALT 3510 U/L, AST 9378 U/L) (Figures 1 and 2). Abdominal imaging was negative for acute pathology including vascular liver disease. He was started on broad-spectrum antibiotics, acyclovir, and N-acetylcysteine.

Additional testing was notable for positive HSV-2 IgM antibody test, HSV-2 detectability by DNA PCR, and genital/oral cultures positive for HSV-2. Based on these results he was diagnosed with HSV hepatitis and treated with acyclovir. Despite initial clinical improvement, his course was further complicated by a recurrent Crohn's flare. He was eventually discharged on high dose oral acyclovir, budesonide, and prednisone. As his HSV viral titer drastically decreased, he was restarted on outpatient vedolizumab infusions. He was continued on lifelong acyclovir for viral suppression due to his immunosuppression.

3. Case 2

An 18-year-old G1P0 woman with no significant past medical history presented to an outside hospital at 26-week gestation with shortness of breath. On presentation, she was febrile and tachycardic with laboratory data significant for aminotransferase elevation (ALT 998 U/L, AST 4559 U/L) and disseminated intravascular coagulopathy (DIC) (Figures 3 and 4). She underwent emergent cesarean section due

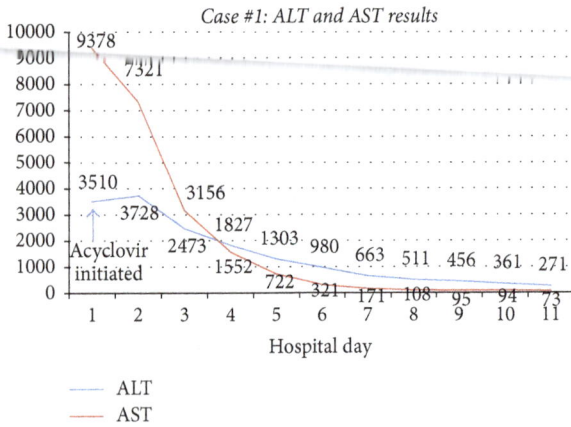

FIGURE 1: Case #1 trend in ALT and AST. ALT: alanine aminotransferase; AST: aspartate aminotransferase.

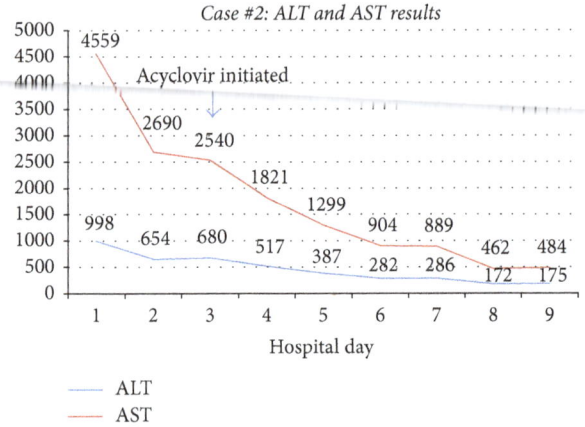

FIGURE 3: Case #2 trend in AST and ALT. ALT: alanine aminotransferase; AST: aspartate aminotransferase.

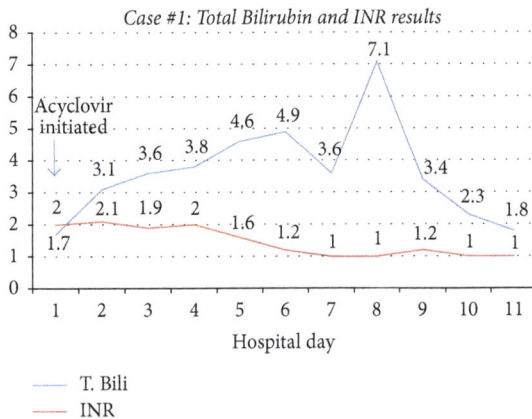

FIGURE 2: Case #1 trend in Total Bilirubin and INR. T. Bili: Total Bilirubin; INR: International Randomized Ratio.

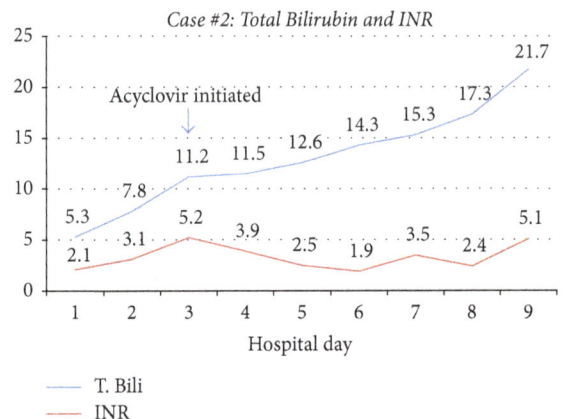

FIGURE 4: Case #2 trend in Total Bilirubin and INR. T. Bili: Total Bilirubin; INR: International Randomized Ratio.

to chorioamnionitis and a male infant was delivered. By day 2, she developed ascites and encephalopathy. A CT scan showed liver findings consistent with fatty infiltration and hemorrhage. She was transferred to our institution for transplant evaluation due to acute liver failure from presumed acute fatty liver of pregnancy. Upon transfer, she required intubation for airway protection and laboratory data revealed worsening multiorgan compromise. Antibiotics were broadened, and empiric acyclovir was initiated on day 3. Continuous venovenous hemofiltration was initiated for management of anasarca and anuria. On day 4 of transfer, her infant reportedly died of HSV-2 sepsis at another hospital. On day 6, our transplant committee determined she was not a transplant candidate due to profound psychosocial concerns. The patient's HSV-2 IgM antibody test and HSV-2 DNA by PCR returned positive and repeat blood cultures grew candida albicans. She subsequently developed septic shock requiring vasopressor support and her family decided on no further escalation of care. On day 9, she died from complications of fulminant liver failure.

4. Case 3

A 65-year-old woman with cirrhosis due to alcohol abuse complicated by refractory hydrothorax and ascites was admitted to the hospital with worsening dyspnea due to hydrothorax. She subsequently underwent uncomplicated liver transplantation with a donor liver from a 29-year-old woman that was IgG antibody positive for Epstein Barr Virus and Cytomegalovirus. She was initiated on immunosuppressive therapy with tacrolimus, mycophenolate mofetil, and a prednisone taper along with prophylactic valganciclovir. Her immediate postoperative course was uncomplicated and liver function tests remained stable. On postoperative day (POD) 8, she had an acute increase in aminotransferases (ALT of 712 U/L, AST of 780 U/L) with all other values within normal limits (Figures 5 and 6); liver ultrasound did not show abnormalities. She complained of worsening abdominal pain as her aminotransferases continued to uptrend and she was started on broad-spectrum antibiotics. CT scan of the abdomen was significant for suspected mesenteric artery pseudoaneurysm not present in past studies. She underwent

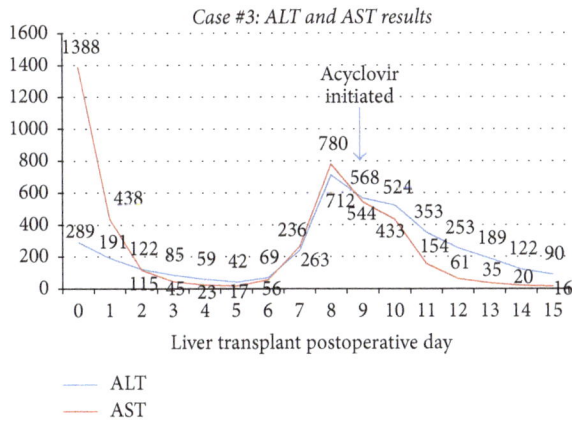

Figure 5: Case #3 trend in AST and ALT. ALT: alanine aminotransferase; AST: aspartate aminotransferase.

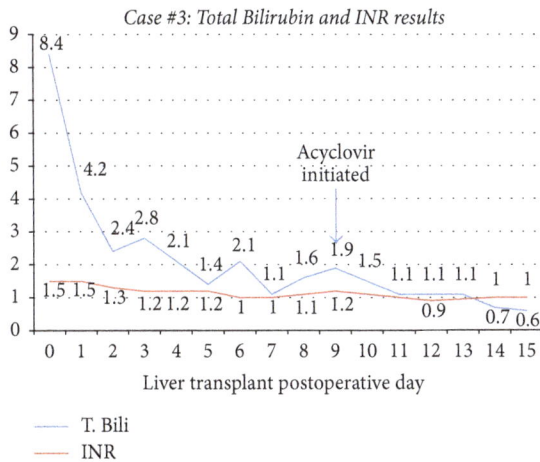

Figure 6: Case #3 trend in Total Bilirubin and INR. T. Bili: Total Bilirubin; INR: International Randomized Ratio.

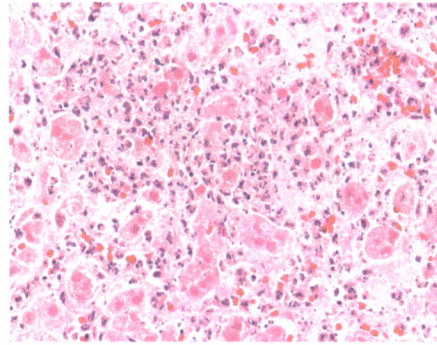

Figure 7: Liver biopsy from patient 3 showing intranuclear viral inclusions within the necrotic areas.

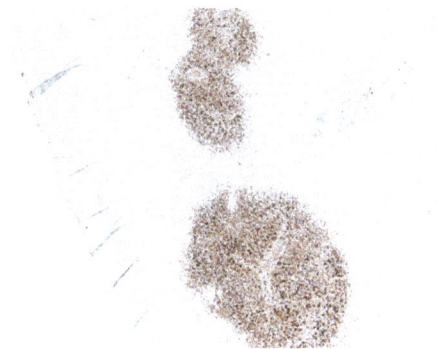

Figure 8: HSV immunostain from liver biopsy (patient 3).

laparotomy for removal of the aneurysm and liver biopsy on POD 8 that showed patchy areas of hepatocyte necrosis (Figures 7 and 8). At this time, her serum HSV-2 IgM antibody and HSV DNA by PCR returned positive and she was initiated on intravenous acyclovir. Of note, she denied prior history of oral or genital HSV infection. Pathology eventually returned as HSV hepatitis with hepatic necrosis. She had complete resolution of transaminase elevation within 5 days of treatment initiation and had an uncomplicated recovery.

5. Discussion and Literature Review

HSV hepatitis is an uncommon cause of acute liver failure, accounting for 0.8% of all cases and only 2% of all viral hepatitis [1, 2]. It is mostly seen in immunocompromised individuals and pregnant women in their third trimester following an orogenital HSV-1 or HSV-2 infection, though previous reports have shown up to 25% of cases in immunocompetent individuals [1]. Due to lack of specific clinical findings, the diagnosis is frequently missed on presentation and can lead to rapid progression to fulminant liver failure and multiorgan collapse if untreated [3]. The patients in all three cases are typical of the population at high risk for HSV hepatitis.

Liver biopsy remains the only gold standard for diagnosis of HSV hepatitis. However the procedure is often not feasible due to coagulopathy or ascites, and it is often necessary to make the diagnosis based on laboratory testing and symptoms [1]. Only the patient in case 3 underwent biopsy that showed histology pathognomonic for HSV infection: hemorrhagic necrosis, inflammation, enlarged ground glass nuclei with marginalized chromatin, and HSV+ immunostaining [4].

Of the presented cases, only the patient in case 1 had oral and genital mucocutaneous lesions, which, while useful in supporting the diagnosis, are absent in up to 50% of cases [3, 5]. Serologic testing is commonly done but carries a high rate of false-negativity and therefore should be used in conjunction with confirmatory PCR testing. All three of the above patients had evidence of disseminated disease with high levels of HSV DNA, and in cases 1 and 3, viral titers dropped after initiation of acyclovir.

Other common features of HSV hepatitis in the absence of a biopsy are aminotransferases >500, fever, coagulopathy, encephalopathy, leukopenia, thrombocytopenia, and acute renal failure (ARF) [2, 4, 6] (see Table 1 for a summary of

TABLE 1: Peak/nadir labs and outcomes of patients presented.

	Predisposing factor	AST (U/L)	ALT (U/L)	Bilirubin (mg/dL)	Platelets ($\times 10^3/\mu L$)[4]	INR	GFR (mL/min/m^2)	Outcome
Case 1	Crohn's- immuno-suppression, steroids	9378	3510	7.4	130	2.1	42	Survived
Case 2	Pregnancy (2nd trimester)	4559	998	21.7	33	5.1	30	Died
Case 3	Liver transplant-immunosuppres-sion, steroids	780	712	1.9	107	1.3	96	Survived

ALT: alanine aminotransferase; AST: aspartate aminotransferase; INR: international normalized ratio; GFR: glomerular filtration rate.

TABLE 2: Epidemiology based on two large literature reviews.

	Norvell et al. Number (%)	Kaufman et al. Number (%)
N	137	52
Age (mean, yrs)	34	N/A
Gender		N/A
(i) Male	51/137 (38)	
(ii) Female	86/137 (62)	
Immunosuppressed	72/137 (53)	35/52 (67)
Pregnant	32/137 (23)	9/52 (17)
Fever	98/100 (98)	42/52 (82)
Herpetic lesions	54/123 (44)	29/52 (57)
Mean peak ALT or AST	4927	N/A
Leukopenia	50/70 (71)	22/52 (43)
Thrombocytopenia	59/63 (93)	23/52 (45)
Coagulopathy	93/111 (83)	10/52 (20)
Acute Renal Failure	34/52 (65)	N/A
Death		
(i) Acyclovir	25/49 (51)	5/9 (55)
(ii) No Acyclovir	74/84 (88)	34/43 (80)

ALT: alanine aminotransferase; AST: aspartate aminotransferase; N/A: not available.

patient data and Table 2 for epidemiologic data from two large literature reviews on HSV hepatitis) [1, 7]. While all of these were evident in cases 1 and 2, the patient in case 3 had a solitary rise in aminotransferases and mild ARF. Additionally, previous reports have noted an anicteric pattern of hepatitis as a commonality in presentation of this disease, though this was not seen in case 1 or 2 in this series [2, 8]. This suggests that these findings and patterns together may support a diagnosis of HSV hepatitis but lack sensitivity and should not be used to rule out the diagnosis.

Previous cases have shown that early initiation of acyclovir (usually within 3 days of presentation) leads to better outcomes due to the cessation of viral replication and spread of infection [1, 6, 8]. While the patients in case 1 and 3 had near complete resolution of hepatitis within 5 days of initiation of acyclovir, unfortunately case 2 had rapid progression to fulminant hepatic failure and death, possibly because

her disease burden was already too great on presentation or that the virus was acyclovir resistant. Though data is sparse, intravenous foscarnet is the agent of choice in cases of acyclovir-resistant herpetic infection; however even dual-agent therapy has proven ineffective in preventing mortality in previous case reports [9]. In general, the data also suggest that acyclovir should be started empirically for high-risk patients with ALF of unknown etiology, pending laboratory confirmation of the diagnosis. However, prospective data on empiric therapy in specific populations are lacking.

In conclusion, there should be a high suspicion for HSV hepatitis as a cause for fulminant liver failure, especially in high-risk patient populations. Though diagnosis with biopsy is the gold standard, HSV PCR with concurrent elevation in aminotransferases can serve as substitute markers for making the diagnosis. HSV hepatitis should not be excluded based on the lack of mucocutaneous lesions, systemic inflammatory reaction markers, ARF, or anicteric hepatitis; however these findings may be used to support a suspected diagnosis. Given the favorable side effect profile of acyclovir, empiric treatment should be initiated early in presentation.

Disclosure

This manuscript was approved by all authors.

References

[1] J. P. Norvell, A. T. Blei, B. D. Jovanovic, and J. Levitsky, "Herpes simplex virus hepatitis: an analysis of the published literature and institutional cases," *Liver Transplantation*, vol. 13, no. 10, pp. 1428–1434, 2007.

[2] K. Ergle, L. Caruso, M. Burt, B. Desai, and R. Patel, "Herpes simplex virus (HSV) in the differential for fulminant hepatic failure," *Case Reports in Clinical Medicine*, vol. 4, no. 2, pp. 63–68, 2015.

[3] L. M. Arkin, L. Castelo-Soccio, and C. Kovarik, "Disseminated herpes simplex virus (HSV) hepatitis diagnosed by dermatology evaluation," *International Journal of Dermatology*, vol. 48, no. 9, pp. 1020-1021, 2009.

[4] L. M. Haag, J. Hofmann, L. I. S. Kredel et al., "Herpes simplex virus sepsis in a young woman with Crohn's disease," *Journal of Crohn's & colitis*, vol. 9, no. 12, pp. 1169–1173, 2015.

[5] R. A. Poley, J. F. Snowdon, and D. W. Howes, "Herpes simplex virus hepatitis in an immunocompetent adult: a fatal outcome due to liver failure," *Case Reports in Critical Care*, vol. 2011, Article ID 138341, 4 pages, 2011.

[6] B. H. Rimawi, J. Meserve, R. H. Rimawi, Z. Min, and J. W. Gnann, "Disseminated herpes simplex virus with fulminant hepatitis," *Case Reports in Hepatology*, vol. 2015, 4 pages, 2015.

[7] B. Kaufman, S. A. Gandhi, E. Louie, R. Rizzi, and P. Illei, "Herpes simplex virus hepatitis: case report and review," *Clinical Infectious Diseases*, vol. 24, no. 3, pp. 334–338, 1997.

[8] R. Nagappan, G. Parkin, I. Simpson, and W. Sievert, "Fulminant hepatic failure from herpes simplex in pregnancy," *Medical Journal of Australia*, vol. 176, no. 12, pp. 595-596, 2002.

[9] C. Herrera, K. Eichelberger, and N. Chescheir, "Antiviral-resistant fulminant herpes hepatitis in pregnancy," *American Journal of Perinatology Reports*, vol. 3, no. 2, pp. 87–90, 2013.

20

Complete Remission after Sequential Therapy of Drug Eluting Beads Transarterial Chemoembolization and Liver Resection in Large Solitary Nodule Hepatocellular Carcinoma

Juferdy Kurniawan,[1] Andri Sanityoso Sulaiman,[1] Sahat Basana Romanti Ezer Matondang,[2] Toar Jean Maurice Lalisang,[3] Ening Krisnuhoni,[4] and Steven Zulkifly[1]

[1]Division of Hepatobiliary, Department of Internal Medicine, Faculty of Medicine, Universitas Indonesia, Cipto Mangunkusumo National General Hospital, Jakarta, Indonesia
[2]Department of Radiology, Faculty of Medicine, Universitas Indonesia, Cipto Mangunkusumo National General Hospital, Jakarta, Indonesia
[3]Department of Surgery, Faculty of Medicine, Universitas Indonesia, Cipto Mangunkusumo National General Hospital, Jakarta, Indonesia
[4]Department of Pathology Anatomy, Faculty of Medicine, Universitas Indonesia, Cipto Mangunkusumo National General Hospital, Jakarta, Indonesia

Correspondence should be addressed to Juferdy Kurniawan; juferdy.k@gmail.com

Academic Editor: Tawesak Tanwandee

Hepatocellular carcinoma (HCC) is the fifth most prevalent and the second highest cause of death among cancer. The treatment of large solitary nodule HCC is still challenging. Transarterial chemoembolization (TACE) and liver resection are two modalities of therapy in HCC management. However, recurrence rate from each therapy is relatively high. We report a case of 46-year-old man diagnosed with large solitary nodule HCC, who was treated with drug eluting bead TACE (DEB-TACE) prior to liver resection. Studies about this combination are still limited and showed various results.

1. Introduction

Transarterial chemoembolization (TACE) is a treatment of choice in hepatocellular carcinoma BCLC Stage B [1, 2]. Drug eluting beads-TACE (DEB-TACE) is a relatively new drug delivery embolization and developed to optimize the delivery of chemotherapeutic agents with minimal systemic toxicity [3, 4]. Complete response (CR) or partial response (PR) after TACE is very dependent on treatment regimen, the amount, and size of the tumor [5]. Large HCC nodule (size $\geq$ 5 cm) had a lower CR percentage. Nodule diameter < 5 cm had 95% CR after first DEB-TACE. Meanwhile, only 13% CR had been found for diameter $\geq$ 5 cm [6].

Liver resection is highly recommended for HCC BCLC Stage A, with single nodule with diameter < 5 cm or multiple nodules (up to 3 nodules) with each diameter < 3 cm (Milan Criteria) [1, 2]. However, many studies reported that liver resection is beneficial for single nodule HCC, without restriction of tumor size. Liver resection of HCC multiple nodules has been associated with lower 5-year survival rates [7, 8]. The median time from resection to recurrence is different from each study. The shortest and longest duration for recurrence are 22 months and 34 months, respectively, after primary resection [9–11].

Lim et al., in 2014, reported that solitary HCC with tumor size > 5 cm was not independent predictors of poor overall survival. The 5-year overall survival and recurrence-free survival rates of size between 5 and 10 cm were 58% and 26%, respectively, and size > 10 cm 53% and 24%, respectively [12]. Retrospective analysis of liver resection for large solitary HCC by Zhao et al. in 2016 showed that 5-year overall survival and disease-free survival were 43% and 47%, respectively [13].

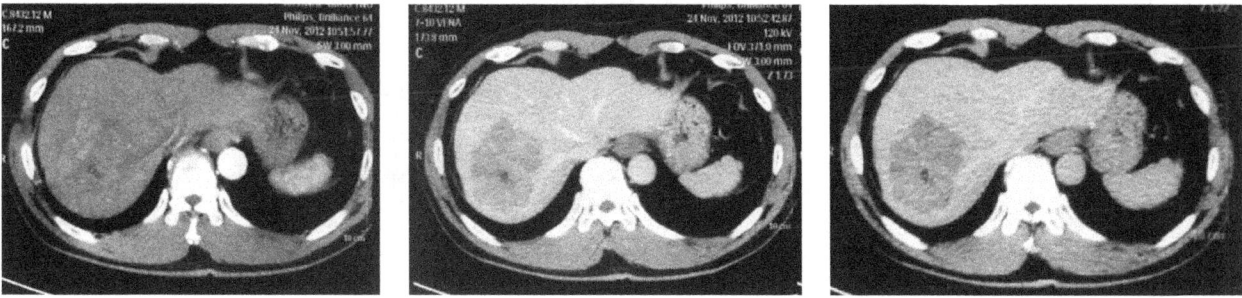

FIGURE 1: Arterial, venous, and delayed phase of Abdominal CT Scan after diagnosis (November 2012).

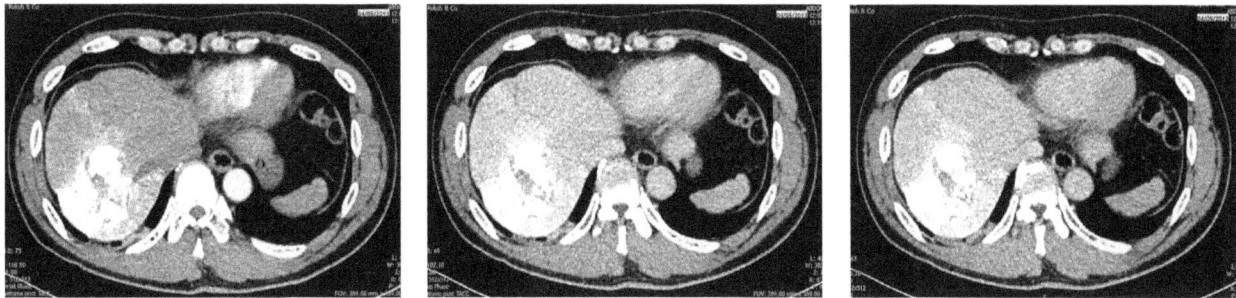

FIGURE 2: Arterial, venous, and delayed phase of Abdominal CT Scan after first DEB-TACE (January 2013).

Zhao et al. also reported the postoperative complications were found in 21% patients, including ascites (21.21%), transient hepatic dysfunction (9.9%), bile leakage (7.7%), and liver failure (4.4%). Thirty-day mortality after resection was 2.2% due to liver failure [13]. Recent study by Chen et al. compared the postoperative complications between solitary HCC < 10 cm and ≥10 cm. Total complications in HCC ≥ 10 cm were 39.1% and higher than HCC < 10 cm (29.8%). Liver failure occurred in 1% (2 patients) and 4% (1 patient), respectively [14].

There are limited studies about postsurgical complication of liver resection of large solitary HCC after TACE. Recent study reported postoperative complications were found in 59.2% (29 patients), including bile leakage (2 patients) and gastrointestinal hemorrhage (1 patient). The alteration of liver function was recovered in 1 month [15].

2. Case Presentation

A man, 46 years old, came to his gastroenterohepatology consultant with chief complaint of abdominal pain on the right upper quadrant. He was diagnosed with hepatocellular carcinoma and chronic hepatitis B. The patient then underwent the 3-phase Abdominal CT Scan examination in November 2012 (Figure 1). The radiologic examination findings revealed an 8 cm solitary nodule HCC in segment 7. He was classified into BCLC Stage B with Child Pugh (CP) score A. The drug eluting bead (DEB) TACE procedure was then planned for the patient. He also received a lamivudine 100 mg once daily for chronic hepatitis B.

The first DEB-TACE was performed in January 2013. Evaluation of the tumor was assessed by using 3-phase

Abdominal CT Scan a month later. It showed minimal hypervascular lesion from middle hepatic artery (Figure 2). DEB-TACE was planned for the patient for the second time. Second DEB-TACE was performed 4 months later in May 2013 and 3-phase Abdominal CT Scan after TACE showed reduction of tumor size to 3 × 4 cm (Figure 3).

In November 2013, liver resection was performed in segments 6, 7, and 8 of the liver. The tissue was sent to pathology anatomy department for histopathological examination. The microscopic findings of resection showed HCC grade III. Radiographic examination of 4 months after liver resection showed no abnormality (Figure 4). Three years after resection, the patient underwent the Abdominal CT Scan examination and no tumor was found. (Figure 5).

3. Discussion

The research about TACE prior to liver resection is very limited. Small trial by Gerunda et al., in 2000, compared 20 HCC patients who underwent resection to TACE prior to resection. Early recurrence (<24 months) and late recurrence (>24 months) were found higher in resection alone group, with 59% and 10% compared to TACE and resection, with 20% and 10%, respectively [16].

Another study reported there are difference of 1-, 2-, and 5-year overall survival rates between the TACE prior to surgery and resection alone group ($p = 0.11$). Contrary to previous study, the 1-, 2-, and 5-year recurrence-free interval were higher in resection alone (97%, 83%, and 45%, resp.) compared to TACE-surgery group (58%, 36%, and 7%, resp.) with $p = 0.01$ [17]. TACE procedure induced tumor downstaging or necrosis and hypothesized to be associated with

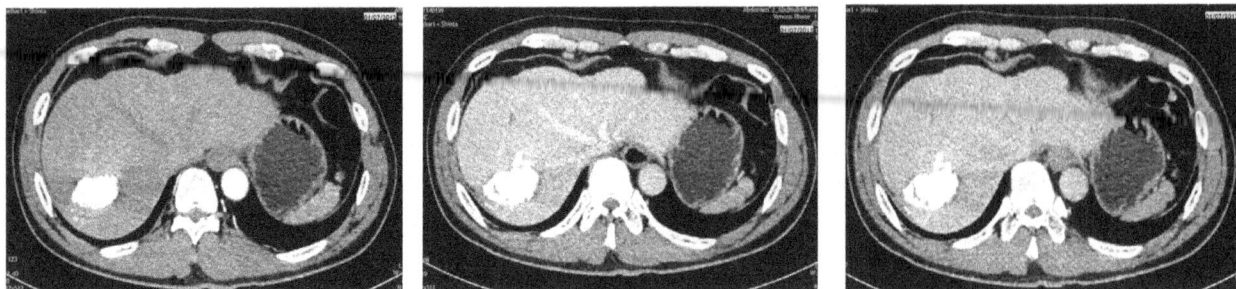

FIGURE 3: Arterial, venous, and delayed phase of Abdominal CT Scan after second DEB-TACE (May 2013).

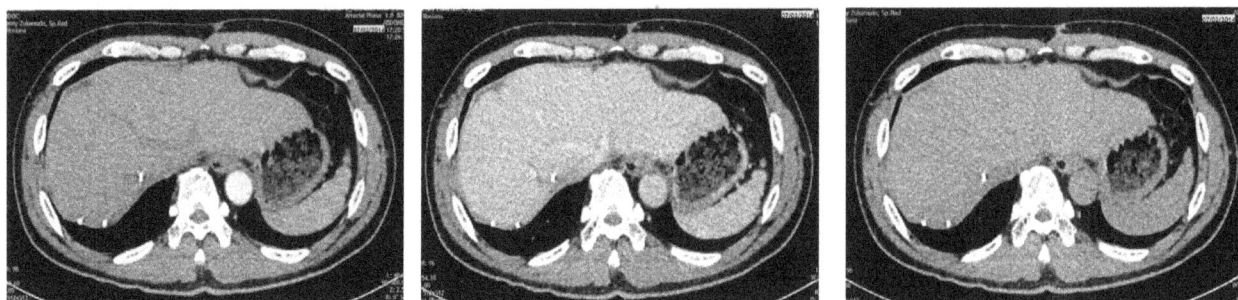

FIGURE 4: Arterial, venous, and delayed phase of Abdominal CT Scan 4 months after surgical resection (February 2014).

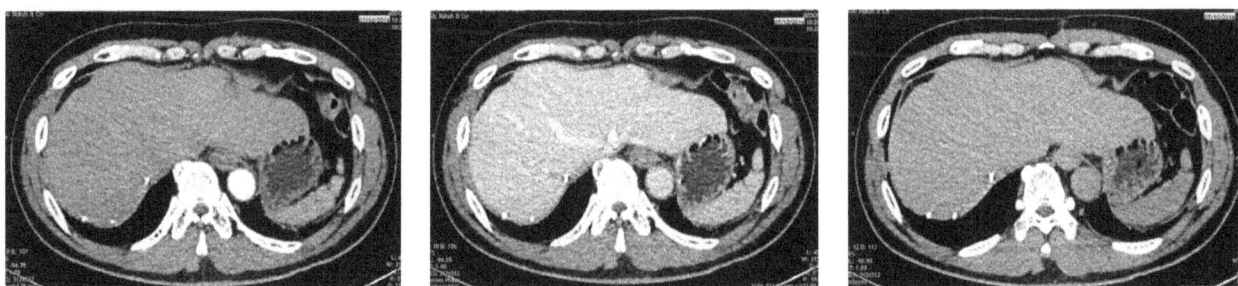

FIGURE 5: Arterial, venous, and delayed phase of Abdominal CT Scan 3 years after surgical resection (November 2016).

improvement of disease-free survival. The higher recurrence rate in TACE-surgical group was especially found in patients with initial resectable HCC. It was suggested that preoperative TACE might induce incomplete necrosis, resulting in hematogenous spread of residual tumor cells after liver resection, and caused recurrences [17, 18].

However, recent study in 2017 compared TACE prior to surgery (49 patients) and TACE alone in large/multifocal HCC (61 patients). All of the patients were classified in BCLC Stage B. The mean initial tumor in TACE + surgery and TACE group is 7.22 ± 3.18 cm and 6.80 ± 3.35 cm, respectively. However, the number of tumors was not limited to solitary tumor. The 1-, 2-, and 3-year overall survival rates in TACE + surgery group were 89.8%, 79.4%, and 59.1%, respectively, and in TACE alone were 75.1%, 61.5%, and 15.1%, respectively. In univariate analysis, solitary tumor was associated with higher overall survival, with $p = 0.012$ [15].

DEB-TACE has been found to be more effective for large nodule (>5 cm) compared to cTACE. In subgroup analysis of Asian patients who received DEB-TACE with size > 5 cm, DEB-TACE was reported to have significantly higher objective response compared to cTACE. The largest tumor size included in this study was 12 cm. Around 16.3% and 66.6% patients with large tumor size achieved CR and PR, respectively, in DEB-TACE group [16].

However, there are no publications that studied about the efficacy of DEB-TACE prior to surgery in large solitary nodule HCC. This case report presents a complete remission after 3 years of solitary large nodule of HCC with sequential therapy of DEB-TACE and liver resection. However, larger studies with longer duration are needed to find the efficacy, survival rates, and tumor recurrence.

For conclusion, the treatment of HCC with solitary large nodule is still challenging for clinicians. HCC patients who underwent TACE before resection have better overall survival, but it might have higher risk for recurrence compared to resection alone. TACE is safe procedure and effective for large HCC. DEB-TACE prior to liver surgery can be suggested for therapy of large solitary nodule of HCC.

References

[1] J. Bruix and M. Sherman, "Management of hepatocellular carcinoma: an update," *Hepatology*, vol. 53, no. 3, pp. 1020–1022, 2011.

[2] European Association for the Study of The Liver, "EASL-EORTC Clinical Practice Guidelines: management of hepatocellular carcinoma," *European Journal of Cancer*, vol. 48, no. 5, pp. 599–641, 2012.

[3] W. Sieghart, F. Hucke, and M. Peck-Radosavljevic, "Transarterial chemoembolization: modalities, indication, and patient selection," *Journal of Hepatology*, vol. 62, no. 5, pp. 1187–1195, 2015.

[4] J. Lammer, K. Malagari, T. Vogl et al., "Prospective randomized study of doxorubicin-eluting-bead embolization in the treatment of hepatocellular carcinoma: results of the PRECISION V study," *CardioVascular and Interventional Radiology*, vol. 33, no. 1, pp. 41–52, 2010.

[5] R. Lencioni and J. M. Llovet, "Modified recist (mRECIST) assessment for hepatocellular carcinoma," *Seminars in Liver Disease*, vol. 30, no. 1, pp. 52–60, 2010.

[6] G. Vesselle, C. Quirier-Leleu, S. Velasco et al., "Predictive factors for complete response of chemoembolization with drug-eluting beads (DEB-TACE) for hepatocellular carcinoma," *European Radiology*, vol. 26, no. 6, pp. 1640–1648, 2016.

[7] A. A. Madkhali, Z. T. Fadel, M. M. Aljiffry, and M. M. Hassanain, "Surgical treatment for hepatocellular carcinoma," *Saudi Journal of Gastroenterology*, vol. 21, no. 1, pp. 11–17, 2015.

[8] H. Nakayama and T. Takayama, "Role of surgical resection for hepatocellular carcinoma based on Japanese clinical guidelines for hepatocellular carcinoma," *World Journal of Hepatology*, vol. 7, no. 2, pp. 261–269, 2015.

[9] P. Tabrizian, G. Jibara, B. Shrager, M. Schwartz, and S. Roayaie, "Recurrence of hepatocellular cancer after resection: patterns, treatments, and prognosis," *Annals of Surgery*, vol. 261, no. 5, pp. 947–955, 2015.

[10] H. Lang, G. C. Sotiropoulos, E. I. Brokalaki et al., "Survival and recurrence rates after resection for hepatocellular carcinoma in noncirrhotic livers," *Journal of the American College of Surgeons*, vol. 205, no. 1, pp. 27–36, 2007.

[11] S. A. Shah, S. P. Cleary, A. C. Wei et al., "Recurrence after liver resection for hepatocellular carcinoma: Risk factors, treatment, and outcomes," *Surgery*, vol. 141, no. 3, pp. 330–339, 2007.

[12] C. Lim, Y. Mise, Y. Sakamoto et al., "Above 5 cm, size does not matter anymore in patients with hepatocellular carcinoma," *World journal of surgery*, vol. 38, no. 11, pp. 2910–2918, 2014.

[13] H. C. Zhao, R. L. Wu, F. B. Liu, Y. Z. Zhao, G. B. Wang, Z. G. Zhang et al., "A retrospective analysis of long term outcomes in patients undergoing hepatic resection for large (>5 cm) hepatocellular carcinoma," *HPB : The Official Journal of The International Hepato Pancreato Biliary Association*, vol. 18, pp. 943–949, 2016.

[14] J.-H. Chen, C.-K. Wei, C.-H. Lee, C.-M. Chang, T.-W. Hsu, and W.-Y. Yin, "The safety and adequacy of resection on hepatocellular carcinoma larger than 10cm: A retrospective study over 10years," *Annals of Medicine and Surgery*, vol. 4, no. 2, pp. 193–199, 2015.

[15] J. Chen, L. Lai, Q. Lin et al., "Hepatic resection after transarterial chemoembolization increases overall survival in large/multifocal hepatocellular carcinoma: A retrospective cohort study," *Oncotarget*, vol. 8, no. 1, pp. 408–417, 2017.

[16] G. E. Gerunda, D. Neri, R. Merenda et al., "Role of transarterial chemoembolization before liver resection for hepatocarcinoma," *Liver Transplantation*, vol. 6, no. 5, pp. 619–626, 2000.

[17] J. Y. Kang, M. S. Choi, S. J. Kim et al., "Long-term outcome of preoperative transarterial chemoembolization and hepatic resection in patients with hepatocellular carcinoma.," *The Korean journal of hepatology*, vol. 16, no. 4, pp. 383–388, 2010.

[18] H. Nishikawa, A. Arimoto, T. Wakasa, R. Kita, T. Kimura, and Y. Osaki, "Effect of transcatheter arterial chemoembolization prior to surgical resection for hepatocellular carcinoma," *International Journal of Oncology*, vol. 42, no. 1, pp. 151–160, 2013.

21

Enteroscopic Management of Ectopic Varices in a Patient with Liver Cirrhosis and Portal Hypertension

G. A. Watson, A. Abu-Shanab, R. L. O'Donohoe, and M. Iqbal

St. Vincent's University Hospital, Dublin 4, Ireland

Correspondence should be addressed to G. A. Watson; geoff_watson7@hotmail.com

Academic Editor: Mario Pirisi

Portal hypertension and liver cirrhosis may predispose patients to varices, which have a propensity to bleed and cause significant morbidity and mortality. These varices are most commonly located in the gastroesophageal area; however, rarely ectopic varices may develop in unusual locations outside of this region. Haemorrhage from these sites can be massive and difficult to control; thus early detection and management may be lifesaving. We present a case of occult gastrointestinal bleeding in a patient with underlying alcoholic liver disease where an ectopic varix was ultimately detected with push enteroscopy.

1. Introduction

Variceal bleeding is a common complication seen in patients diagnosed with liver cirrhosis and portal hypertension, and it is associated with high mortality rates. The origin of bleeding can often be detected by direct visualization using endoscopic procedures or radiologically. However, in rare instances the source of bleeding may not be immediately apparent, and it is important to consider the possibility of ectopic varices, located in an area outside of the more common gastroesophageal region. Clinical awareness and suspicion are paramount as bleeding from these sites may be life-threatening and immediate intervention is critical. We present a case of gastrointestinal bleeding in a patient with underlying alcoholic liver disease where the source of bleeding was initially unclear; however, push enteroscopy detected an ectopic varix at the site of a previous hepaticojejunostomy.

2. Case Report

A 44-year-old gentleman was transferred to our specialist liver unit from a peripheral hospital with ongoing melaena on a background of alcoholic cirrhosis with portal hypertension. He initially presented with generalised abdominal pain and nausea. His haemoglobin on admission to the peripheral hospital was found to be 7.5 g/dL. His background was significant for chronic pancreatitis and subsequent type 2 diabetes mellitus. Furthermore, three years ago he developed a biliary stricture after laparoscopic cholecystectomy that required multiple biliary stents and ultimately a hepaticojejunostomy.

Physical examination was unremarkable except for mild pallor, palmar erythema, and moderate ascites. Routine blood tests on transfer to our unit are shown in Table 1.

He received multiple blood transfusions throughout his admission (eight in the peripheral hospital, requiring a further twenty-six units in our unit). He was also treated with octreotide and terlipressin due to a high suspicion of portal hypertension induced gastrointestinal haemorrhage.

An oesophagogastroduodenoscopy (OGD) was performed on admission to the peripheral hospital and showed mild oesophagitis and grade 1 varices. CT angiogram the following day reported no active bleeding. A repeat OGD after transfer to our unit confirmed grade 1 oesophageal varices and portal hypertensive gastropathy, with no source of bleeding identified. A CT four-phase liver examination was performed and showed a nodular liver and occlusion of the main portal vein with cavernous transformation (Figure 1).

During this period the patient continued to have intermittent melaena, up to four times daily, passing circa 500 mL of fresh blood. Haemoglobin levels continued to fall and dropped to 5.4 g/dL on day 10 of admission; however, the patient remained haemodynamically stable. A radiolabeled red blood cell nuclear imaging scan was performed during

TABLE 1: Blood panel. WCC (white cell count), Hb (haemoglobin), MCV (mean corpuscular volume), Hct (haematocrit), Plts (platelets), INR (international normalised ratio), Na+ (sodium), K+ (potassium), Cl– (chloride), Ca2+ (calcium), Inorg PO^4 (inorganic phosphate), Mg2+ (magnesium), Alb (albumin), BR (bilirubin), Alk Phos (alkaline phosphatase), GGT (gamma glutamyl transpeptidase), ALT (alanine transaminase), AST (aspartate aminotransferase), and CRP (C-reactive protein).

Blood panel			
WCC 15.6 × 10^9/L	Na+ 124 mmol/L	Alb 19 g/L	Ca2+ 1.8 mmol/L
Hb 8.1 g/dL	K+ 4.2 mmol/L	BR 7 μmol/L	Inorg PO^4 0.95 mmol/L
MCV 83 fL	Cl– 92 mmol/L	Alk Phos 5 iu/L	Mg2+ 0.66 mmol/L
Hct 0.227 L/L	Urea 5.8 mmol/L	GGT 8 iu/L	
Plts 134 × 10^9/L	Creatinine 54 μmol/L	ALT 15 iu/L	CRP 23.4 mg/L
INR 0.91		AST 16 U/L	

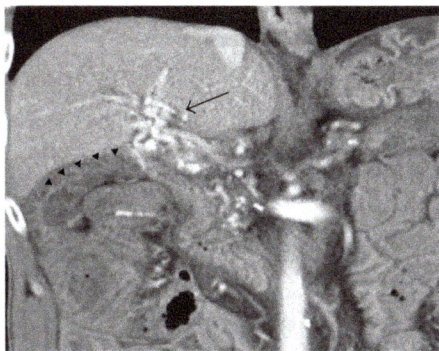

FIGURE 1: Coronal reformat of the portal venous phase of a multiphase CT liver examination shows an occluded main portal vein with cavernous transformation (arrow). The efferent limb of the hepaticojejunostomy (arrowheads) can be seen extending away from the lateral aspect of the venous collaterals.

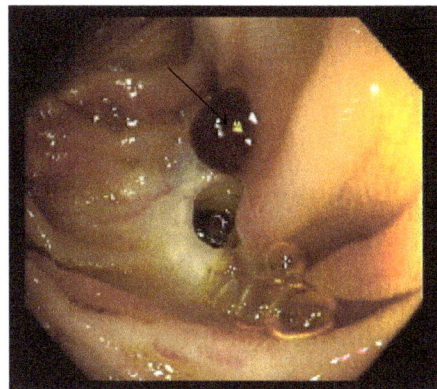

FIGURE 2: Nipple sign of the ectopic varix at the site of the hepaticojejunostomy (arrow).

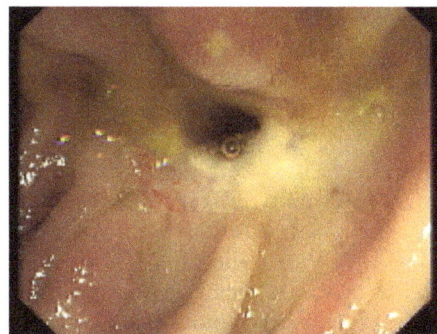

FIGURE 3: Healed ectopic varix at the site of the hepaticojejunostomy with signs of injection.

this period of active haemorrhage; however, the origin of bleeding remained elusive.

The following day a push enteroscopy was attempted using a pediatric colonoscope and was successfully passed to the jejunal loop as far as the hepaticojejunostomy. An area of mucosal erythema with prominent vessels as well as a fresh clot was seen adjacent to the hepaticojejunostomy, features consistent with an ectopic varix.

The case was discussed at length at our multidisciplinary team (MDT) meeting. As the option of TIPS (transjugular intrahepatic portosystemic shunt) was ruled out due to portal vein thrombosis, the feasibility of embolization for presumably ectopic variceal bleed was discussed with our interventional radiologists; however, as there was no obvious source of bleeding identified on previous scans it was difficult to decide on the optimal course of management.

Ultimately the overall consensus was that push enteroscopy could be attempted again with the intention of injecting Histoacryl into this ectopic varix at the site of the hepaticojejunostomy. Four days later the procedure was performed and the ectopic varix which was the source of bleeding was finally visualized and identified in the form of a nipple sign at the site of hepaticojejunostomy (Figure 2). Due to its difficult position, the site was injected with Histoacryl and lipiodol. An X-ray of the abdomen was requested and

displayed a radiopaque density in the right upper quadrant consistent with filling of the contour of the ectopic varix adjacent to the surgical clips and represented the site of injection (Figure 3).

A repeat enteroscopy was performed the following week and clearly displayed a healed ectopic varix at the site of hepaticojejunostomy with signs of injection (Figure 4). Prior to discharge, management options in the case of future rebleeding were discussed at our multidisciplinary meeting (MDM). The general consensus was that while surgical intervention would be an option in the future, it would be associated

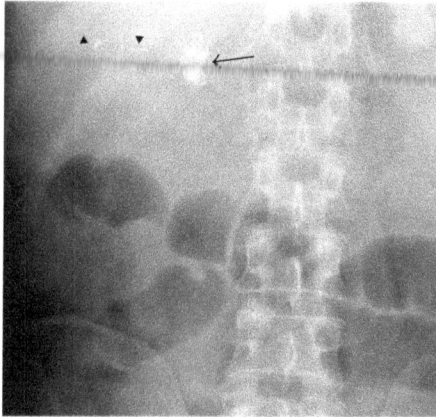

FIGURE 4: Plain radiograph of the abdomen following injection of the ectopic varix shows radiopaque embolic material (arrow) medial to surgical clips (arrowheads) positioned inferiorly to the right lobe of the liver.

with a significant risk of morbidity and mortality. It was thus decided that in the case of recurrent bleeding we would again consider endoscopic management.

3. Discussion

Portal hypertension and liver cirrhosis may predispose patients to varices, most commonly located in the gastroesophageal area. Ectopic varices may be described as abnormally dilated submucosal vessels located in unusual locations outside of this area. These rare portosystemic collaterals are responsible for 5% of all variceal bleeds [1]. Haemorrhage can be massive with mortality reaching up to 40% [2]; thus clinical awareness and suspicion are crucial in early detection and management in cases where the source of bleeding remains uncertain.

Norton and colleagues reviewed 169 cases of bleeding ectopic varices from different origins. In 26% of cases the source of bleeding was a peristomal varix. Another 17% were duodenal, 17% were jejunal and ileal, 14% were colonic, 9% were peritoneal, 8% were rectal, and a small minority of bleeding varices originated from rare sites such as the ovary and vagina [3]. In another study of 37 patients with liver cirrhosis who underwent capsule endoscopy, 8.1% of patients were found to have small bowel varices [4]. Anorectal varices have been reported in approximately 44% of patients with cirrhosis; however, only a small number become symptomatic [5].

Risk factors for developing varices in locations outside of the more common zones include prior abdominal surgery, and varices have been known to develop in unusual locations such as the urinary bladder, ovaries, and bare area of the liver due to adhesions and in cases of extrahepatic portal hypertension [1, 2, 6, 7]. Ectopic varices may also develop in the absence of portal hypertension due to congenital anomalous portosystemic anastomoses, abnormal vessel structures, arteriovenous fistulae, and rare familial conditions or in relation to thrombosis [8–12].

Patients usually present with hematemesis, melaena, or lower gastrointestinal bleeding, which may range from mild spotting to gross, life-threatening haemorrhage [13]. While initial medical management aims to stabilise the patient haemodyamically with blood transfusions and splanchnic vasoconstrictors such as terlipressin, emergent upper gastrointestinal endoscopy has been the cornerstone of first-line management in patients presenting with gross upper gastrointestinal bleeding. Endoscopic band ligation (EBL) and endoscopic injection sclerotherapy (EIS) have been successfully used in controlling haemorrhage from duodenal [14, 15], jejunal [16], colonic [17], anorectal [18], and stomal varices [19].

To date there are no set guidelines for managing bleeding ectopic varices. Various factors may influence decision-making such as the location of haemorrhage, clinical presentation, and the underlying medical disorder. Akhter and Haskal [2] provided a comprehensive review of the current therapeutic modalities available and recent advances in managing ectopic variceal bleeding, including double balloon enteroscopy and transcatheter embolization or sclerotherapy, with or without portosystemic decompression, that is, transjugular intrahepatic portosystemic shunts (TIPS) [2].

In addition, other modalities outside of the acute setting have proven to be valuable adjuncts. Capsule endoscopy has been successful in visualizing jejunal and small bowel varices [2, 4, 20] while push enteroscopy can also navigate the small bowel and allow for intervention, as was the case in our patient [1, 2, 16, 21]. CT, CT angiography, and CT enteroclysis have all been used for successful diagnosis of duodenal [22, 23] and colonic varices [24]. While technetium TC-99m red blood cell scintigraphy was explored in this case and in previous settings [25], its definitive role in management remains uncertain.

The role of TIPS in the management of bleeding ectopic varices in cirrhotics caused by intrahepatic portal hypertension has frequently been publicised [20, 26]. TIPS have been shown to be more effective in preventing rebleeding from oesophageal varices than endoscopic methods [27, 28]. This means of intervention is often reserved for patients without a history of decompensation (e.g., high MELD (Model of End Stage Liver Disease) score, encephalopathy, and ischaemic liver disease).

Finally, surgical intervention remains an option that is employed less often due to the high risk of morbidity and mortality in patients with liver disease but may be considered a salvage option in a select cohort of patients where previous management strategies have failed.

4. Conclusion

Variceal haemorrhage is a feared complication in cirrhotic patients. Its origin is often restricted to the gastroesophageal region; however, development of ectopic varices may occur and clinical suspicion is critical when presented with a patient with obscure haemorrhage with a prior history of hepaticojejunostomy.

Management of ectopic variceal bleed remains uncertain and has only been described in small case reviews and reports to date. We recommend a multidisciplinary approach, which is crucial in guiding decisions regarding management, both in the short term and in the long term. Interventional radiology and surgery should be considered in the event of massive haemorrhage; however, alternative techniques, such as push enteroscopy, can have a big role as an adjunct outside of the acute setting.

References

[1] M. Kinkhabwala, A. Mousavi, S. Iyer, and R. Adamsons, "Bleeding ileal varicosity demonstrated by transhepatic portography," *American Journal of Roentgenology*, vol. 129, no. 3, pp. 514–516, 1977.

[2] N. M. Akhter and Z. J. Haskal, "Diagnosis and management of ectopic varices," *Gastrointestinal Intervention*, vol. 1, no. 1, pp. 3–10, 2012.

[3] I. D. Norton, J. C. Andrews, and P. S. Kamath, "Management of ectopic varices," *Hepatology*, vol. 28, no. 4, pp. 1154–1158, 1998.

[4] G. D. De Palma, M. Rega, S. Masone et al., "Mucosal abnormalities of the small bowel in patients with cirrhosis and portal hypertension: a capsule endoscopy study," *Gastrointestinal Endoscopy*, vol. 62, no. 4, pp. 529–534, 2005.

[5] S. W. Hosking, A. G. Johnson, H. L. Smart, and D. R. Triger, "Anorectal varices, haemorrhoids, and portal hypertension," *The Lancet*, vol. 333, no. 8634, pp. 349–352, 1989.

[6] A. Helmy, K. Al Kahtani, and M. Al Fadda, "Updates in the pathogenesis, diagnosis and management of ectopic varices," *Hepatology International*, vol. 2, no. 3, pp. 322–334, 2008.

[7] D. Lebrec and J.-P. Benhamou, "Ectopic varices in portal hypertension," *Clinics in Gastroenterology*, vol. 14, no. 1, pp. 105–121, 1985.

[8] M. Feldman, V. M. Smith, and C. G. Warner, "Varices of the colon: report of three cases," *Journal of the American Medical Association*, vol. 179, pp. 729–730, 1962.

[9] J. P. Iredale, P. Ridings, F. P. McGinn, and M. J. P. Arthur, "Familial and idiopathic colonic varices: an unusual cause of lower gastrointestinal haemorrhage," *Gut*, vol. 33, no. 9, pp. 1285–1288, 1992.

[10] H. B. Wheeler and R. Warren, "Duodenal varices due to portal hypertension from arteriovenous aneurysm," *Annals of surgery*, vol. 146, no. 2, pp. 229–238, 1957.

[11] L. Zaman, J. R. Bebb, S. P. Dunlop, J. C. Jobling, and K. Teahon, "Familial colonic varices—a cause of 'polyposis' on barium enema," *The British Journal of Radiology*, vol. 81, no. 961, pp. 17–19, 2008.

[12] S.-H. Ryu, H.-S. Chang, S.-J. Myung, and S.-K. Yang, "Rectal varices caused by thrombosis of intra-abdominal vessels," *Gastrointestinal Endoscopy*, vol. 55, no. 3, p. 409, 2002.

[13] M. Q. Khan, S. Al-Momen, and A. Alghssab, "Duodenal varices causing massive lower gastrointestinal hemorrhage," *Annals of Saudi Medicine*, vol. 19, no. 5, pp. 440–443, 1999.

[14] Y. Akazawa, I. Murata, T. Yamao et al., "Successful management of bleeding duodenal varices by endoscopic variceal ligation and balloon-occluded retrograde transvenous obliteration," *Gastrointestinal Endoscopy*, vol. 58, no. 5, pp. 794–797, 2003.

[15] Y. Yoshida, Y. Imai, M. Nishikawa et al., "Successful endoscopic injection sclerotherapy with N-butyl-2- cyanoacrylate following the recurrence of bleeding soon after endoscopic ligation for ruptured duodenal varices," *American Journal of Gastroenterology*, vol. 92, no. 7, pp. 1227–1229, 1997.

[16] H. Hekmat, A. Al-Toma, M. P. J. H. Mallant, C. J. J. Mulder, and M. A. J. M. Jacobs, "Endoscopic N-butyl-2-cyanoacrylate (Histoacryl) obliteration of jejunal varices by using the double balloon enteroscope," *Gastrointestinal Endoscopy*, vol. 65, no. 2, pp. 350–352, 2007.

[17] W.-C. Chen, M.-C. Hou, H.-C. Lin, F.-Y. Chang, and S.-D. Lee, "An endoscopic injection with N-butyl-2-cyanoacrylate used for colonic variceal bleeding: a case report and review of the literature," *American Journal of Gastroenterology*, vol. 95, no. 2, pp. 540–542, 2000.

[18] R. Shudo, Y. Yazaki, S. Sakurai et al., "Combined endoscopic variceal ligation and sclerotherapy for bleeding rectal varices associated with primary biliary cirrhosis: a case showing a long-lasting favorable response," *Gastrointestinal Endoscopy*, vol. 53, no. 6, pp. 661–665, 2001.

[19] H. C. Wolfsen, R. A. Kozarek, J. E. Bredfeldt, L. F. Fenster, and L. L. Brubacher, "The role of endoscopic injection sclerotherapy in the management of bleeding peristomal varices," *Gastrointestinal Endoscopy*, vol. 36, no. 5, pp. 472–474, 1990.

[20] L.-G. Lim, Y.-M. Lee, L. Tan, S. Chang, and S.-G. Lim, "Percutaneous paraumbilical embolization as an unconventional and successful treatment for bleeding jejunal varices," *World Journal of Gastroenterology*, vol. 15, no. 30, pp. 3823–3826, 2009.

[21] S. Getzlaff, C. A. Benz, D. Schilling, and J. F. Riemann, "Enteroscopic cyanoacrylate sclerotherapy of jejunal and gallbladder varices in a patient with portal hypertension," *Endoscopy*, vol. 33, no. 5, pp. 462–464, 2001.

[22] D. Weishaupt, T. Pfammatter, P. R. Hilfiker, U. Wolfensberger, and B. Marincek, "Detecting bleeding duodenal varices with multislice helical CT," *American Journal of Roentgenology*, vol. 178, no. 2, pp. 399–401, 2002.

[23] T. P. Jain, M. S. Gulati, G. K. Makharia, and S. B. Paul, "Case of the season: detection of duodenal varices by CT enteroclysis," *Seminars in Roentgenology*, vol. 40, no. 3, pp. 204–206, 2005.

[24] T. R. Smith, "CT demonstration of ascending colon varices," *Clinical Imaging*, vol. 18, no. 1, pp. 4–6, 1994.

[25] S. Bykov, A. Becker, L. Koltun, E. Yudko, and I. Garty, "Massive bleeding from jejunal varices in a patient with thalassemia major detected by Tc-99m red blood cell scintigraphy," *Clinical Nuclear Medicine*, vol. 30, no. 6, pp. 457–459, 2005.

[26] M. Vangeli, D. Patch, N. Terreni et al., "Bleeding ectopic varices—treatment with transjugular intrahepatic portosystemic shunt (TIPS) and embolisation," *Journal of Hepatology*, vol. 41, no. 4, pp. 560–566, 2004.

[27] G. V. Papatheodoridis, J. Goulis, G. Leandro, D. Patch, and A. K. Burroughs, "Transjugular intrahepatic portosystemic shunt compared with endoscopic treatment for prevention of variceal rebleeding: a meta-analysis," *Hepatology*, vol. 30, no. 3, pp. 612–622, 1999.

[28] J. C. García-Pagán, K. Caca, C. Bureau et al., "Early use of TIPS in patients with cirrhosis and variceal bleeding," *The New England Journal of Medicine*, vol. 362, no. 25, pp. 2370–2379, 2010.

22

Hepatic Iron Overload following Liver Transplantation from a C282Y/H63D Compound Heterozygous Donor

E. Veitsman ⓘ,[1] E. Pras,[2,3] O. Pappo,[4] A. Arish,[5] R. Eshkenazi,[5] C. Feray,[6,7] J. Calderaro,[7,8] D. Azoulay,[7,9] and Z. Ben Ari[1,3]

[1]*Liver Disease Center, Sheba Medical Center, Ramat Gan, Israel*
[2]*Institute of Genetics, Sheba Medical Center, Ramat Gan, Israel*
[3]*Sackler School of Medicine, Tel Aviv University, Tel Aviv, Israel*
[4]*Department of Pathology, Sheba Medical Center, Ramat Gan, Israel*
[5]*Hepato-Biliary-Pancreatic Surgery Department, Sheba Medical Center, Ramat Gan, Israel*
[6]*Department of Hepatology, Henri Mondor Hospital, Créteil, France*
[7]*Unite Inserm 955, France*
[8]*Department of Pathology, Henri Mondor Hospital, Créteil, France*
[9]*Department Hepato-Pancreato-Biliary Surgery and Liver Transplantation, Henri Mondor Hospital, Créteil, France*

Correspondence should be addressed to E. Veitsman; e_veitsman@rambam.health.gov.il

Academic Editor: Ned Snyder

Hereditary hemochromatosis (HH) is a genetic disease associated with progressive iron overload, eventually leading in some cases to damage of parenchymal organs, such as the liver, pancreas, and heart. Although the gene had been identified (HFE), HH pathogenesis remains to be fully elucidated. We report here, for the first time, a case of inadvertent transplantation of a liver from a donor with C282Y/H63D compound heterozygosity into a nonhemochromatotic 19-year-old Caucasian male recipient with primary sclerosing cholangitis. Progressive iron overload occurred over 1.5 years, as observed in liver biopsies and iron studies, after ruling out secondary causes of iron overload. This case strengthens the hypothesis that the liver, rather than the small intestine, plays a primary role in the maintenance of iron homeostasis.

1. Introduction

Hereditary hemochromatosis (HH) is an autosomal recessive iron metabolism disorder, characterized by increased intestinal iron absorption and deposition in the parenchyma of liver, pancreas, heart, and other organs ([1], Pietrangelo A). HH remains the most commonly identified genetic disorder in Caucasians ([2], Bacon BR). C282Y homozygotes account for 80%-85% of HH patients. H63D and S65C mutations are also commonly detected but are generally only associated with iron overload in C282Y/H63D or C282Y/S65C compound heterozygotes ([2], Bacon BR). Recently mutations of other genes encoding iron regulatory proteins, such as hepcidin, hemojuvelin, transferrin receptor 2, and ferroportin, have been implicated in inherited iron overload syndromes [2].

There are four main pathophysiological mechanisms involved in iron overload: increased absorption of dietary iron in the upper intestine, decreased expression of iron regulatory hormone hepcidin, altered function of HFE, and iron-elicited tissue injury with fibrogenesis [2]. Yet, the exact pathophysiological mechanism of iron overload in HH remains elusive. In addition, the precise site of the main metabolic defect in HH patients has been a subject of controversy for many years. Duodenal cells, hepatocytes, and/or macrophages have been proposed to be targeted by HH.

The study in HFE-knockout mice reported by Vujic Spasic et al. [3] showed that conditional deletion of HFE in the liver induces a hemochromatosis phenotype, while its conditional deletion in duodenal cells or macrophages does not have the same effect on iron metabolism. Liver transplantation provides a unique opportunity to elucidate the role of the liver and the intestine in the pathogenesis of iron overload in HH ([4] **Dwyer JP**). Here, we report the development of iron overload in a nonhemochromatotic patient following liver transplantation from a donor with compound C282Y/H63D heterozygosity.

2. Case Report

A 19-year-old Caucasian male presenting with severe primary sclerosing cholangitis underwent orthotopic liver transplantation and required a retransplant 5 weeks later due to a liver insufficiency caused by ligation of ruptured arterial pseudoaneurysm. He received more than 40 blood transfusions. The second donor was a 76-year-old male without a history of liver disease. The patient's postoperative course after retransplant included prolonged hemodialysis (8 weeks) due to acute kidney injury, cytomegalovirus (CMV) infection, hepatitis E infection, and hepatic artery stenosis in the anastomosis area, treated by angioplasty and stent insertion. Of note, hepatic artery stenosis resulted in ischemic-like cholangiopathy and prolonged cholestasis.

The patient's condition stabilized eight months after transplantation. Cyclosporin and Myfortic were administered for immunosuppression, in addition to aspirin and ursodeoxycholic acid. A liver biopsy performed at that period revealed numerous hypertrophic, iron-loaded macrophages and severe bile duct damage and loss, consistent with early mild chronic rejection (Figure 1). Hemosiderosis was attributed to secondary iron overload, considering the numerous risk factors for this complication presenting before and after the retransplant (multiple blood transfusions, kidney injury, and CMV infection).

Eight months later, elevation of liver enzymes was observed: alanine transaminase (ALT), 127 IU/L, aspartate transaminase (AST), 61 IU/L, alkaline phosphatase, 209 IU/L, and gamma-glutamyl-transpeptidase (GGT), 222 IU/L. Extensive laboratory and radiologic evaluations showed no abnormalities, aside from iron-related parameters: serum iron, 110 ng/ml, ferritin, 3170 mg/dl (versus 29 mg/dL before transplant), transferrin, 119 mg/dL, and transferrin saturation, 66%. Repeated liver biopsy revealed sinusoidal fibrosis with mild cholangiolar proliferation. Iron staining showed significant accumulation of iron in macrophages and hepatocytes, consistent with marked hemosiderosis (Figure 2).

The combination of abnormal laboratory iron parameters and biopsy findings showing clear worsening of iron accumulation, without apparent new risk factors for secondary iron overload, led us to suspect primary rather than secondary hemosiderosis. Genetic testing of the patient's DNA ruled out preexisting HH and did not show any common HFE mutations (C282Y or H63D). Genetic high-resolution melt curve analysis of a biopsy sample revealed compound C282Y/H63D heterozygosity, confirming a genetic defect in the donor tissue, which elicited hereditary hemochromatosis in a recipient without any known HFE mutation.

Magnetic Resonance Imaging (MRI) performed or iron assessment revealed mild hepatic iron overload, consistent

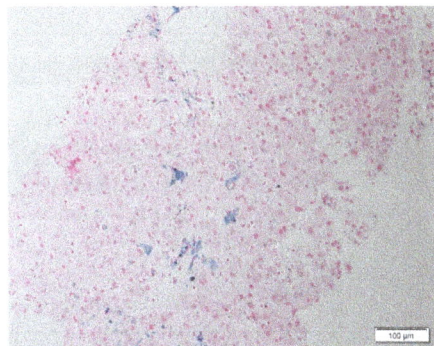

FIGURE 1: Liver biopsy 6 months after OLT showing hypertrophic macrophages containing iron and slight accumulation of hemosiderin in hepatocytes (Perls' stain).

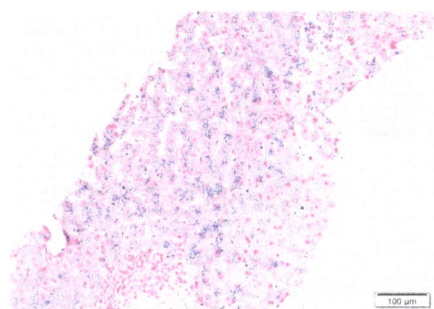

FIGURE 2: Liver biopsy 18 months after OLT demonstrating heavy granular iron deposition in hepatocytes and macrophages corresponding to hemosiderosis (Perls' stain).

with 5 mg/gr, and did not show accumulation of iron in other organs: pancreas, adrenals, spleen, and heart.

Following the confirmation of the diagnosis, the patient was enrolled in a phlebotomy program.

3. Methods

Liver biopsies were fixed in 10% formalin, embedded in paraffin, and stained with hematoxylin-eosin, trichrome, reticulin, periodic acid Schiff (PAS), and iron stains, according to standard methods.

3.1. Molecular Analyses. The C282Y and H63D mutations were detected by Sanger sequencing using the primers: F-ACACAGCTGATGGTATGAGTTGAT and R-ATGAAAA-GATGAAAAGCTCTGACAA; F-AGAAGGAAGTGAA-AGTTCCAGTCTT and R-ATCTCACTGCCATAATTAC-CTCCTC, respectively. Amplification was carried out in a 25 μL reaction containing 50 ng DNA, 10 ng of each primer, and 12.5 μL RM (Thermo Scientific). After an initial denaturation of 2 min at 95°C, 30 cycles were performed (95°C, 60°C and 72°C, for 30 sec each), followed by a final extension of 10 min at 72°C and sequencing, using an automated ABI Prism 3100 Genetic Analyzer (Perkin Elmer).

TABLE 1

Reference #	Year of publication	Donor	Recipient	Reason for transplant	Time from OLT to HH development (months)	Outcome
[5]	1999	C282Y homozygote liver & intestine	Non-HH	Cholestatic liver disease & short bowel syndrome	21	Biochemical abnormalities consistent with HH
[6]	2003	C282Y heterozygote liver	new missense mutation R6S	Alcoholic cirrhosis	49	Treated with phlebotomy
[7]	2009	C282Y homozygote liver	H63D heterozygote	HBV+HCV +ethanol	60	Died due to lung cancer
[4]	2011	C282Y homozygote liver	Non-HH	Fulminant HBV reactivation	24	Treated with phlebotomy
Present case	2016	C282Y/H63D compound heterozygote	Non-HH	PSC and Crohn's disease	18	Planned for phlebotomy

4. Discussion

Here, we present a first report of inadvertent transplantation of a liver from a donor with C282Y/H63D compound heterozygosity into a nonhemochromatotic recipient. The number of cases shed light onto current knowledge (Table 1) of HH pathogenesis, which remains to be fully elucidated.

The possible role of the liver versus the intestine in the pathogenesis of HH has been the subject of long existing controversy. The "tale of two sites" began long before the development of HFE genetic studies and liver transplantation has become the greatest contributor in the understanding of HH pathophysiology. In the early 1990s, evidence ruling out an exclusively intrahepatic defect began to accumulate. Adams et al. [8] described a biopsy-proven rapid decline of hepatic iron levels in a hemochromatosis liver, which was inadvertently transplanted into a recipient suffering from acute liver failure. A few years later, when genetic analyses became available, the same team presented an even more informative case when both the liver and the intestine from a C282Y homozygous patient were transplanted into a normal recipient [5]. Twenty-one months later, the recipient developed the biochemical abnormalities typical of early hemochromatosis (increased transferrin saturation with still normal hepatic iron concentration and normal serum ferritin). The authors concluded that both cases supported their hypothesis regarding existence of a site-specific fundamental defect in the intestine of hemochromatosis patients [5, 8]. Further support of this theory was provided by several case reports of non-HH recipients who received livers from HH donors [9] and development of a decrease in iron overload after transplant in the majority of these patients.

Strong arguments against this hypothesis were presented in early 2000s, with claims that if HH is due to an intestinal defect, liver transplantation would not cure the hemochromatosis and iron would be expected to reaccumulate [10]. Yet, a number of studies failed to observe any long-term (up to 12 years) reaccumulation of iron after liver transplantation for

HH [11–13]. In 2003, Wigg AJ et al. [6] described, for the first time, the development of phenotypic hereditary hemochromatosis in a non-HH liver transplant recipient following transplantation of a liver from a C282Y heterozygous donor. In their case, a novel pathogenic missense mutation of the HFE gene, R6S, was discovered in the recipient. The authors hypothesized that an interaction between R6S heterozygosity in the recipient and C282Y heterozygosity in the donor liver drove development of iron overload in the patient. In essence, the authors suggested that a hepatic defect is required for expression of HH and that the intestinal HFE genotype can impact but is not the exclusive determinant of iron metabolism [6].

Since then, a growing body of evidence has supported the hypothesis that the liver, rather than the intestine, plays a primary role in the maintenance of iron homeostasis. Ismail MK et al. [7] presented another case of posttransplant iron overload following transplantation of a C282Y homozygous liver into an H63D heterozygous recipient. The authors suggested involvement of hepcidin, a relatively newly discovered iron flow regulator [14, 15]. They also speculated that heterozygosity for the H63D mutation in the presence of a liver with the C282Y mutation may be much more consequential, as in the case of Wigg et al. [6].

Finally, Dwyer JP et al. [4] reported a case of inadvertent transplantation of a liver with C282Y homozygosity from an HH donor into a C282Y wild type (no hemochromatosis and no HFE mutations) recipient with fulminant hepatic failure due to hepatitis B reactivation. The development of clinically significant hemochromatosis was detected in a recipient two years following the transplant. In this case, only C282Y homozygosity (without any mutation in a recipient) was sufficient to trigger hemochromatosis in the recipient. In the present case, several risk factors for secondary iron overload presented immediately after transplantation (multiple blood transfusions and hemodialysis), but no additional risk factors accumulated between the first and the second biopsy. Thus, transfer of the genetic defect of hemochromatosis from the donor liver to the recipient is the most probable explanation for iron overload development with features of primary hemochromatosis. We hypothesize that C282Y/H63D heterozygosity in the donor liver triggered development of the HH phenotype in the recipient who did not have any evidence of pathogenic HFE mutations. This case provides support for the hypothesis that the liver plays the most critical role in iron homeostasis.

Our case study has a few limitations. First, hepcidin, as a well-established and key regulator of iron flow from duodenal hepatocytes to the liver, was not evaluated in our patient. The use of hepcidin assays is limited for research purposes only and is still not available in any medical institution in Israel. Second, the occurrence of clinical iron overload in compound C282Y/H63D heterozygosity according to the recent data is extremely rare [16]. The concomitant existence of an additional unknown genetic defect in the recipient (coding the HH genes or other genes involved in iron metabolism), which possibly triggered iron overload, was considered but was not evaluated. In addition, there is a possibility of contribution of nongenetic factors such as the multiple transfusions and renal dialysis.

In conclusion, we presented the first report of inadvertent transplantation of a liver from a donor with C282Y/H63D compound heterozygosity into a nonhemochromatotic recipient. The case strengthens the hypothesis that the liver, rather than the small intestine, plays a primary role in the maintenance of iron homeostasis.

References

[1] A. Pietrangelo, "Hereditary hemochromatosis: pathogenesis, diagnosis, and treatment," *Gastroenterology*, vol. 139, no. 2, pp. 393–408, 2010.

[2] B. R. Bacon, P. C. Adams, K. V. Kowdley, L. W. Powell, and A. S. Tavill, "Diagnosis and management of hemochromatosis: 2011 practice guideline by the American Association for the study of liver diseases," *Hepatology*, vol. 54, no. 1, pp. 328–343, 2011.

[3] M. Vujić Spasić, J. Kiss, T. Herrmann et al., "HFE acts in hepatocytes to prevent hemochromatosis," *Cell Metabolism*, vol. 7, no. 2, pp. 173–178, 2008.

[4] J. P. Dwyer, S. Sarwar, B. Egan, N. Nolan, and J. Hegarty, "Hepatic iron overload following liver transplantation of a C282y homozygous allograft: A case report and literature review," *Liver International*, vol. 31, no. 10, pp. 1589–1592, 2011.

[5] P. C. Adams, G. Jeffrey, K. Alanen et al., "Transplantation of haemochromatosis liver and intestine into a normal recipient," *Gut*, vol. 45, no. 5, p. 783, 1999.

[6] A. J. Wigg, H. Harley, and G. Casey, "Heterozygous recipient and donor HFE mutations associated with a hereditary haemochromatosis phenotype after liver transplantation," *Gut*, vol. 52, no. 3, pp. 433–435, 2003.

[7] M. K. Ismail, A. Martinez-Hernandez, S. Schichman, S. Chaudhry, and B. Waters, "Transplantation of a liver with the C282Y mutation into a recipient heterozygous for H63D results in iron overload," *The American Journal of the Medical Sciences*, vol. 337, no. 2, pp. 138–142, 2009.

[8] P. C. Adams, C. N. Ghent, D. R. Grant, J. V. Frei, and W. J. Wall, "Transplantation of a donor liver with haemochromatosis: Evidence against an inherited intrahepatic defect," *Gut*, vol. 32, no. 9, pp. 1082-1083, 1991.

[9] D. J. Brandhagen, "Liver transplantation for hereditary hemochromatosis," *Liver Transplantation*, vol. 7, no. 8, pp. 663–672, 2001.

[10] D. Brandhagen, "Can liver transplantation improve our understanding of the pathophysiology of iron overload?" *Liver Transplantation*, vol. 10, no. 9, pp. 1218–1220, 2004.

[11] D. H. G. Crawford, L. M. Fletcher, S. G. Hubscher et al., "Patient and graft survival after liver transplantation for hereditary hemochromatosis: Implications for pathogenesis," *Hepatology*, vol. 39, no. 6, pp. 1655–1662, 2004.

[12] F. S. Dar, W. Faraj, M. B. Zaman et al., "Outcome of liver transplantation in hereditary hemochromatosis," *Transplant International*, vol. 22, no. 7, pp. 717–724, 2009.

[13] M.-P. Bralet, J.-C. Duclos-Vallee, D. Castaing et al., "No hepatic iron overload 12 years after liver transplantation for hereditary hemochromatosis (multiple letters)," *Hepatology*, vol. 40, no. 3, article 762, 2004.

[14] T. Ganz, "Hepcidin in iron metabolism," *Current Opinion in Hematology*, vol. 11, no. 4, pp. 251–254, 2004.

[15] P. C. Adams, V. McAlister, S. Chakrabarti, M. Levstik, and P. Marotta, "Is serum hepcidin causative in hemochromatosis? Novel analysis from a liver transplant with hemochromatosis," *Canadian Journal of Gastroenterology & Hepatology*, vol. 22, no. 10, pp. 851–853, 2008.

[16] S. F. Leitman, "Hemochromatosis: the new blood donor," *International Journal of Hematology*, vol. 2013, no. 1, pp. 645–650, 2013.

23

Resolution of Crizotinib-Associated Fulminant Hepatitis following Cessation of Treatment

Gregory W. Charville ⓘ,[1] Sukhmani K. Padda,[2] Richard K. Sibley,[1] Ajithkumar Puthillath,[3] and Paul Y. Kwo[4]

[1]Department of Pathology, Stanford University School of Medicine, Stanford, CA 94305, USA
[2]Department of Medicine, Division of Oncology, Stanford University School of Medicine, Stanford, CA 94305, USA
[3]Stockton Hematology Oncology Medical Group, Stockton, CA 95204, USA
[4]Department of Medicine, Division of Gastroenterology and Hepatology, Stanford University School of Medicine, Stanford, CA 94305, USA

Correspondence should be addressed to Gregory W. Charville; gwc@stanford.edu

Academic Editor: Sorabh Kapoor

Targeted cancer treatments offer the prospect of precise inhibition of tumor growth without the untoward off-target toxicity of traditional chemotherapies. Still, unintended, often idiosyncratic side effects, such as drug-induced liver injury, can occur. We discuss the case of a 26-year-old female with a history of *ROS1*-rearranged lung adenocarcinoma, undergoing treatment with the tyrosine kinase inhibitor crizotinib, who presented to our hospital with abdominal pain and scleral icterus. Liver chemistries were notable for hyperbilirubinemia (5 mg/dL total) and marked transaminasemia (AST 1736 U/L, ALT >3500 U/L); liver biopsy demonstrated acute hepatitis with extensive necrosis. There was no evidence of an infectious or autoimmune etiology. It was discovered that the patient was taking a 500 mg once daily dose of crizotinib, in lieu of the intended dose of 250 mg twice daily. After immediate cessation of crizotinib therapy upon hospital admission, there was complete biochemical resolution of the hepatitis. This case highlights the potential reversibility of fulminant crizotinib-associated hepatoxicity, possibly related to supratherapeutic dosing, when managed with abrupt stoppage of the drug and initiation of supportive care.

1. Introduction

Crizotinib is a small-molecule inhibitor of the protooncogene receptor tyrosine kinases anaplastic lymphoma kinase (ALK), ROS1, and MET. As a targeted therapy, crizotinib has received approval for treatment of a distinct subgroup of non-small-cell lung cancers mediated by rearrangements of *ALK* or *ROS1* [1, 2]. Most patients with *ALK*- or *ROS1*-rearranged lung cancers show an objective response to tyrosine kinase inhibition, which now represents a first-line approach to the treatment of these unique tumors [3]. The most common side effects of crizotinib include nausea, diarrhea, visual disturbances, fatigue, anorexia, constipation, abdominal pain, and upper respiratory tract infection, among others [3]. Elevated aminotransferases of varying degree have been reported as a side effect in trials of crizotinib. A much less common, and

sometimes irreversible, side effect of crizotinib is fulminant hepatitis.

2. Case Report

A 26-year-old female presented to our hospital with a primary complaint of intermittent, progressive right upper quadrant abdominal pain of one week's duration, which coincided with the onset of darkened urine and yellowing of the eyes. There was mild nausea, but no emesis. The patient had no subjective fever or rashes. She perceived no significant swelling or unusual bleeding. She had no chest pain or myalgia. Her appetite was normal.

The past medical history was notable for a diagnosis of primary lung adenocarcinoma by bronchoscopic biopsy of a right lower lobe radiographic consolidation four months prior to this presentation. By immunohistochemistry, the adenocarcinoma expressed cytokeratin 7, thyroid transcription factor-1 (TTF-1), and napsin-A, but did not express cytokeratin 20, GATA-3, or PAX8, findings consistent with adenocarcinoma of lung origin. Fluorescence in situ hybridization (FISH) analysis of the primary tumor showed cytogenetic evidence of a *ROS1* gene rearrangement. No actionable mutations were detected by exon-targeted sequencing. Staging positron emission tomography-computed tomography studies revealed a fludeoxyglucose- (FDG-) avid right lower lobe lung mass with additional consolidation/nodularity in the right middle lobe, left upper lobe, and lingula, and no evidence of mediastinal or hilar lymphadenopathy; however, endobronchial ultrasound-guided biopsy of a level ten lymph node showed involvement by metastatic disease. MRI of the brain showed no evidence of intracranial metastasis.

Given the presence of a *ROS1* gene rearrangement, the patient was started on oral crizotinib therapy (250 mg twice daily) 10 weeks prior to her presentation. One week after the initiation of crizotinib therapy, the patient was admitted to another hospital with chest pain, subjective fever, and emesis. She was diagnosed with a bacterial pneumonia and discharged from the hospital with instructions to complete seven-day courses of levofloxacin and metronidazole and a ten-day course of fluconazole, while decreasing her crizotinib dose to 250 mg once daily. One week after discharge from this preceding hospitalization, the patient's liver chemistries were normal: total bilirubin 0.2 mg/dL, AST (SGOT) 15 U/L, ALT (SGPT) 25 U/L, and alkaline phosphatase 58 U/L. Five weeks and two days prior to the current presentation, after the resolution of the abovementioned symptoms, the patient was instructed to increase the crizotinib dose back to the original 250 mg twice per day. However, on admission to our hospital, the patient reported restarting crizotinib at one dose of 500 mg daily, as she found the side effects of gastrointestinal upset more tolerable with this self-imposed regimen. The patient denied other new medications, toxin exposures, or drug/alcohol use. There were no known sick contacts or significant travel.

On physical examination, the vital signs were normal with blood pressure 107/69, heart rate 75 beats per minute, temperature 36.8°C (oral), respiratory rate 12 per minute, and oxygen saturation 96% on room air. The patient was not in distress. The eyes showed mild scleral icterus and the oropharynx was without lesions. Both the rate and rhythm of the heart were regular; there were no heart murmurs. The lungs were bilaterally clear to auscultation: there were no wheezes or rales. The patient exhibited mild epigastric and right upper quadrant abdominal pain on examination, but there was no palpable mass or organomegaly. Examination of the extremities showed no cyanosis or edema. The skin itself was not jaundiced and did not display spider angiomata or palmar erythema. There was no asterixis.

Liver chemistries at the time of admission showed total bilirubin 4.5 mg/dL (3.5 mg/dL conjugated, 1.5 mg/dL unconjugated), AST 1736 U/L, ALT >3500 U/L, and alkaline phosphatase 144 U/L. The INR was above the threshold of normal at 2.2. The white blood cell count was 10.6 K/μL. The platelet count was 195 K/μL. PCR studies of the serum for hepatitis B virus, hepatitis C virus, herpes simplex viruses- (HSV-) 1 and 2, and Epstein-Barr virus (EBV) were negative. Serologic studies for anti-hepatitis A virus antibody (IgM), anti-hepatitis C virus antibody (IgG), anti-hepatitis B virus core antibody (IgM), and hepatitis B surface antigen were all negative. Anti-varicella zoster virus IgG antibody was present, while IgM antibody was not. Analysis of the serum for antinuclear antibody was negative (titer <1:80), as were studies for anti-liver-kidney-microsomal antibody and anti-smooth muscle antibody. Serum acetaminophen levels were below the limit of detection (<2.0 μg/mL). Ceruloplasmin was normal at 27.7 mg/dL.

Computed tomography imaging with the aid of intravenous contrast was notable for periportal edema with a small amount of perihepatic fluid and gallbladder mural edema. There were no intra- or extrahepatic mass lesions. Significant interval decrease in the radiographic burden of disease in the right lung was noted with minimal ongoing ground-glass opacities in the right upper and right middle lobes.

Given suspicion of crizotinib-associated hepatotoxicity, targeted therapy was discontinued on admission to our hospital. A continuous infusion of N-acetylcysteine was started (6.25 mg/kg/hr). The AST showed immediate improvement, peaking on the first day of admission (Figure 1). The ALT remained at the maximum limit of detection until the third day of admission and then precipitously declined. Six days after admission, results of serologic studies showed mildly elevated anti-HSV IgM (1.35; normal <1.10); anti-HSV-1 IgG was also present, while anti-HSV-2 IgG was not. With this information, intravenous acyclovir (10 mg/kg every eight hours) was initiated.

On the seventh day of hospitalization, a transjugular liver biopsy was performed. Histologic sections of the liver biopsy were notable for a predominantly lymphohistiocytic panlobular inflammatory infiltrate accompanied by swaths of parenchymal dropout (Figures 2(a) and 2(b)). The inflammatory infiltrate included abundant pigment-laden macrophages and the occasional plasma cell. Granulocytes, including the rare eosinophil, were also seen. The sampled portal tracts showed the appropriate constellation of artery, vein, and interlobular bile duct without evidence of ductopenia. The inflammation was not centered on the portal tracts and the bile ducts themselves showed no obvious intraepithelial infiltrate or reactive-type epithelial changes. Numerous degenerating and necrotic hepatocytes were seen. Those hepatocytes that remained showed reactive cytoplasmic vacuolization and mitotic activity suggestive of a regenerative response. Periodic acid-Schiff (PAS) stain with diastase pretreatment drew attention to the ceroid pigment-laden Kupffer cells indicative of the significant hepatocyte death that must have preceded this biopsy (Figure 2(c)). The PAS-positive intracytoplasmic aggregates of alpha-1-antitrypsin deficiency were not seen. Cholestasis was also prominent. Reticulin and trichrome stains highlighted areas of hepatocyte loss and parenchymal collapse (Figure 2(d)). There was no significant fibrosis by trichrome stain. Hepatic stores of copper and iron were not significantly increased on special stains for each element. The periportal copper deposition of chronic cholestasis

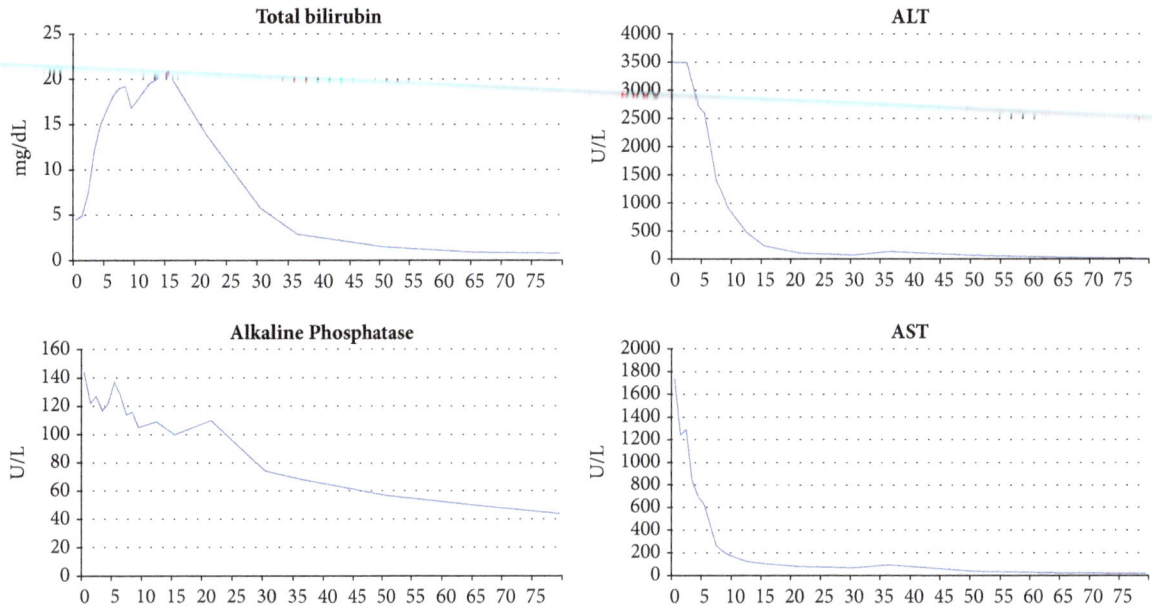

FIGURE 1: Time-course of liver function studies. The x-axis spans from Day 0 (day of admission and cessation of crizotinib therapy) to Day 79.

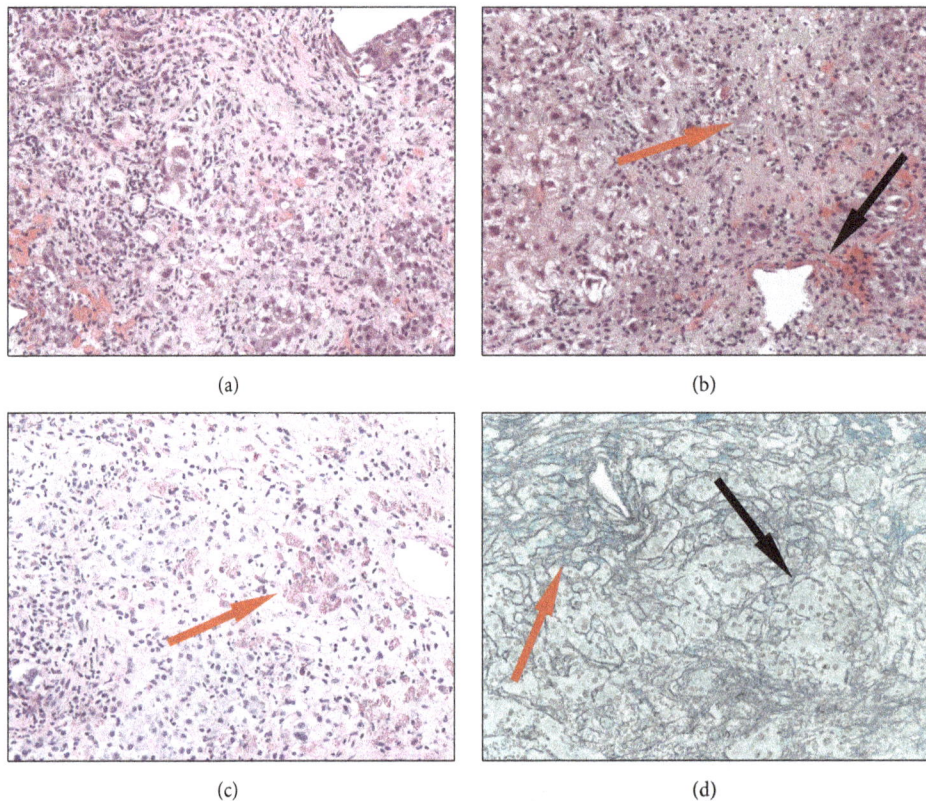

(a)

(b)

(c)

(d)

FIGURE 2: (a) H&E-stained histologic section of the liver biopsy demonstrating severe acute hepatitis characterized by a panlobular mixed inflammatory infiltrate with extensive hepatocyte necrosis (200x magnification). (b) H&E-stained histologic section of the liver biopsy demonstrating bridging parenchymal necrosis (red arrow) and cholestasis (black arrow) (200x magnification). (c) Periodic acid-Schiff stained histologic section of the liver biopsy with diastase pretreatment highlighting numerous ceroid pigment-laden macrophages (red arrow) (200x magnification). (d) Reticulin-stained histologic section of the liver biopsy demonstrating areas of parenchymal collapse (red arrow) and regenerative thickening of the hepatocyte plates (black arrow) (100x magnification).

was not present. No viral cytopathic effects were identified; immunohistochemical stains for HSV and adenovirus were both negative. Furthermore, analysis of biopsied tissue by PCR showed no evidence of varicella zoster virus, HSV-1/2, cytomegalovirus, or EBV. Nonspecific viral culture of the liver biopsy also showed no viral cytopathic effect.

Acyclovir was discontinued eight days after admission (two days following its initiation), at which time the total bilirubin also peaked. N-acetylcysteine was discontinued and the patient was discharged to home nine days after admission with continually downtrending liver chemistries. She developed edema and ascites post discharge and required furosemide 40 mg daily and spironolactone 100 mg daily for three weeks until these symptoms resolved. Despite this, the liver tests continued to normalize during the patient's subsequent outpatient treatment. She never developed hepatic encephalopathy. All liver chemistries had normalized at follow-up 79 days after admission (Figure 1). Computed tomography studies at that time showed an interval increase in the right lower lobe ground-glass opacity, along with small nodules throughout the remainder of the bilateral lungs; the radiographic appearance of the liver was improved. Given evidence of residual cancer burden, a chemotherapeutic regimen of carboplatin and pemetrexed was initiated.

3. Discussion

Liver injury of varying degree is a documented side effect of crizotinib anticancer therapy. In 171 patients receiving first-line crizotinib, Solomon et al. observed elevated aminotransferases in 61 (36%), with 14% of patients showing Grades 3-4 transaminasemia [3]. Of these 24 patients with Grades 3-4 aminotransferase increases, all but four were successfully managed with dose interruptions or reductions. Those four outstanding cases required complete cessation of therapy. In a phase 1 study of crizotinib therapy in 79 pediatric patients (aged 1-22 years) with various malignancies, ALT elevations were seen in 62% and AST elevations in 56% [4]. Although none of the 899 patients with "definite, highly likely, or probable" drug-induced liver injury in the Drug-Induced Liver Injury Network's prospective study were attributed to crizotinib, these studies largely preceded the widespread implementation of the drug [5].

In addition to these more commonplace and modest aminotransferase abnormalities, individual cases of fulminant hepatic failure in the setting of crizotinib therapy have been reported. Sato et al. describe the case of a 54-year-old female presenting with fulminant hepatitis 29 days following the initiation of crizotinib therapy [6]. The patient died seven days after presentation despite cessation of crizotinib. Although the patient was also taking sitagliptin and rabeprazole, crizotinib was the only new medication. The history was notable in this case for chronic inactive hepatitis C infection. A similar case involved a 62-year-old female who presented with markedly elevated serum aminotransferase 17 days after starting crizotinib; therapy was stopped a week later (24 days after initiation), but the patient's clinical status continued to decline and the patient ultimately died of liver failure 40 days after first taking crizotinib [7]. Liver biopsy findings were not presented in these cases.

The histologic findings in this case were notable for a severe lobular hepatitis with submassive parenchymal dropout. The inflammatory infiltrate was not portal-based and the bile ducts themselves were relatively spared. The inflammation was predominantly lymphohistiocytic, but there were no frank granulomata. Neutrophils outnumbered both eosinophils and plasma cells, though the latter two could be identified without much searching. Features to suggest a robust regenerative response—proliferation of residual hepatocytes and widening of the hepatocyte plates—were readily apparent. This finding may have predicted the clinical recovery of liver function seen in this case after the cessation of crizotinib. Paralleling the biochemical evidence of hyperbilirubinemia, there was marked cholestasis that was mostly canalicular and hepatocellular.

This case is also of interest because of the complete resolution of such severe hepatitis, in contrast to the fatal cases described above. Although the exact timing of the onset of liver injury was unknown in the present case, the serum transaminases precipitously declined following the cessation of therapy, suggesting that this intervention was key to the resolution of the injury process. Earlier case reports have shown normalization of more modestly elevated aminotransferases following the withdrawal of crizotinib [8]. A patient with a maximal ALT 1096 IU/L on crizotinib was initially taken off the drug and subsequently underwent successful oral desensitization, tolerating a second course of therapy until the cancer progressed [9].

One salient aspect of this case is the patient-initiated dosing regimen of 500 mg once daily that deviated from the recommended dose during the period preceding the hospitalization for fulminant hepatitis. This regimen reportedly relieved the patient's perceived gastrointestinal discomfort in the setting of reinitiation of crizotinib at 250 mg twice daily following a brief cessation of therapy in the context of pneumonia. In the earliest dose-escalation studies of crizotinib, studied doses ranged from 50 mg once daily to 300 mg twice daily [1]. The effective mean plasma trough concentration of 120 ng per mL, established in preclinical studies, was achieved by dosing regimens of 200 mg or more twice daily. In the cohort receiving 300 mg twice daily, dose-limiting fatigue was noted, leading to the selection of 250 mg twice daily as the maximum tolerated dose. To our knowledge, crizotinib dose-dependent hepatotoxicity has not been observed. It is possible that the 500 mg once daily dosing regimen contributed to the remarkable hepatotoxicity in this case, as well as the favorable clinical response to discontinuation of the drug.

Alternative differential diagnostic considerations in this case included drug/toxin-induced liver injury secondary to another offending agent, although eosinophils did not feature prominently in the inflammatory infiltrate. Furthermore, the patient did not endorse recent exposure to drugs or potential hepatotoxins, aside from crizotinib. Autoimmune hepatitis was also a consideration; the negative anti-smooth muscle, anti-liver-kidney-microsomal, and anti-nuclear antibody studies, and the overall lack of a plasma cell-rich infiltrate, provided no support for an autoimmune etiology. We did not see histologic features to suggest hepatotropic or nonhepatotropic viral infection; also, correlation with viral

PCR and serologic studies gave no support for a viral etiology. Notably, the hepatitis resolved without immunosuppression; acyclovir was only briefly given in the face of a positive anti-HSV IgM titer. Taken together, the constellation of findings points to drug-induced liver injury secondary to crizotinib.

This case highlights the potential for complete clinical and biochemical resolution of a fulminant hepatitis arising in association with crizotinib therapy for non-small-cell lung cancer when managed with abrupt cessation of the drug in combination with supportive care, including N-acetylcysteine. Patients should be monitored closely on all chemotherapeutic regimens, such as crizotinib, with prompt evaluation if significant elevations of liver tests are noted; querying whether doses of chemotherapeutic regimens were altered by patients or the treating team may be particularly relevant.

References

[1] E. L. Kwak, Y-J. Bang, D. R. Camidge, A. T. Shaw, B. Solomon, R. G. Maki et al., "Anaplastic lymphoma kinase inhibition in non-small-cell lung cancer," *The New England Journal of Medicine*, vol. 363, no. 18, pp. 1693–1703, 2010.

[2] A. T. Shaw, S.-H. I. Ou, and Y.-J. Bang, "Crizotinib in *ROS1*-re-arranged non-small-cell lung cancer," *The New England Journal of Medicine*, vol. 371, no. 2030-2031, pp. 1963–1971, 2014.

[3] B. J. Solomon, T. Mok, and D.-W. Kim, "First-line crizotinib versus chemotherapy in ALK-positive lung cancer," *The New England Journal of Medicine*, vol. 371, no. 23, pp. 2167–2177, 2014.

[4] Y. P. Mossé, M. S. Lim, S. D. Voss et al., "Safety and activity of crizotinib for paediatric patients with refractory solid tumours or anaplastic large-cell lymphoma: A Children's Oncology Group phase 1 consortium study," *The Lancet Oncology*, vol. 14, no. 6, pp. 472–480, 2013.

[5] N. Chalasani, H. L. Bonkovsky, R. Fontana, W. Lee, A. Stolz, J. Talwalkar et al., "Features and Outcomes of 899 Patients With Drug-Induced Liver Injury: The DILIN Prospective Study," *Gastroenterology*, vol. 148, no. 7, pp. 1340–1352.e7, Jun 2015.

[6] Y. Sato, D. Fujimoto, Y. Shibata et al., "Fulminant hepatitis following crizotinib administration for ALK-positive non-small-cell lung carcinoma," *Japanese Journal of Clinical Oncology*, vol. 44, no. 9, pp. 872–875, 2014.

[7] R. M. J. M. van Geel, J. J. M. A. Hendrikx, J. E. Vahl et al., "Crizotinib-induced fatal fulminant liver failure," *Lung Cancer*, vol. 93, pp. 17–19, 2016.

[8] M.-P. Ripault, V. Pinzani, V. Fayolle, G.-P. Pageaux, and D. Larrey, "Crizotinib-induced acute hepatitis: First case with relapse after reintroduction with reduced dose," *Clinics and Research in Hepatology and Gastroenterology*, vol. 37, no. 1, pp. e21–e23, 2013.

[9] Y. Yasuda, Y. Nishikawa, Y. Sakamori et al., "Successful oral de-sensitization with crizotinib after crizotinib-induced hepatitis in an anaplastic lymphoma kinase-rearranged non-small-cell lung cancer patient: A case report," *Molecular and Clinical Oncology*, vol. 7, no. 2, pp. 295–297, 2017.

24

Rupture of Hepatocellular Carcinoma after Transarterial Chemoembolization followed by Massive Gastric Bleeding

Kazuhiro Nishida [ID],[1] **Alan Kawarai Lefor,**[2] **and Tomohiro Funabiki**[1]

[1]*Department of Emergent and Critical Care Medicine, Saiseikai Yokohamashi Tobu Hospital, 3-6-1, Shimosueyoshi, Tsurumi, Yokohama-city, Kanagawa 230-8765, Japan*
[2]*Department of Surgery, Jichi Medical University, 3311-1 Yakushiji, Shimotsuke, Tochigi 329-0498, Japan*

Correspondence should be addressed to Kazuhiro Nishida; pandadebanda4@gmail.com

Academic Editor: Dario Lorenzin

Introduction. Transarterial chemoembolization (TACE) is the first-line therapy for patient with unresectable hepatocellular carcinoma (HCC). Although TACE is a generally safe procedure, major complications can be occurred. We describe a patient with rupture of HCC after TACE followed by gastric bleeding. *Case Presentation.* An 81-year-old man presented with worsening epigastric pain. He had been diagnosed with multiple HCC with nonalcoholic steatohepatitis and underwent TACE 19 days previously. A contrast enhanced computed tomography (CT) scan of the abdomen showed rupture of an HCC. He was treated nonoperatively and discharged on hospital day 18. Five weeks after TACE, he was emergently admitted with massive hematochezia and shock. A contrast enhanced CT scan demonstrated extrinsic gastric compression by an HCC lesion with extravasation of contrast into the stomach. Emergent upper gastrointestinal endoscopy showed a bleeding gastric ulcer with extraluminal compression which was successfully controlled by hypertonic saline-epinephrine injection. Due to tumor progression, he was discharged for palliative care and died six weeks after TACE. *Conclusion.* Rupture of HCC is a life-threatening complication after TACE with mortality rates up to 50%. After treatment of a ruptured HCC, extragastric compression and bleeding can occur due to direct compression by a primary lesion or intraperitoneal dissemination.

1. Background

Transarterial chemoembolization (TACE) is the first-line therapy for patients with an unresectable hepatocellular carcinoma (HCC) and hepatic metastases. Although TACE is a generally safe, major complications such as tumor rupture, liver abscess, bile leak, hepatic failure, gastrointestinal hemorrhage/ulceration, and pulmonary embolism can occur [1–5]. The major complication rate is reported to be 2.1-2.5% with a mortality rate up to 16.7% [2, 4]. Especially for the patients with an HCC larger than 10 cm, the major complication rate is as high as 4.9% [3]. The incidence of ruptured HCC after TACE is very low, with few published reports. In the 1990s, Liu reported 391 patients who underwent 1443 sessions of TACE, with rupture of an HCC occurring in only six patients (1.5% per patient and 0.4% per procedure) [5]. Two decades later, Tu reported on 1120 patients who underwent 2863 sessions of TACE. Six patients suffered rupture of the HCC (0.5% per patient and 0.2-0.4% per procedure) and two of them died [2]. HCC rupture after TACE is rare but can be a fetal complication.

2. Case Presentation

An 81-year-old man presented with abdominal discomfort and distention. His medical history was remarkable for hypertension and type 2 diabetes mellitus. He and his family denied alcohol abuse. Physical examination revealed hepatomegaly without jaundice, ascites, or hepatic encephalopathy. Laboratory data included platelet count 101,000/mm^3, total bilirubin 0.9 mg/dl, AST 33 IU/L, ALT IU/L, and PT-INR 1.15. The serum AFP and PIVKA-II levels were 1081.0 ng/ml and 43 mAU/ml. Serologic tests for hepatitis B and C virus were negative. The diagnosis of nonalcoholic steatohepatitis with Child-Pugh A liver cirrhosis was made and four HCC

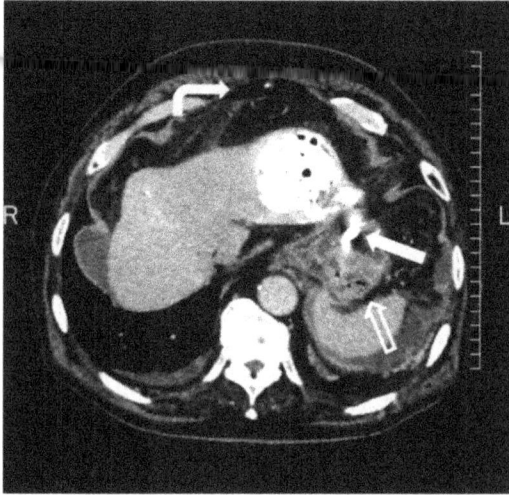

FIGURE 1: A contrast enhanced computed tomography scan of the abdomen showed iodized oil (arrow) and intraperitoneal free (curved arrow) air with a rupture of the HCC in segment II into the peritoneal cavity adjacent to the gastric wall (open arrow).

lesions were found in segments II, VI, and VIII on the imaging. The largest one was located near the liver capsule in segment II measuring 6.5 cm in diameter. The other three lesions were less than 2 cm with one in segment VI and two in segment VIII. Segmental TACE with epirubicin and iodized oil was performed and he was discharged uneventfully.

He was doing well until he developed abdominal pain 15 days after TACE which was gradually getting worse emergency transport to the hospital. His temperature was 37.7°C, blood pressure 102/41 mmHg, and pulse rate 79/minute. On physical examination, the abdomen was distended and hard to palpation without rebound tenderness. His hemoglobin was 12.6 g/dl. A contrast enhanced computed tomography (CT) scan of the abdomen showed iodized oil and intraperitoneal free air with a rupture of the HCC in segment II into the peritoneal cavity adjacent to the gastric wall (Figure 1). Extravasation of contrast medium was not seen. Emergent upper gastrointestinal endoscopy confirmed no gastric mucosal lesions or a site of perforation. Without evidence of septic shock or hemorrhage, surgical drainage and transcatheter arterial embolization (TAE) are considered less effective. He was treated nonoperatively with piperacillin and tazobactam. Although an abdominal abscess formed, he was discharged on hospital day 18 with continued antimicrobial therapy.

Five weeks after undergoing TACE, he was readmitted with hematochezia and hemorrhagic shock. The hemoglobin level was dropped to 6.6 g/dl. A contrast enhanced CT scan demonstrated gastric extraluminal compression by an HCC lesion with extravasation of contrast medium into the stomach (Figure 2). Emergent upper gastrointestinal endoscopy showed a submucosal tumor with central ulceration located on the anterior wall of the gastric body, corresponding to extraluminal compression by a HCC (Figure 3). The hemorrhage from the ulcer was successfully controlled by

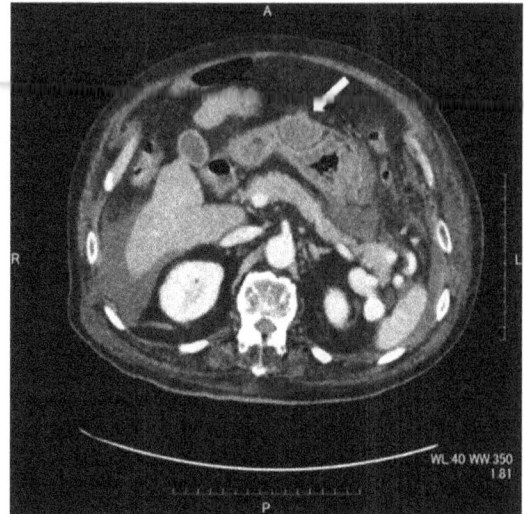

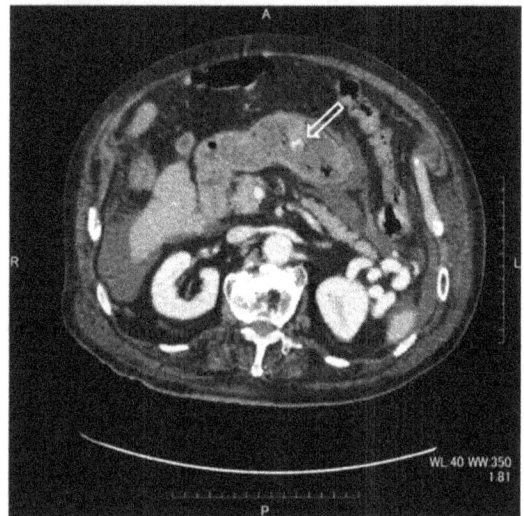

FIGURE 2: A contrast enhanced computed tomography scan demonstrated gastric extraluminal compression by hepatocellular carcinoma (arrow) and extravasation of contrast medium into the stomach (open arrow).

hypertonic saline-epinephrine injection. Another submucosal tumor was found in the gastric fundus without ulcer formation (Figure 4). The patient's condition stabilized and he was discharged for palliative care and died six weeks after undergoing TACE.

3. Discussion

The incidence rate of ruptured HCC after TACE is low with few cases reported. An extensive search was conducted (http://www.pubmed.com) for articles related to this topic, using the following search terms: "ruptured hepatic carcinoma" and "TACE" or "transarterial chemoembolization." A total of 21 previously reported patients were identified and are summarized in Table 1 [2, 6–16].

Fourteen patients were reported from Asia where it is known that hepatitis C virus infection is relatively common.

TABLE 1: Previously reported cases of HCC rupture after TACE.

No.	Author	Year	Country	Age	Gender	Etiology	Cirrhosis	Tumor size (cm)	Location	Interval	Treatment	Outcome	Cause of death,
1	Tu [2], Jia [6]	2016, 2013	China	45	M	HBV	Present	9	Right	10	Conservative	Died	N.A
2				61	M	N.A.	Absent	13	Right	6	TAE	Alive	N.A.
3				53	M	HBV	Present	11	Right+Left	7	Conservative	Died	
4				57	M	HBV	Absent	14	Right+Left	9	TAE	Alive	
5				64	M	N.A.	Absent	16	Right+Left	17	Conservative	Alive	
6				67	F/M	N.A.	Absent	16	Right+Left	13	Conservative	Alive	
7	Singh Bhinder [7]	2015	USA	67	M	alcohol, HCV	Present	4	VII	1	TAE	Alive	
8	Park [8]	2011	Korea	52	M	HBV, alcohol	Present	12.3	VII	30	Conservative	Died	Hepatic failure, more than 1 year after TACE
9	Bruls [9]	2011	Belgium	78	M	alcohol	Present	7	II, IV	3 weeks	Conservative	Died	Tumor rupture, 2 month after TACE
10	Ritter [10]	2011	Germany	74	M	alcohol	Present	16	III, IVb	14 hours	Conservative	Died	Few hours after tumor rupture
11	Sun [11]	2010	China	28	F	N.A.	N.A.	13	Right	1 month	TAE	Alive	
12				42	F	N.A.	N.A.	11	Right	3	TAE	Alive	
13				83	F	N.A.	N.A.	14	Right	5 month	TAE	Died	Respiratory failure, 1 week after rupture
14				51	M	N.A.	N.A.	7	Right	16 hours	TAE	Alive	
15				47	M	N.A.	N.A.	10	Right	7 months	TAE	Alive	
16	Nawawi [12]	2010	Malaysia	66	M	alcohol	Present	3.5	N.A.	N.A.	N.A.	Died	Tumor rupture, 2 month after TACE
17	Reso [13]	2009	Canada	90	M	N.A.	N.A.	11	Right	4 hours	Conservative	Died	Respiratory failure, 16 days after TACE
18	Reichman [14]	2009	USA	53	M	HBV	Present	6	VII, VIII	6 hours	Laparotomy	Died	Shortly after tumor rupture
19	Battula [15]	2007	UK	61	M	N.A.	Present	11	Right	2	Laparotomy	Died	Tumor rupture, 2 days after TACE
20				69	M	N.A.	Present	13	Right	24	Conservative	Alive	
21	Yeh [16]	2002	Taiwan	45	M	HCV	Present	N.A.	IV-VIII	2 month	Laparotomy	Died	Hepatic failure, one month after surgery

HBV: hepatitis B virus: HCV: hepatitis C virus: HCC: hepatocellular carcinoma: TAE: transarterial embolization: TACE: transarterial chemoembolization: USA: the United States of America: UK: United Kingdom.

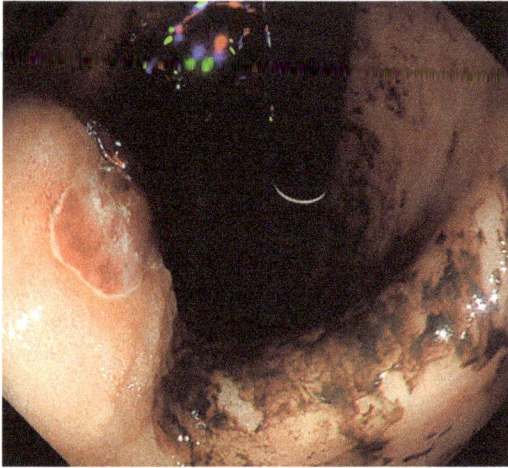

FIGURE 3: Emergent upper gastrointestinal endoscopy showed a submucosal tumor with central ulceration located on the anterior wall of the gastric body, corresponding to extraluminal compression by the hepatocellular carcinoma.

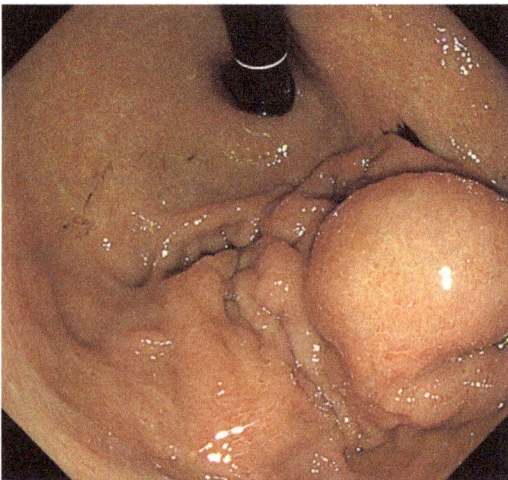

FIGURE 4: Another submucosal tumor was found in the gastric fundus without ulcer formation.

The age ranges from 28 to 90 with a mean of 60 years old. Male gender was 17/20, except for one patient (Number 6 in Table 1) reported as a female by Tu and as a male by Jia [2, 6]. Fourteen of 20 patients had a tumor over 10 cm in diameter. Some case reports suggest that a large tumors increase the risk of rupture [2, 6, 7, 15]. The cause of rupture after TACE is unknown, but fragility of the tumor wall and increased intratumoral pressure are thought to contribute to this complication. Occlusion of the feeding artery leads to necrosis of the tumor which results in wall fragility. Necrosis also leads to increased intratumoral pressure and secondary infection, especially by anaerobic gas forming organisms. In the present patient, the tumor size was 6.5 cm but located near the liver surface. Thin normal liver parenchyma might easily rupture if the tumor wall becomes necrotic with an increase in the intratumoral pressure. An anaerobic infection may have played an important role in the rupture because gas was seen

in the tumor and intraperitoneally on the CT obtained at admission in the same location that an abscess later formed.

Treatment for rupture of an HCC after TACE rupture is either nonoperative or exploratory laparotomy. In the last 20 years, TAE has been increasingly used to control bleeding. If there are no signs of peritonitis or active bleeding; nonoperative therapy may be the treatment of choice. If concomitant hemorrhage is evident and hemostasis is necessary, TAE may be better tolerated than laparotomy. The interval between TACE and rupture has been reported 4-6 hours to 5-7 months. A shorter interval seemed to be associated with shorter survival. Since the mortality rate reached 52.4% (11/21) in previously reported patients who suffered HCC rupture, this is a high mortality complication after TACE.

None of the patients with a ruptured HCC had gastric compression or gastrointestinal bleeding except for the present patient. Generally, extragastric compression is rare. Chen et al. performed endoscopic ultrasonography on 55 patients with extragastric compression and found five with malignant etiologies, one of which was HCC [17]. Direct compression by a primary lesion may have resulted in gastric wall extension with erosion which progressed to bleeding.

4. Conclusion

HCC rupture is a life-threatening complication after TACE with a mortality rate up to 50%. After treatment of HCC rupture, extragastric compression with subsequent gastric bleeding can occur due to direct compression by a primary lesion or disseminated disease.

Authors' Contributions

Kazuhiro Nishida gathered patient's date, designed the case report, and drafted manuscript. Alan Kawarai Lefor supervised the report. Tomohiro Funabiki conceived of the study and participated in its design and coordination. All authors read and approved the final manuscript.

References

[1] A. Basile, G. Carrafiello, A. M. Ierardi, D. Tsetis, and E. Brountzos, "Quality-improvement guidelines for hepatic transarterial chemoembolization," *CardioVascular and Interventional Radiology*, vol. 35, no. 4, pp. 765–774, 2012.

[2] J. Tu, Z. Jia, X. Ying et al., "The incidence and outcome of major complication following conventional TAE/TACE for hepatocellular carcinoma," *Medicine (United States)*, vol. 95, no. 49, p. e5606, 2016.

[3]   T. Xue, F. Le, R. Chen et al., "Transarterial chemoembolization for huge hepatocellular carcinoma with diameter over ten centimeters: a large cohort study," *Medical Oncology*, vol. 32, no. 3, 2015.

[4]   J. Xia, Z. Ren, S. Ye et al., "Study of severe and rare complications of transarterial chemoembolization (TACE) for liver cancer," *European Journal of Radiology*, vol. 59, no. 3, pp. 407–412, 2006.

[5]   C.-L. Liu, H. Ngan, C. M. Lo, and S. T. Fan, "Ruptured hepatocellular carcinoma as a complication of transarterial oily chemoembolization," *British Journal of Surgery*, vol. 85, no. 4, pp. 512–514, 1998.

[6]   Z. Jia, F. Tian, and G. Jiang, "Ruptured hepatic carcinoma after transcatheter arterial chemoembolization," *Current Therapeutic Research, Clinical and Experimental*, vol. 74, pp. 41–43, 2013.

[7]   N. Singh Bhinder and S. M. Zangan, "Hepatocellular carcinoma rupture following transarterial chemoembolization," *Seminars in Interventional Radiology*, vol. 32, no. 1, pp. 49–53, 2015.

[8]   Y. H. Park, S. H. Kang, S. U. Kim et al., "A Case of Hepaticoduodenal Fistula Development after Transarterial Chemoembolization in Patient with Hepatocellular Carcinoma," *The Korean Journal of Gastroenterology*, vol. 58, no. 3, pp. 149–152, 2011.

[9]   S. Bruls, J. Joskin, R. Chauveau, J. Delwaide, and P. Meunier, "Ruptured hepatocellular carcinoma following trans catheter arterial chemoembolization," *Journal Belge de Radiologie - Belgisch Tijdschrift voor Radiologi*, vol. 94, no. 2, pp. 68–70, 2011.

[10] C. O. Ritter, M. Wartenberg, A. Mottok et al., "Spontaneous liver rupture after treatment with drug-eluting beads," *CardioVascular and Interventional Radiology*, vol. 35, no. 1, pp. 198–202, 2012.

[11] JH. Sun, LG. Wang, HW. Bao, JL. Lou, LX. Cai, and C. Wu, "Emergency embolization in the treatment of ruptured hepatocellular carcinoma following transcatheter arterial chemoembolization," *Hepatogastroenterology*, vol. 201, no. 57, pp. 616–619.

[12] O. Nawawi, M. Hazman, B. Abdullah et al., "Transarterial embolisation of hepatocellular carcinoma with doxorubicin-eluting beads: single centre early experience," *Biomedical Imaging and Intervention Journal*, vol. 6, no. 1, 2010.

[13] A. Reso, C. G. Ball, F. R. Sutherland, O. Bathe, and E. Dixon, "Rupture and intra-peritoneal bleeding of a hepatocellular carcinoma after a transarterial chemoembolization procedure: A case report," *Cases Journal*, vol. 2, no. 1, 2009.

[14] T. W. Reichman, T. Anthony, J. M. Millis, and G. Testa, "Uncharacteristically early fatal intraperitoneal rupture of hepatocellular carcinoma following transarterial chemoembolization," *Digestive and Liver Disease*, vol. 41, no. 2, pp. 175-176, 2009.

[15] N. Battula, M. Madanur, O. Priest et al., "Spontaneous rupture of hepatocellular carcinoma: a Western experience," *The American Journal of Surgery*, vol. 197, no. 2, pp. 164–167, 2009.

[16] C.-N. Yeh, H.-M. Chen, M.-F. Chen, and T.-C. Chao, "Peritoneal implanted hepatocellular carcinoma with rupture after TACE presented as acute appendicitis," *Hepato-Gastroenterology*, vol. 49, no. 46, pp. 938–940, 2002.

[17] T. K. Chen, C. H Wu, C. L. Lee, Y. C. Lai, S. S. Yang, and T. C. Tu, "Endoscopic ultrasonography to study the causes of extragastric compression mimicking gastric submucosal tumor," *J Formos Med Assoc*, vol. 100, pp. 100–758, 2001.

25

Refractory Hepatic Hydrothorax: A Rare Complication of Systemic Sclerosis and Presinusoidal Portal Hypertension

Gary A. Abrams [ID],[1] **Robert Chapman,**[1] **and Samuel R. W. Horton**[2]

[1]*Gastroenterology & Liver Center, Greenville Health System, University of South Carolina School of Medicine Greenville, Greenville, SC, USA*
[2]*Department of Pathology, Greenville Health System, University of South Carolina School of Medicine Greenville, Greenville, SC, USA*

Correspondence should be addressed to Gary A. Abrams; gabrams@ghs.org

Academic Editor: Julio M. F. Chebli

We report on a rare case of refractory hepatic hydrothorax in an individual with Scleroderma/CREST syndrome and noncirrhotic portal hypertension. Portal pressure measurements revealed a normal transjugular hepatic venous portal pressure gradient, mild pulmonary hypertension, and an unremarkable liver biopsy except for mild sinusoidal dilation. Pulmonary hypertension, cardiac diastolic dysfunction, and chronic kidney disease were determined to be the causes of his refractory pleural effusions and ascites. Over the year, he underwent 50 thoracenteses and 20 paracenteses averaging 10–12 liters/week. Repeat pulmonary evaluation determined his pulmonary pressures to be normal and a secondary review of the "unremarkable" liver biopsy noted mild venous outflow obstruction and possibly Nodular Regenerative Hyperplasia (NRH). Repeat portal pressures indirectly and directly confirmed the existence of presinusoidal portal hypertension that has been associated with NRH. A transjugular intrahepatic portal systemic shunt (TIPS) was placed and he has not required thoracentesis or paracentesis over the past 18 months.

1. Introduction

Idiopathic noncirrhotic portal hypertension (INCPH) has many etiologies, but a common denominator is vascular resistance at various locations that include the intrahepatic sinusoidal and presinusoidal as well as extrahepatic portal and hepatic veins [1]. Schistosomiasis is a common worldwide illness and the most frequent cause of INCPH [2]. Nodular Regenerative Hyperplasia (NRH) was first described in 1959 [3]; however this is a histological diagnosis that can often be overlooked. We describe a complicated rare case of refractory right-sided pleural effusions and ascites due to NRH and presinusoidal portal hypertension that was successfully treated with a transjugular intrahepatic portal systemic shunt (TIPS).

2. Case Report

A 59-year-old Caucasian male was referred to our liver center for refractory right-sided pleural effusion and abdominal ascites. His history is significant for Scleroderma/CREST syndrome and chronic kidney disease (CKD). He had 12 paracenteses in 2015 and starting from February 2016 was undergoing thoracentesis 3 times weekly (about 8-9 liters/week) and a single weekly paracentesis up to 5 liters. Medications included Spironolactone 50 mg and Furosemide 20 mg, which were limited dosages due to CKD. In February 2016, prior to our visit, he underwent a liver transplant evaluation: Na 138 mg/dL, Cr 4.4 mg/dL, eGFR 31 mL/min, INR 1.0, Hb 13 g/dL, Platelets 342 Th/mm^3, TB 0.5 g/dL, AlkPhos 278 IU/L, ALT/AST 46/40 IU/L, albumin 2.7 mg/dL, negative viral serology, ANA 1 : 320, SMA and AMA negative, C282Y/H63D, and MELD-Na score 14. Abdominal ultrasound revealed a heterogeneous liver and ascites. A thoracentesis demonstrated a SAAG 1.9 and total protein 3.3 gm/dL suggesting posthepatic portal hypertension. A right heart catheterization was notable for RA 5 mmHg, PA 31/15 mm/Hg, mean 22 mmHg, normal Echo LV function, and grade 1 diastolic dysfunction. At this juncture, the etiology of his presumed cirrhosis had not been determined and a liver biopsy with portal pressures was to be scheduled but he wanted a second opinion and presented to us in March.

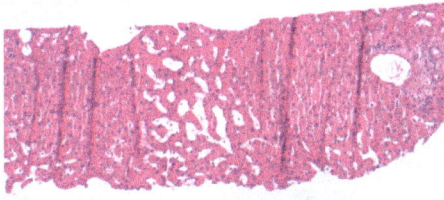

FIGURE 1: (H&E, 100x) needle core biopsy of hepatic parenchyma demonstrating central vein and sinusoidal dilatation.

TABLE 1: Cardiac and portal pressure measurements.

Right cardiac catherization (mmHg)	
Initial	RA 5, PA 31/15 (mean 22)
After albumin	RA 13, PA 57/30 (mean 39), PWP 20, CO 5.5 L/min
PFTs	DLco 9.33 L, VC 2.75 L
Portal pressure measurements (mmHg)	
Initial after albumin	FHVP 16, WHVP 17, HVPG 1
Pre-TIPS without albumin	FHVP 2, WHVP 4, HVPG 5, PVP 15, PPG 11
Post-TIPS	FHVP 5, WHVP 7, HVPG 2, PVP 14, PPG 7

RA: right atrial pressure, PWP: pulmonary wedge pressure, CO: cardiac output, FHVP: free hepatic vein pressure, WHVP: wedge hepatic vein pressure, HVPG: hepatic vein pressure gradient, PVP: direct portal venous pressure measurement, PPG: portal pressure gradient (PVP minus WHVP), PFTs: pulmonary function tests, DLco: diffusion capacity of carbon dioxide, VC: vital capacity, TIPS: transjugular intrahepatic portosystemic shunt.

The physical exam revealed a pleasant frail appearing gentleman with stable vital signs: B/P 87/58, HR 80, and BMI 24.5 kg/m^2; labs demonstrated TB 0.5 md/dL, AlkPhos 462 IU/L, ALT/AST 62/65 IU/L, total protein 5.7 IU/L, albumin 3.2 mg/dL, and Cr 2.4 mg/dL (spironolactone had been discontinued one month earlier). A large right-sided-pleural effusion with moderate abdominal ascites was noted on examination. He underwent a transjugular intrahepatic portal systemic shunt study (TIPS) and liver biopsy after 100 gm of IV albumin (given for renal dysfunction) with the following results: RA 13 mmHg, FHVP 16 mmHg, WHVP 17 mmHg, and HVPG 1 mmHg (Table 1). The TIPS was aborted due to the normal sinusoidal portal pressure gradient and elevated right-sided pressures. A right heart catheterization 5 hours later revealed RA 13 mm/Hg, PA 57/30 mm/Hg, mean 39 mm/Hg, PWP 20, and C.O 5.5 L/min. Presumptive diagnosis was mild/moderate mixed arterial and venous pulmonary hypertension. The liver biopsy revealed mild sinusoidal dilatation, no inflammation or fibrosis, trace iron deposition and was considered unremarkable, other than mild outflow obstruction (Figure 1). The patient was subsequently referred for a pulmonary work-up as well as a dysphagia evaluation. Pulmonary function tests demonstrated a low DLco 9.33 L, vital capacity 2.75 L, and a repeat heart catheterization after a thoracentesis and paracentesis without albumin: RA 3 mm/Hg, PA 30/10 mm/Hg, mean 18 mm/Hg,

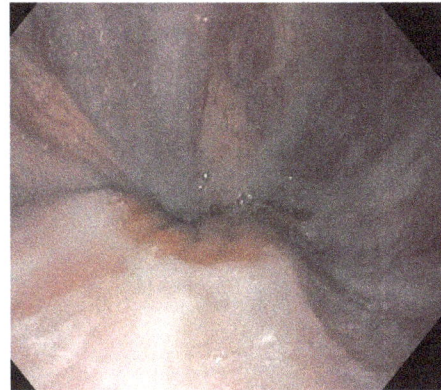

FIGURE 2: Endoscopic view of a trace varix.

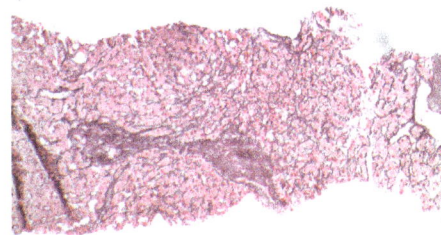

FIGURE 3: (Reticulin, 100x) hepatic parenchyma exhibiting subtle nodularity without significant fibrosis.

and PWP 12 mm/Hg (Table 1). An EGD demonstrated trace esophageal varices (Figure 2). A second interpretation of the liver biopsy noted mild venous outflow obstruction and possibly Nodular Regenerative Hyperplasia (NRH, Figures 3 and 4). Taken together, in the setting of normal right heart pressures and a possible diagnosis of NRH, the patient could have portal hypertension due to a presinusoidal obstruction. He underwent a repeat shunt study this time with direct and indirect portal pressures: RA 2 mm/Hg, FHVP 4 mm/Hg, WHVP 5 mm/Hg, PVP 15 mm/Hg, and portal pressure gradient (PPG = PVP minus FHVP) 11 mm/Hg (Table 1). He successfully underwent a TIPS shunt with a post-TIPS PPG of 7 mm/Hg. Prior to TIPS, the patient underwent 50 thoracenteses and 20 paracenteses over that past year and after TIPS he had 1 thoracentesis/paracentesis 10 days after and none over the past 18 months. Other than mild hepatic encephalopathy, controlled on medication, no other adverse effects have been reported.

3. Discussion

Idiopathic noncirrhotic portal hypertension (INCPH) has been proposed to unify the obliterated vasculopathy that links various etiologies [4]. Five diagnostic criteria must be met to diagnose INCPH: (1) clinical evidence of portal hypertension, (2) absence of cirrhosis or advanced fibrosis on liver biopsy, (3) intrahepatic etiologies of liver disease such as viral hepatitis and fatty liver disease, (4) Sarcoidosis, Schistosomiasis, and congenital hepatic fibrosis, and (5)

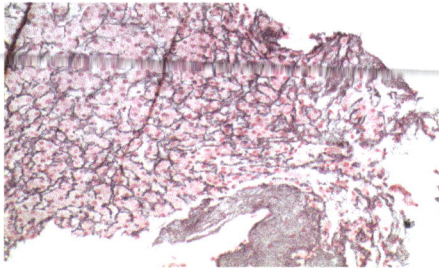

FIGURE 4: (Reticulin, 200x) hepatic plate thinning and compression adjacent to an area of nodularity.

patent portal and hepatic veins [4]. Nodular Regenerative Hyperplasia (NRH) is one subtype of INCPH histologically characterized by liver nodularity, hyperplasia, and no fibrosis [5]. NRH has been associated with many rheumatologic and vascular disorders [6] suggesting a myriad of autoimmune, inflammatory, or neoplastic mechanisms of injury. To date, only 22 cases of Systemic Sclerosis/CREST associated with NRH have been published in a recent systematic review [7].

An initial assessment of ascites and pleural effusions includes a simple diagnostic paracentesis testing the serum-albumin-ascites-gradient (SAAG) and total protein content. In our subject, the SAAG was 1.9 consistent with portal hypertension, and together with a total protein of 3.1 mg/dL both are suggestive for a posthepatic etiology of the ascites [8]. Pulmonary hypertension has been commonly reported in subjects with Systemic Sclerosis [9] and this led to the subject's pulmonary and cardiac evaluation. Why were the posthepatic portal and right heart catheterization pressures on the same day spuriously elevated? We speculate that the albumin infusion immediately prior to these measurements temporarily increased the vascular pressures. Albumin infusions are used prior to a large volume paracentesis to prevent postparacentesis circulatory renal dysfunction especially in subjects with baseline renal impairment [10]. We have recently become aware of two other individuals, in our practice, which had elevated right-sided portal pressures after albumin infusions that were normal without a prior colloid transfusion. Hence, we have altered our practice whereby patients scheduled for portal pressure measurements for refractory ascites warranting prophylactic albumin infusions will undergo a large volume paracentesis several days prior to pressure assessments.

Portal pressure measurements are the primary diagnostic approach to establish the anatomic pathogenesis of portal hypertension [11]. The FHVP should be within a couple of mmHg higher than the RA pressure. The WHVP indirectly estimates the portal pressure and if the difference between the two measurements, called the HVPG, is greater than 6 mmHg, this signifies sinusoidal portal hypertension. Postsinusoidal portal hypertension is defined by an elevated FHVP and WHVP but a normal HVPG. In comparison, presinusoidal portal hypertension cannot be diagnosed by these indirect portal pressure measurements alone, requiring direct calculation of the portal venous system. A clinically significant HVGP is considered $\geq$ 10 mmHg and predicts

the development of ascites or esophageal varices and clinical decompensation in subjects with compensated cirrhosis [12].

The patient's initial portal pressures were consistent with posthepatic portal hypertension. The liver biopsy did not reveal cirrhosis; therefore pulmonary hypertension and mild diastolic dysfunction were determined to be the culprits of the pleural effusions and ascites. However, a subsequent pulmonary evaluation revealed mild pulmonary dysfunction and normal right heart pressures. During this period he had an EGD for dysphagia, and trace esophageal varices were noted. Finally, a repeat interpretation of the liver biopsy suggested NRH. Taking these together, we were suspicious of a presinusoidal etiology for his effusions/ascites and directly measured the portal vein along with indirect measurements. The portal pressure was 15 mmHg and the PPG was 11 mmHg, consistent with portal hypertension; therefore we proceeded with TIPS placement. Ten days after TIPS he needed a single 3-liter thoracentesis and subsequently has not warranted any further thoracentesis or paracentesis over the past 1.5 years. A recent review investigated the outcome of TIPS in 25 subjects with NCPH [13]. NRH was identified in 12 subjects and associated with Scleroderma in only 1 person in this study. Eight of nine NRH individuals had a normal WHVP; all 12 had elevated portal pressures and 9/10 had an elevated HVPG. Indications for TIPS included either esophageal varices or ascites; none of the NRH subjects had hepatic hydrothorax listed as an indication. The long-term outcome over 3 years was very good with 80% functioning TIPS and hepatic encephalopathy was the most common adverse effect.

An international working definition of liver nodules defined NRH in 1995 [14]. It is postulated that the underlying pathogenesis for presinusoidal portal hypertension is obliteration of the small portal venules [15] and abnormal electron dense deposits within the hepatic microcirculation [16]. The immunologic or immunogenetic risk factors for these microvasculopathies are unknown. The association of NRH and Scleroderma has been limited to case reports but the recent systemic review does suggest common clinical manifestations including Raynaud's phenomenon in 19/19 individuals (as did our case), ascites in 6/8, and varices in 10/13 of individuals [7]. Pulmonary information was limited to only 9 subjects with dyspnea; however the exact etiology is unclear and pulmonary hypertension or fibrosis was mentioned. To our knowledge, there are no reported cases of refractory hepatic hydrothorax in the literature as a complication of Systemic Sclerosis and NRH.

In conclusion, this case highlights an unusual presentation of refractory hepatic hydrothorax and ascites due to the combination of Systemic Sclerosis/CREST syndrome causing NRH and presinusoidal portal hypertension that was successfully treated with a TIPS shunt. This case also brings forth the diagnostic awareness that both indirect and direct portal vein measurements are warranted to diagnose presinusoidal portal hypertension.

References

[1] S. Sarin and R. Khanna, "Non-cirrhotic portal hypertension," *Clinics in Liver Disease*, vol. 18, no. 2, pp. 451–476, 2014.

[2] K. M. De Cock, "Hepatosplenic schistosomiasis: A clinical review," *Gut*, vol. 27, no. 6, pp. 734–745, 1986.

[3] P. E. Steiner, "Nodular regenerative hyperplasia of the liver," *American Journal of Pathology*, pp. 943-935, 1959.

[4] J. N. Schouten, J. C. Garcia-Pagan, D. C. Valla, and H. L. A. Janssen, "Idiopathic noncirrhotic portal hypertension," *Hepatology*, vol. 54, no. 3, pp. 1071–1081, 2011.

[5] I. W. Wanless, "Micronodular transformation (nodular regenerative hyperplasia) of the liver: a report of 64 cases among 2,500 autopsies and a new classification of benign hepatocellular nodules," *Hepatology*, vol. 11, no. 5, pp. 787–797, 1990.

[6] M. Hartleb, K. Gutkowski, and P. Milkiewicz, "Nodular regenerative hyperplasia: Evolving concepts on under diagnosed cause of portal hypertension," *World Journal of Gastroenterology*, vol. 17, no. 11, pp. 1400–1409, 2011.

[7] L. Graf, R. Dobrota, S. Jordan, L. M. Wildi, O. Distler, and B. Maurer, "Nodular regenerative hyperplasia of the liver: a rare vascular complication in systemic sclerosis," *The Journal of Rheumatology*, vol. 45, no. 1, pp. 103–106, 2018.

[8] B. A. Runyon, A. A. Montano, E. A. Akriviadis, M. R. Antillon, M. A. Irving, and J. G. McHutchison, "The serum-ascites albumin gradient is superior to the exudate-transudate concept in the differential diagnosis of ascites," *Annals of Internal Medicine*, vol. 117, no. 3, pp. 215–220, 1992.

[9] R. Aithala, A. G. Alex, and D. Danda, "Pulmonary hypertension in connective tissue diseases: an update," *International Journal of Rheumatic Diseases*, vol. 20, no. 1, pp. 5–24, 2017.

[10] F. Wong, "Management of ascites in cirrhosis," *Journal of Gastroenterology and Hepatology*, vol. 27, no. 1, pp. 11–20, 2012.

[11] R. Groszmann, J. D. Vorobioff, and H. Gao, "Measurement of portal pressure: when, how, and why to do it," *Clinics in Liver Disease*, vol. 10, no. 3, pp. 499–512, 2006.

[12] C. Ripoll, R. Groszmann, G. Garcia-Tsao et al., "Hepatic venous pressure gradient predicts clinical decompensation in patients with compensated cirrhosis," *Gastroenterology*, vol. 133, no. 2, pp. 481–488, 2007.

[13] D. Regnault, L. d' Alteroche, and C. Nicolas, "Ten-year experience of transjugular intrahepatic portosystemic shunt for noncirrhotic portal hypertension," *European Journal of Gastroenterology and Hepatology*, 2018.

[14] International Working Party, "Terminology of nodular hepatocellular lesions," *Hepatology*, vol. 22, no. 3, pp. 983–993, 1995.

[15] K. A. Al-Mukhaizeem, A. Rosenberg, and A. H. Sherker, "nodular regenerative hyperplasia of the liver: an under-recognized cause of portal hypertension in hematological disorders," *American Journal of Hematology*, vol. 75, no. 4, pp. 225–230, 2004.

[16] M. L. Russell and H. J. Kahn, "Nodular regenerative hyperplasia of the liver associated with progressive systemic sclerosis: A case report with ultrastructural observation," *The Journal of Rheumatology*, vol. 10, no. 5, pp. 748–752, 1983.

26

Liver Metastases in Pancreatic Acinar Cell Carcinoma Treated with Selective Internal Radiation Therapy with Y-90 Resin Microspheres

Felipe Nasser,[1] Joaquim Maurício Motta Leal Filho,[1] Breno Boueri Affonso,[1] Francisco Leonardo Galastri,[1] Rafael Noronha Cavalcante,[1] Diego Lima Nava Martins,[1] Vanderlei Segatelli,[2] Lilian Yuri Itaya Yamaga,[3] Rene Claudio Gansl,[4] Bernardino Tranchesi Junior,[5] and Antônio Luiz de Vasconcellos Macedo[6]

[1]*Interventional Radiology Unit, Hospital Israelita Albert Einstein, Av. Albert Einstein 627/701, Morumbi, 05652-900 São Paulo, SP, Brazil*
[2]*Pathology Department, Hospital Israelita Albert Einstein, Av. Albert Einstein 627/701, Morumbi, 05652-900 São Paulo, SP, Brazil*
[3]*Nuclear Medicine Unit, Hospital Israelita Albert Einstein, Av. Albert Einstein 627/701, Morumbi, 05652-900 São Paulo, SP, Brazil*
[4]*Oncology Department, Hospital Israelita Albert Einstein, Av. Albert Einstein 627/701, Morumbi, 05652-900 São Paulo, SP, Brazil*
[5]*Cardiology Department, Hospital Israelita Albert Einstein, Av. Albert Einstein 627/701, Morumbi, 05652-900 São Paulo, SP, Brazil*
[6]*General and Oncological Surgery, Hospital Israelita Albert Einstein, Av. Albert Einstein 627/701, Morumbi, 05652-900 São Paulo, SP, Brazil*

Correspondence should be addressed to Joaquim Maurício Motta Leal Filho; jotamauf@yahoo.com.br

Academic Editor: Melanie Deutsch

Background. Pancreatic acinar cell carcinoma (PACC) is a rare tumor. Surgical resection is the treatment of choice when feasible, but there are no clear recommendations for patients with advanced disease. Liver-directed therapy with Y-90 selective internal radiation therapy (SIRT) has been used to treat hepatic metastases from pancreatic tumors. We describe a case of PACC liver metastases treated with SIRT. *Case Report.* 59-year-old man was admitted with an infiltrative, solid lesion in pancreatic tail diagnosed as PACC. Lymph nodes in the hepatic hilum were enlarged, and many metastatic liver nodules were observed. After partial pancreatectomy, the left and right lobes of the liver were separately treated with Y-90 resin microspheres. Follow-up imaging revealed that all hepatic nodules shrank by at least 50%, and 3 nodules disappeared completely. Lipase concentration was 8407 U/L at baseline, rose to 12,705 U/L after pancreatectomy, and declined to 344 U/L after SIRT. Multiple rounds of chemotherapy in the subsequent year shrank the hepatic tumors further; disease then progressed, but a third line of chemotherapy shrank the tumors again, 16 months after SIRT treatment. *Conclusion.* SIRT had a positive effect on liver metastases from PACC. In conjunction with systemic therapy, SIRT can achieve sustained disease control.

1. Introduction

Pancreatic acinar cell carcinoma (PACC) is a rare tumor that accounts for approximately 1% of malignant pancreatic neoplasms [1]. Surgery is the treatment of choice in these patients, particularly for early-stage disease. Chemotherapy and radiotherapy have been used in locally advanced or metastatic disease, but their efficacy has not been studied in controlled, prospective studies, and there are no definitive guidelines for treating advanced PACC [2–4].

Selective internal radiation therapy (SIRT) with yttrium-90 (Y-90) resin microspheres is an alternative treatment for patients with primary or secondary liver malignancies not amenable to resection [5, 6]. During SIRT, radiotherapy is delivered directly to the liver by superselective intra-arterial catheterization. Several studies have reported the safety

TABLE 1: Laboratory examinations of an asymptomatic 59-year-old man with pancreatic acinar cell carcinoma treated with selective internal radiation therapy with Y-90 resin microspheres.

Laboratory measures	Timing of measurement*			
	Before pancreatectomy 08/01/2015	After pancreatectomy 08/13/2015	After first SIRT 09/15/2015	After second SIRT 10/30/2015
Alpha-Fetoprotein, IU/mL (normal range 0.0 to 5.8 IU/mL)	7.1	5.8	11.5	10.3
CEA, ng/mL (normal range 0.52 to 8.90 ng/mL)	1.39	0.78	1.04	2.06
CA 19-9, U/mL (normal range 2.50 to 34.0 U/mL)	1.61	0.60	1.65	1.25
Lipases, U/L (normal range 31 to 186 U/Lg)	8407	12,705	6387	344

CEA, carcinoembryonic antigen; CA, carbohydrate antigen; SIRT, selective internal radiation therapy. *Pancreatectomy was performed on 8/03/2015, first SIRT was performed on 8/14/2015, and second SIRT was performed on 9/18/2015.

and efficacy of SIRT in treating hepatocellular carcinoma, metastatic colorectal cancers, and neuroendocrine tumors [7–9]. SIRT may also benefit patients with other primary or secondary liver tumors, such as cholangiocarcinoma; sarcoma; and metastases from breast, cervical, pancreatic, and lung cancers [10].

In the context of pancreatic cancer, SIRT has been used as a salvage therapy [11, 12] or in combination with systemic therapy [13] to treat hepatic metastases from pancreatic exocrine tumors and neuroendocrine tumors [14, 15]. There are few cases reported in the literature, most of them using SIRT to treat pancreatic adenocarcinoma liver metastases. The response rate (complete or partial response according to mRECIST) described is around 40% and the median overall survival is around 9 months after SIRT [16]. Here, we describe the case of a patient with liver metastases from PACC treated with SIRT. This study was approved by the Institutional Review Board of our Hospital.

2. Case Presentation

A 59-year-old man underwent a transabdominal ultrasound to investigate persistent postprandial abdominal pain and was admitted to the hospital with liver nodules of unknown cause. Most laboratory values were close to normal, including the tumor markers alpha-fetoprotein, carcinoembryonic antigen, and carbohydrate antigen 19-9; however, serum lipase concentrations were elevated (Table 1).

An abdominal, contrast-enhanced computed tomography (CT) scan and magnetic resonance imaging (MRI) showed multiple, unresectable hypovascular liver nodules in both lobes (Figures 1(a) and 1(d)). The largest, in segment V, was 5.3 cm in diameter (Table 2). The scans also showed an infiltrating, poorly delimited, solid lesion in the pancreatic tail that was invading and causing thrombosis of the splenic vein. Lymph nodes in the hepatic hilum were enlarged.

Positron emission tomography- (PET-) CT with 18-fluorodeoxyglucose (18-FDG) showed that the pancreatic and hepatic lesions were hypermetabolic, with a maximum standardized uptake value of 8.5. An ultrasound-guided biopsy of

the largest hepatic nodule was performed on the same day as the PET-CT, and the histopathologic analysis was suspicious for PACC. Whole-body PET-CT with a somatostatin analog (68Ga-DOTATATE) revealed no lesion suggestive of a tumor highly expressing somatostatin receptors, which excluded a diagnosis of well-differentiated neuroendocrine tumors. No extrahepatic metastases were evident.

The tumor board (composed of a clinical oncologist, oncological surgeon, and interventional radiologist) decided to resect the primary tumor and treat the liver metastases with SIRT. Systemic chemotherapy was contraindicated because the patient was living abroad and would not be able to attend follow-up appointments in our country. Pathologic (microscopic examination) analysis of the resected pancreatic body and tail showed that the tumor was characterized by marked cellularity and a paucity of fibrous stroma. The neoplastic cells were arranged in solid nests and in some areas formed an acinar arrangement (Figure 2(a)), with round or oval nuclei, moderate pleomorphism, prominent nucleoli, and eosinophilic granular cytoplasm. The neoplastic cells were focally positive for periodic acid-Schiff (PAS) stain and resistant to diastase digestion. In an immunohistochemical study, the tumor cells were diffusely immunoreactive for CK18 and focally positive for CK7, alpha-1-antitrypsin (Figure 2(b)), and alpha-1-antichymotrypsin. Scattered cells were positive for synaptophysin and chromogranin A. The neoplastic cells were not immunopositive for alpha-fetoprotein.

The patient then underwent SIRT to control the secondary liver lesions. Because of the extent of the liver lesions, SIRT was performed in 2 stages. First, Y-90 resin microspheres (20 to 60 μm, SIR-Spheres; Sirtex Medical Limited, North Sydney, Australia) were delivered to the right hepatic lobe, and 1 month later microspheres were delivered to the left hepatic lobe and a right hepatic artery branch to segments IV/VIII.

In the first SIRT treatment, a pulmonary shunt of 6.5% was detected. We used the Dose Activity Calculator (http://apps01.sirtex.com/smac/) [17, 18] to calculate the appropriate dose and administered a Y-90 dose of 1.36 GBq (37 mCi equivalent) through the right hepatic artery and a

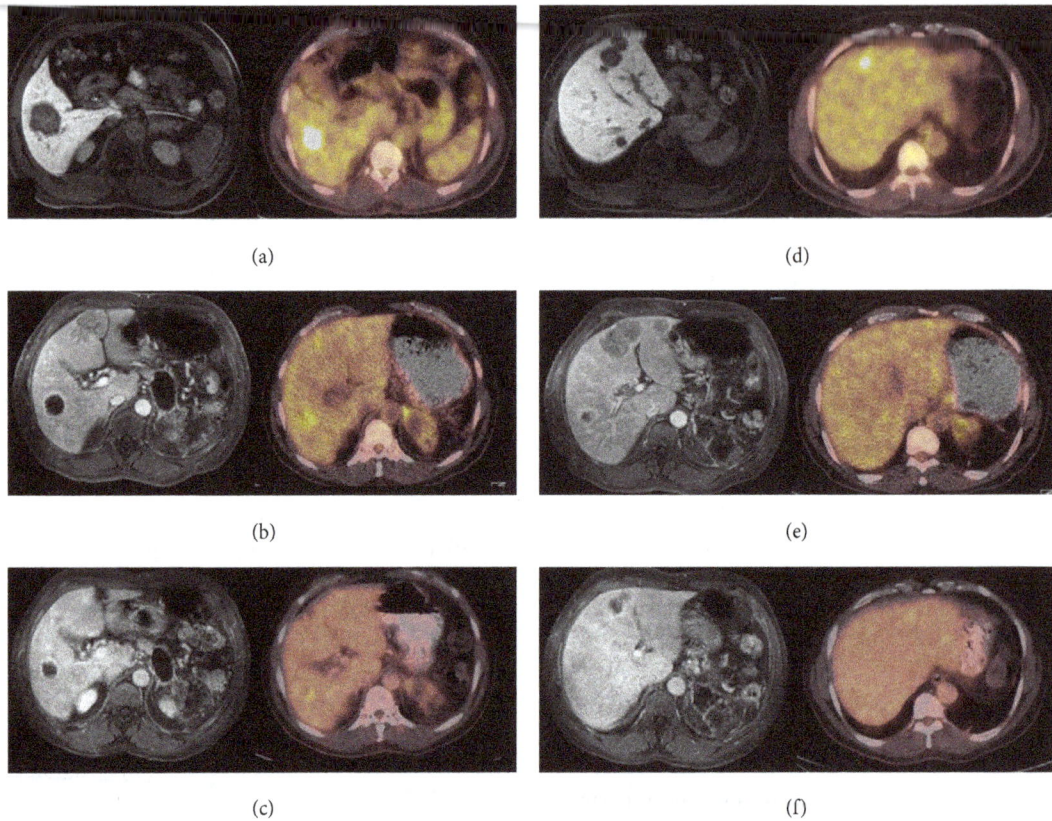

FIGURE 1: Magnetic resonance (MR) and positron emission tomography-computed tomography with 18-fluorodeoxyglucose (18-FDG PET-CT) imaging. (a–c) Axial MR images in the portal phase (left column) and axial 18-FDG PET-CT images (right column) showing the evolution of the largest hypovascular and hypermetabolic liver nodule in the *right lobe*: (a) at admission, (b) 30 days after the first SIRT session, and (c) 45 days after the second SIRT session. (d–f) Axial MR images in the portal phase (left column) and axial 18-FDG PET-CT (right column) showing evolution of the largest hypovascular and hypermetabolic liver nodules in the *left lobe*: (d) at admission, (e) 30 days after the first SIRT session (note that the lesions had grown), and (f) 45 days after the second SIRT session.

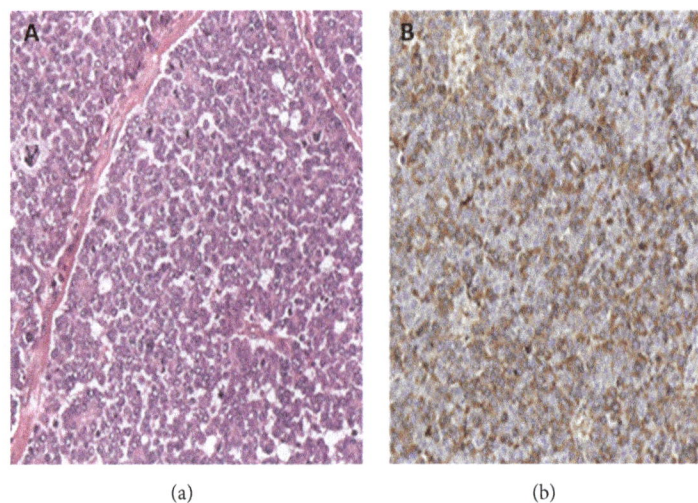

FIGURE 2: Histopathology of the resected pancreas. (a) Neoplasm with a solid acinar architectural microscopic pattern (hematoxylin and eosin, 20x); (b) positive immunostaining (brown; counterstained with hematoxylin and eosin) for alpha-1-antitrypsin in neoplastic cells.

TABLE 2: Measurement of liver nodules on magnetic resonance images before and after selective internal radiation therapy (SIRT) with Y-90 resin microspheres.

Segment & nodules (N)	Nodule size, cm			Reduction in nodule diameter after both SIRT treatments, %
	08/01/2015	09/15/2015	10/30/2015	
Right lobe				
V				
N1	5.3	3.0	2.2	58
VI				
N1	3.2	2.5	1.4	56
VII				
N1	1.1	0.4	0.0	100
N2	1.8	0.7	0.0	100
Left lobe				
IV				
N1	1.3	2.4	1.2	50
N2	2.5	4.2	1.8	57
N3	3.0	4.6	2.4	48
II				
N1	0.5	1.5	0.4	73
N2	0.8	1.2	0.0	100
N3	1.0	2.3	0.9	61
N4	2.7	4.5	2.0	55

dose of 0.34 GBq through the artery branch for segment VIII (part of the nodule in segment IV was being fed by this branch) (Figures 3(a), 3(b), and 3(c)). A follow-up MRI 30 days after the first administration of SIRT showed that the nodules in the treated right lobe of the liver had shrunk, whereas the lesions in the untreated left lobe had grown (Figures 1(b) and 1(e), Table 2).

In the second SIRT treatment, a pulmonary shunt of 5% was detected, and a dose of 0.25 GBq (6.7 mCi) was delivered through the right hepatic artery branch to segments IV and VIII (to treat the remaining portion of segment IV), and 0.65 GBq (17.5 mCi) was delivered through the left hepatic artery (Figures 3(d) and 3(e)). A PET-CT scan 45 days later showed only a slight heterogeneous distribution of 18-FDG in the region of the previously observed lesions (Figures 1(c) and 1(f)), and the maximum standardized uptake value had declined to 4.2 from the pretreatment value of 8.5. A new abdominal MRI performed on the same day showed that the nodules had shrunk in both the right and left lobes (Table 2) [19]. All hepatic nodules were reduced in size by at least 50%, and 3 nodules disappeared, partial response according to mRECIST criteria.

After both SIRT treatments, the patient presented with Grade 1 fatigue that lasted approximately 1 week. Measurement of liver enzymes indicated that no liver damage had occurred (data not shown). Serum lipase concentrations progressively decreased from a high of 12,705 U/L to 344 U/L (Table 1), indicating control of the disease.

The patient returned to the United States, where he has been under the care of an oncologist at the M. D. Anderson Cancer Center in Houston, Texas. Beginning 6 weeks after the second SIRT (November 3, 2015), he was treated with folinic acid-fluorouracil-oxaliplatin (FOLFOX) chemotherapy every 2 weeks for 6 cycles. Imaging on April 7, 2016, showed improvement in the hepatic lesions that did not reach the criteria for a partial response, and the FOLFOX treatment was continued. In July 2016, the hepatic lesions progressed; FOLFOX was discontinued, and chemotherapy with capecitabine was initiated. An abdominal MRI 82 days later showed hepatic lesions of 3.3 cm, 1.2 cm, and 1.0 cm in segment II and a 1.5 cm lesion in segment VII. The volume of the right hepatic lobe had decreased from April 7, and multiple millimeter-sized subcapsular and peritoneal lesions were evident. Chemotherapy with capecitabine was continued. Three weeks later, PET-CT confirmed the hepatic lesions and further indicated peritoneal carcinomatosis and involvement of the abdominal and retroperitoneal lymph nodes. A few days later, a CT-guided biopsy was performed, after which the chemotherapy regimen was changed to chronomodulated bevacizumab plus irinotecan with fluorouracil and folinic acid (FOLFIRI). To date, 2 cycles of bevacizumab plus FOLFIRI have been administered. CT images obtained on December 16, 2016 (490 days after the initial SIRT), indicated that the tumors had shrunk considerably (Figure 4). The patient is still alive today.

3. Discussion

Pancreatic acinar cell carcinoma is a rare neoplasm, representing 1% to 2% of exocrine pancreatic neoplasms in

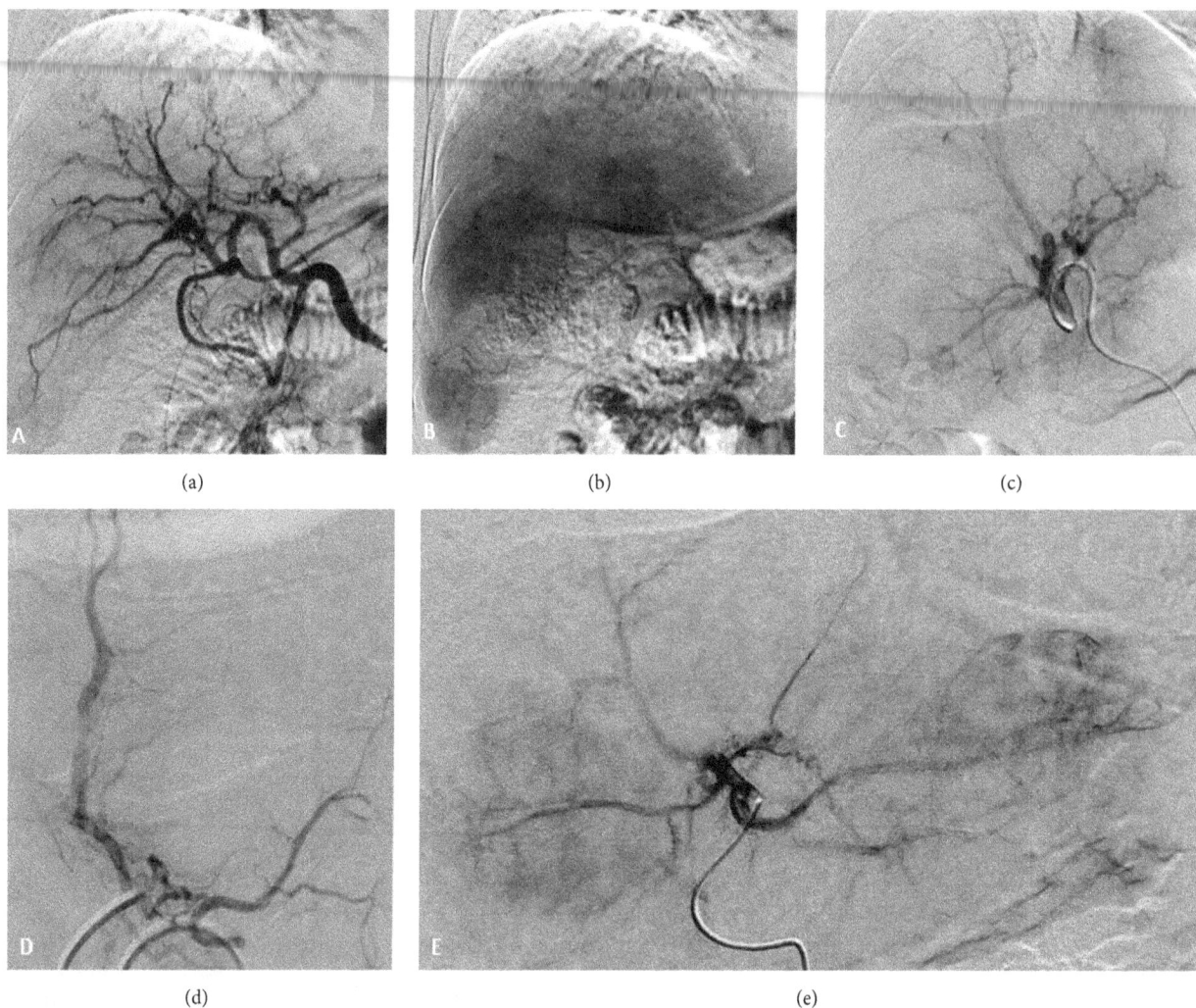

(a)   (b)   (c)

(d)   (e)

FIGURE 3: Digital subtraction angiography: (a) Angiogram showing the anatomy of the common hepatic artery. (b) Late phase showing some of the nodules. (c) Angiogram of the right hepatic artery before SIRT. (d) Catheterization of the arterial branch feeding segments IV/VIII. (e) Angiogram of the left hepatic artery before SIRT.

adults [2]. It occurs more frequently in men, with a peak incidence in the seventh decade of life [2, 3, 20]. Although survival is typically longer with PACC (median 18 to 30 months; 17 months for metastatic disease treated with chemotherapy) than it is with pancreatic ductal adenocarcinoma (a median of 6 months) [3, 20], metastasis is common; indeed, metastases are already present in half of patients at diagnosis, and recurrence has been reported in up to 72% of patients [3, 4].

In PACC, the tumor cells bear a morphological resemblance to acinar cells and express pancreatic enzymes such as trypsin, lipase, chymotrypsin, and amylase [1, 2]. The most common symptoms are abdominal pain and bloating, and 10% to 15% of patients develop lipase hypersecretion syndrome, which elevates blood lipase concentrations and can produce symptoms such as subcutaneous nodules resulting from fat necrosis and polyarthralgia from sclerotic lesions in cancellous bone [1, 2]. In our case, the patient had abdominal

pain, and a diagnostic ultrasound found hepatic nodules of unknown origin. The patient also presented with a high serum lipase concentration of 8407 U/L (Table 1), despite not having clinical symptoms of lipase hypersecretion syndrome.

Surgical resection is associated with longer survival and is therefore always recommended when feasible, although it is rarely curative [3]. In our case, surgical resection of the primary tumor was possible despite the metastatic disease, and the patient underwent partial pancreatectomy (body plus tail). There are no clear recommendations for treating advanced PACC (metastases or locally unresectable tumors). Chemotherapy and radiotherapy have been used, but their effectiveness has been evaluated in only a small number of patients, with mixed results [2–4].

SIRT with Y-90 resin microspheres is a relatively new treatment modality that has been effective in treating liver metastases from several locations, such as the cervix, breast, lung, colon, rectum, and pancreas [7–10]. In 19 patients with

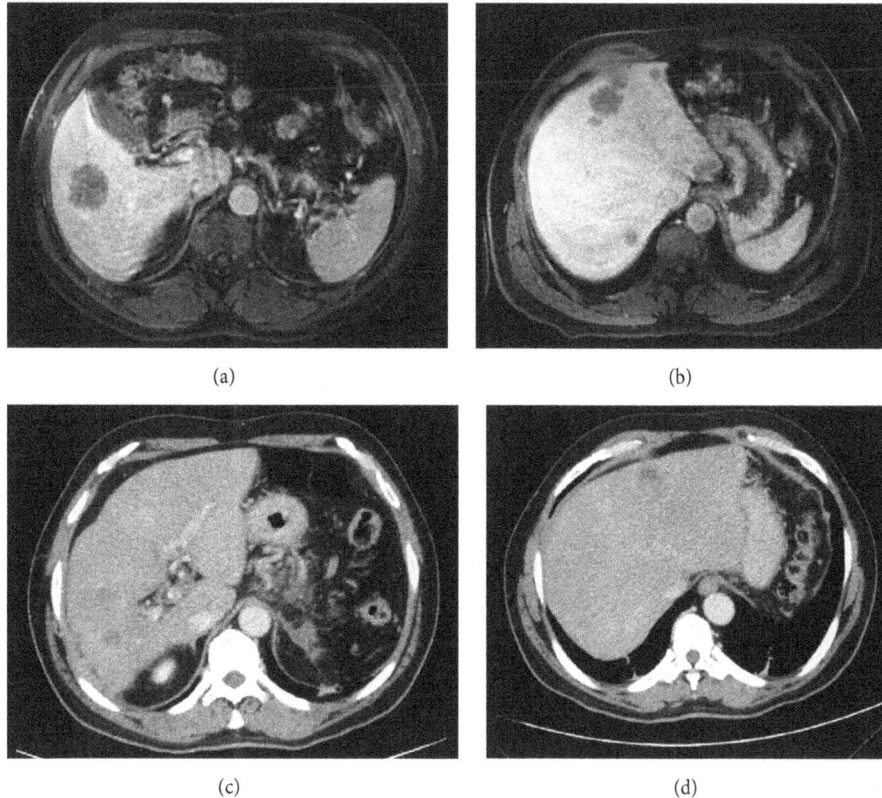

FIGURE 4: Comparison of baseline magnetic resonance imaging (MRI) (August 1, 2015) with computed tomography (CT) imaging performed on December 16, 2016. (a, b) Axial MRI images, portal phase, showing the hepatic nodules in the right (a) and left (b) lobes at admission. (c, d) Axial CT images, portal phase, showing regression of the hepatic nodules in the right (c) and left (d) lobes 15 months after the second SIRT and after several lines of chemotherapy.

liver metastases from pancreatic cancer, SIRT, used as salvage therapy, was associated with an objective response in the liver of 47% and a median overall survival of 9 months after treatment [11]. SIRT combined with systemic chemotherapy demonstrated 31% of partial response and 38% stable disease in the liver assessed using mRECIST; the median overall survival was 12.5 months after SIRT [13]. Fidelman and colleagues in a series of 3 cases of pancreatic tumors treated with SIRT verified that a patient with solid and papillary epithelial neoplasm (SAPEN) of the pancreas with hypervascular hepatic lesions at angiography got partial response assessed using mRECIST. On the other hand, patient with pancreatic adenocarcinoma did not respond to SIRT [15]. Recently, Michl et al. evaluated (pancreatic adenocarcinoma liver metastases treated with SIRT) tumor response according to PET Response Criteria In Solid Tumors (PERCIST). They found 35% of complete response, 6% of partial response, and 59% of disease progression. And the median overall survival was 8.8 months [21]. However, none of these patients had PACC.

In our patient, imaging showed multiple hypovascular liver nodules in both lobes, with no extrahepatic metastases, suggesting that he would be a good candidate for SIRT to attempt control of the liver disease. Follow-up imaging after SIRT revealed that the treatment was effective: all hepatic nodules were reduced in size by at least 50%, and 3 nodules disappeared (partial response according to mRECIST criteria).

Lipase hypersecretion syndrome occurs in a minority of patients with PACC, often in association with hepatic metastases, but can resolve with treatment [2]. Our patient's serum lipase concentrations decreased markedly after treatment with SIRT (Table 1). Considering that the lipase concentrations rose rather than fell after partial pancreatectomy, we attribute this finding to the efficacy of SIRT with Y-90 resin microspheres in reducing the burden of the liver metastases.

Chemotherapy with FOLFOX initiated after the SIRT initially shrank the tumors further, but the patient's disease subsequently progressed. Capecitabine treatment did not reverse the progression; however, 2 cycles of chronomodulated bevacizumab plus FOLFIRI dramatically shrank the tumors again, as shown with CT imaging 16 months after the first SIRT treatment.

SIRT was successful in reducing the burden of hepatic metastases from PACC; however multiple lines of systemic chemotherapy were needed to sustain the improvement as to treat also the lymph nodes at the hepatic hilum.

Acknowledgments

The authors thank Naomi Ruff, Ph.D., of Eubio Medical Communications LLC for providing medical editing support, funded and provided by Sirtex Medical Ltd.

References

[1] A. L. Mulkeen, P. S. Yoo, and C. Cha, "Less common neoplasms of the pancreas," *World Journal of Gastroenterology*, vol. 12, no. 20, pp. 3180–3185, 2006.

[2] P. Chaudhary, "Acinar cell carcinoma of the pancreas: a literature review and update," *Indian Journal of Surgery*, vol. 77, no. 3, pp. 226–231, 2015.

[3] K. D. Holen, D. S. Klimstra, A. Hummer et al., "Clinical characteristics and outcomes from an institutional series of acinar cell carcinoma of the pancreas and related tumors," *Journal of Clinical Oncology*, vol. 20, no. 24, pp. 4673–4678, 2002.

[4] M. A. Lowery, D. S. Klimstra, J. Shia et al., "Acinar cell carcinoma of the pancreas: New genetic and treatment insights into a rare malignancy," *Oncologist*, vol. 16, no. 12, pp. 1714–1720, 2011.

[5] L. Bester, B. Meteling, N. Pocock, A. Saxena, T. C. Chua, and D. L. Morris, "Radioembolisation with Yttrium-90 microspheres: An effective treatment modality for unresectable liver metastases," *Journal of Medical Imaging and Radiation Oncology*, vol. 57, no. 1, pp. 72–80, 2013.

[6] R. J. Lewandowski, J.-F. Geschwind, E. Liapi, and R. Salem, "Transcatheter intraarterial therapies: Rationale and overview," *Radiology*, vol. 259, no. 3, pp. 641–657, 2011.

[7] S. A. Gulec, K. Pennington, J. Wheeler et al., "Yttrium-90 microsphere-selective internal radiation therapy with chemotherapy (Chemo-SIRT) for colorectal cancer liver metastases: An in vivo double-arm-controlled phase II trial," *American Journal of Clinical Oncology: Cancer Clinical Trials*, vol. 36, no. 5, pp. 455–460, 2013.

[8] E. W. Lee, A. S. Thakor, B. A. Tafti, and D. M. Liu, "Y90 Selective Internal Radiation Therapy," *Surgical Oncology Clinics of North America*, vol. 24, no. 1, pp. 167–185, 2015.

[9] A. Saxena, T. C. Chua, L. Bester, A. Kokandi, and D. L. Morris, "Factors predicting response and survival after yttrium-90 radioembolization of unresectable neuroendocrine tumor liver metastases: A critical appraisal of 48 cases," *Annals of Surgery*, vol. 251, no. 5, pp. 910–916, 2010.

[10] N. Khajornjiraphan, N. A. Thu, and P. K. Chow, "Yttrium-90 microspheres: a review of its emerging clinical indications," *Liver Cancer*, vol. 4, no. 1, pp. 6–15, 2015.

[11] M. Michl, A. R. Haug, T. F. Jakobs et al., "Radioembolization with yttrium-90 microspheres (SIRT) in pancreatic cancer patients with liver metastases: efficacy, safety and prognostic factors," *Oncology*, vol. 86, no. 1, pp. 24–32, 2014.

[12] T. X. Yang, T. C. Chua, and D. L. Morris, "Radioembolization and chemoembolization for unresectable neuroendocrine liver metastases - A systematic review," *Surgical Oncology*, vol. 21, no. 4, pp. 299–308, 2012.

[13] A. Y. Kim, K. Unger, H. Wang, and M. J. Pishvaian, "Incorporating Yttrium-90 trans-arterial radioembolization (TARE) in the treatment of metastatic pancreatic adenocarcioma: a single center experience," *BMC Cancer*, vol. 16, no. 1, article 492, 2016.

[14] J. M. Loree, T. Hiruki, and H. F. Kennecke, "Case report of cirrhosis following yttrium-90 radioembolization for pancreatic neuroendocrine liver metastases," *Case Reports in Oncology*, vol. 9, no. 1, pp. 76–82, 2016.

[15] N. Fidelman, R. K. Kerlan, R. A. Hawkins et al., "Radioembolization with 90Y glass microspheres for the treatment of unresectable metastatic liver disease from chemotherapy-refractory gastrointestinal cancers. Final report of a prospective pilot study," *Journal of Gastrointestinal Oncology*, vol. 7, no. 6, pp. 860–874, 2016.

[16] A. Gordon, O. Uddin, A. Riaz, R. Salem, and R. Lewandowski, "Making the case: intra-arterial therapy for less common metastases," *Seminars in Interventional Radiology*, vol. 34, no. 02, pp. 132–139, 2017.

[17] A. Kennedy, S. Nag, and R. Salem, "Recommendations for radioembolization of hepatic malignancies using yttrium-90 microsphere brachytherapy: a consensus panel report from the radioembolization brachytherapy oncology consortium," *International Journal of Radiation Oncology, Biology, Physics*, vol. 68, no. 1, pp. 13–23, 2007.

[18] *SIR-Spheres® microspheres (Yttrium-90 Microspheres)*, Sirtex Medical Limited, North Sydney, New South Wales, Australia, 2014.

[19] E. A. Eisenhauer, P. Therasse, J. Bogaerts et al., "New response evaluation criteria in solid tumours: revised RECIST guideline (version 1.1)," *European Journal of Cancer*, vol. 45, no. 2, pp. 228–247, 2009.

[20] L. Tian, X. F. Lv, J. Dong et al., "Clinical features and CT/MRI findings of pancreatic acinar cell carcinoma," *International Journal of Clinical and Experimental Medicine*, vol. 8, no. 9, pp. 14846–14854, 2015.

[21] M. Michl, S. Lehner, P. M. Paprottka et al., "Use of PERCIST for prediction of progression-free and overall survival after radioembolization for liver metastases from pancreatic cancer," *Journal of Nuclear Medicine*, vol. 57, no. 3, pp. 355–360, 2016.

27

Retrospective Identification of Herpes Simplex 2 Virus-Associated Acute Liver Failure in an Immunocompetent Patient Detected Using Whole Transcriptome Shotgun Sequencing

Atsushi Ono,[1,2] **C. Nelson Hayes,**[1,2] **Sakura Akamatsu,**[1,2] **Michio Imamura,**[1,2] **Hiroshi Aikata,**[1,2] **and Kazuaki Chayama**[1,2,3]

[1]*Department of Gastroenterology and Metabolism, Applied Life Sciences, Institute of Biomedical & Health Science,
 Hiroshima University, Hiroshima, Japan*
[2]*Liver Research Project Center, Hiroshima University, Hiroshima, Japan*
[3]*Laboratory for Digestive Diseases, SNP Research Center, The Institute of Physical and Chemical Research (RIKEN), Hiroshima, Japan*

Correspondence should be addressed to Kazuaki Chayama; chayama@hiroshima-u.ac.jp

Academic Editor: Fumio Imazeki

Acute liver failure (ALF) is a severe condition in which liver function rapidly deteriorates in individuals without prior history of liver disease. While most cases result from acetaminophen overdose or viral hepatitis, in up to a third of patients, no clear cause can be identified. Liver transplantation has greatly reduced mortality among these patients, but 40% of patients recover without liver transplantation. Therefore, there is an urgent need for rapid determination of the etiology of acute liver failure. In this case report, we present a case of herpes simplex 2 virus- (HSV-) associated ALF in an immunocompetent patient. The patient recovered without LT, but the presence of HSV was not suspected at the time, precluding more effective treatment with acyclovir. To determine the etiology, stored blood samples were analyzed using whole transcriptome shotgun sequencing followed by mapping to a panel of viral reference sequences. The presence of HSV-DNA in blood samples at the time of admission was confirmed using real-time polymerase chain reaction, and, at the time of discharge, HSV-DNA levels had decreased by a factor of 10^6. *Conclusions.* In ALF cases of undetermined etiology, uncommon causes should be considered, especially those for which an effective treatment is available.

1. Introduction

Acute liver failure (ALF), also called fulminant hepatic failure, is a rare but life-threatening condition characterized by sudden deterioration of liver function and associated with coagulopathy (international normalized ratio ≥ 1.5) and hepatic encephalopathy [1, 2]. Mortality among ALF patients is high, often resulting from multiorgan failure and brain stem decompression due to cerebral edema [3]. ALF implies that the patient had no prior history of liver disease or cirrhosis [2], providing few clues to the underlying etiology, and the rapid onset and difficulty of identification at the earliest stages may lead to delays in the start of treatment. Nonspecific treatments have limited effectiveness, and ALF accounts for

about 7% of liver transplantations [1]. However, spontaneous recovery is observed in up to 45% of ALF patients, and specific treatments for known etiologies can be effective [3]. Acetaminophen overdose is the most common cause of ALF in the United States and Europe, whereas viral hepatitis is more common in Asia and Africa, but numerous other causes have been reported, including drug-induced liver injury, viral hepatitis, ischemic liver injury, Wilson's disease, and acute presentation of autoimmune hepatitis [4, 5]. Aside from hepatitis viruses A, B, and E, other viruses including parvovirus B19, SEN virus, echovirus 18, and several members of the Herpesviridae (e.g., herpes simplex, herpes zoster, Epstein-Barr, and cytomegalovirus) have been reported to cause ALF in rare cases [6–9]. Optimal treatments can differ widely among these etiologies, but, in at least 15% of cases, the etiology cannot be adequately determined, and treatment choices must made based on incomplete information [3]. However, treatment of ALF could be improved by retrospective analysis of cases of ALF with uncertain etiology to establish the risk factors and clinical presentation of these etiologies to aid in future diagnosis. Improvements in rapid sequencing methodology might soon even make it possible to use real-time benchtop sequencing as a diagnostic tool [10, 11]. In this report, we describe an instructive case in which a more effective treatment could have been selected if less common etiologies had been considered upon admission.

Herpes simplex virus (HSV) infection is an uncommon cause of ALF that typically occurs following reactivation as a result of pregnancy or immunosuppression [13–15]. Therefore, it is rarely identified until after death or liver transplantation (LT) [13]. Here, we present a case of HSV-associated ALF in an immunocompetent patient who recovered without LT. We also suggest the usefulness of next generation RNA sequencing and real-time polymerase chain reaction of stored blood samples for retrospective identification of pathogens causing ALF from stored blood samples.

2. Case Presentation

A previously healthy 18-year-old Japanese female initially presented to her local hospital with fever and pharyngodynia. She reported that she had not had sexual intercourse within the previous 6 months. Based on physical findings, including fever and presence of swollen tonsils with white pus-filled spots, as well as laboratory findings that revealed liver dysfunction (AST: 373 IU/L, ALT: 461 IU/L) and inflammatory status (white blood cell count: 18600 μ/L, CRP: 5.4 mg/dL), a diagnosis of infectious mononucleosis was made. She was hospitalized, and treatment with 200 mg/day of minocycline and 300 mg/day of hydrocortisone was started. The next day, she exhibited symptoms of right abdominal pain, and computed tomography (CT) scan revealed ascites. The diagnosis of Fitz-Hugh-Curtis Syndrome was suspected, and treatment of 2 g/day of azithromycin was initiated. However, she presented with worsening of liver function. Drug-induced liver injury was suspected, and all antibiotics were discontinued. After withdrawal of the drugs, she presented with coagulopathy and further worsening of liver function tests, wherein she was transferred to our hospital.

On admission to our hospital, the patient's mental status was Glasgow coma scale (GCS) 13 (eye opening: 3; verbal response: 4; best motor response: 6), hepatic encephalopathy grade 2, and her body temperature was 38.1°C. Other vital signs were stable as follows: blood pressure 114/67 mmHg, heart rate 88 bpm, SpO2 99% in room air, and respiratory rate 17/min. No skin abnormalities were identified. A laboratory analysis revealed severe liver dysfunction, coagulopathy, inflammation, thrombocytopenia, and anemia (Table 1).

An abdominal and chest dynamic contrast-enhanced CT scan revealed periportal collar sign, splenomegaly, and a small amount of ascites and pleural effusion (Figure 1). No obvious hepatic atrophy was observed. The patient was diagnosed with ALF based on criteria published by the Ministry

TABLE 1: Laboratory data at time of admission.

Hematologic test	
White blood cells (/μL)	3740
Neutrophils (%)	80
Lymphocytes (%)	6
Monocytes (%)	4
Eosinophils (%)	0
Basophils (%)	0
Red blood cells ($\times 10^4$/μL)	3.12
Hemoglobin (g/dL)	9.3
Platelet count ($\times 10^4$/μL)	1.1
Coagulation	
Prothrombin time (%)	17
Prothrombin time-INR	2.92
Chemistry	
Aspartate aminotransferase (IU/L)	8676
Alanine aminotransferase (IU/L)	5114
Total bilirubin (mg/dL)	4.3
Direct bilirubin (mg/dL)	2.7
Alkaline phosphatase (IU/L)	480
Lactate dehydrogenase (IU/L)	9120
γ-Glutamyltranspeptidase (IU/L)	206
Blood urea nitrogen (mg/dL)	6
Creatinine (mg/dL)	0.5
C-reactive protein (mg/dL)	3.06
Procalcitonin (ng/mL)	0.15
Total protein (g/dL)	5.3
Albumin (g/dL)	2.7
Sodium (mmol/L)	136
Chloride (mmol/L)	92
Potassium (mmol/L)	3.4
Ferritin (ng/mL)	34780
Copper (μg/dL)	53
Ceruloplasmin (mg/dL)	19
Ammonia (μmol/L)	17
IgG (mg/dL)	1028
IgM (mg/dL)	210
IgA (mg/dL)	206
Anti-nuclear antibodies (<)	×80
Hepatitis B surface antigen (IU/mL)	0.02
Hepatitis B core antibodies (COI)	0.1
Hepatitis C virus antibodies (COI)	0.1
IgM-hepatitis A virus antibodies	<0.4
Epstein-Barr virus	
Anti-VCA IgG	80
Anti-VCA IgM	<10
Anti-VCA IgA	<10
Anti-EBNA antibodies	40
Cytomegalovirus	
IgG (−)	26
IgM (−)	(−)
HIV-1,2 antibodies	(−)

COI: cut-off index; INR: international normalized ratio.

of Health, Labour, and Welfare of Japan [5, 16], although the etiology was unknown (drug-induced ALF was suspected).

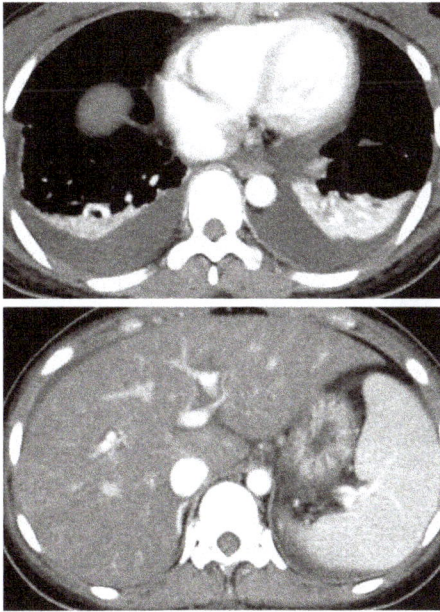

FIGURE 1: Dynamic contrast-enhanced CT scan.

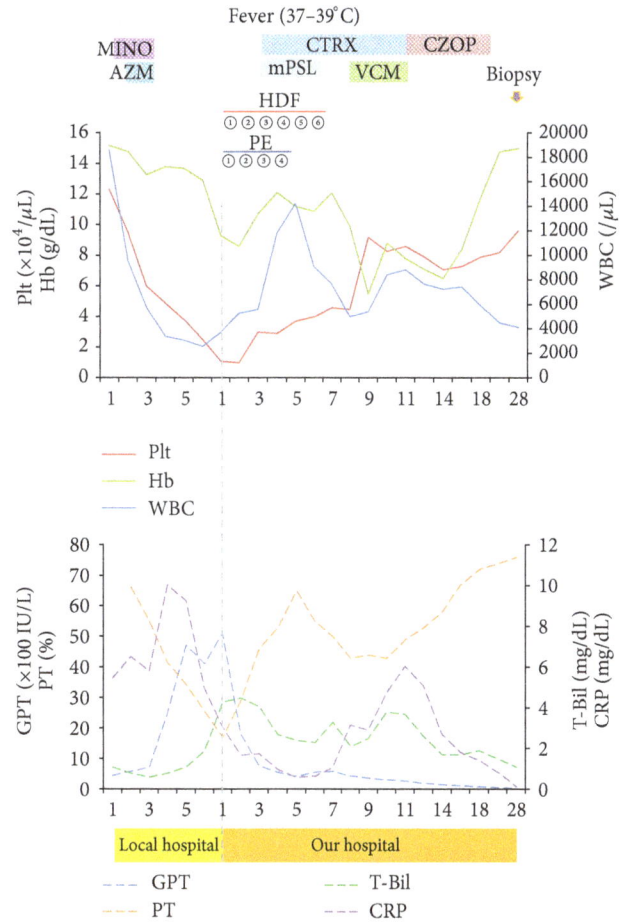

FIGURE 2: The patient's clinical course. MINO: minocycline, AZM: azithromycin, CTRX: ceftriaxone, VCM: vancomycin, CZOP: cefozopran; mPSL: methylprednisolone sodium succinate.

The patient was treated six times with hemodialysis filtration (HDF) and four times with peritoneal dialysis (Figure 2). Although the origin of the fever was not determined, infectious disease was suspected, and the patient was treated with antibiotics as shown in Figure 2. Liver needle biopsy was performed on day 29. Histopathological findings showed piecemeal necrosis and nuclear inclusion bodies (Figure 3(a)). Neither extensive necrosis nor obvious parenchymal hepatocytes or liver fibrosis was observed. The pathological diagnosis of a fragment of liver tissue indicated periportal hepatocellular loss and regenerative bile duct (Figure 3(b)). Focal necrosis accompanied by lymphocyte infiltration and eosinophilic body is scarcely recognized in the hepatocytes in the lobule. Some of the hepatocytes around the Gleason sheath are accompanied by piecemeal necrosis and show extensive shedding, but the reconstructed image is poor. The appearance of multinucleated hepatocytes is observed at another site in the leaflet. The Gleason sheath is fibrillary in part with mild infiltration of chronic inflammatory cells and mild neutrophil infiltration. Aggregation of regenerated bile ducts was observed. No cholestasis was apparent in hepatocytes or bile ducts. These findings appear to be consistent with acute liver injury.

The patient recovered from ALF and was discharged from the hospital on day 30.

2.1. RNA Sequencing.
In order to reveal the cause of her liver failure, we retrospectively screened her stored blood samples by RNA sequencing for the presence of viral RNA. The patient provided written informed consent, and the study was performed in accordance with the World Medical Association Declaration of Helsinki and with the approval of the local ethics committee. RNA-Seq, also called whole transcriptome shotgun sequencing, involves isolation of sample RNA, depletion of ribosomal RNA, and synthesis of cDNA, which is then sequenced using next generation sequencing technology. RNA was extracted from stored blood samples, and fragmented RNA was linked with RNA $3'$ adapter. Reverse transcription and polymerase chain reaction were performed using single-stranded cDNA templates. Sequencing was performed using the HiSEQ 2500 platform (Illumina, Tokyo, Japan) using paired end reads. Reads were trimmed using Trimmomatic (version 0.36), and quality scores were examined before and after trimming using FastQC (version 0.11.3). Bowtie2 [17] was used to map the RNA reads against 7,195 sequences from the viral RefSeq collection downloaded from the National Center for Biotechnology Information (downloaded on April 17, 2016). All sequence analysis was performed on the Shirokane 3 supercomputer at the University of Tokyo.

2.2. Results of RNA Mapping.
Results of Bowtie2 mapping revealed matches against three viral RefSeq sequences: NC_022518.1 (human endogenous retrovirus K113: 164 reads), NC_023677.1 (chimpanzee alpha-1 herpesvirus strain 105650: 264 reads), and NC_001798.2 (human herpesvirus 2 strain HG52: 270,696 reads). After remapping, 1,216,468 out of a total of 139,632,418 reads (0.87%) mapped to the NC_001798.2

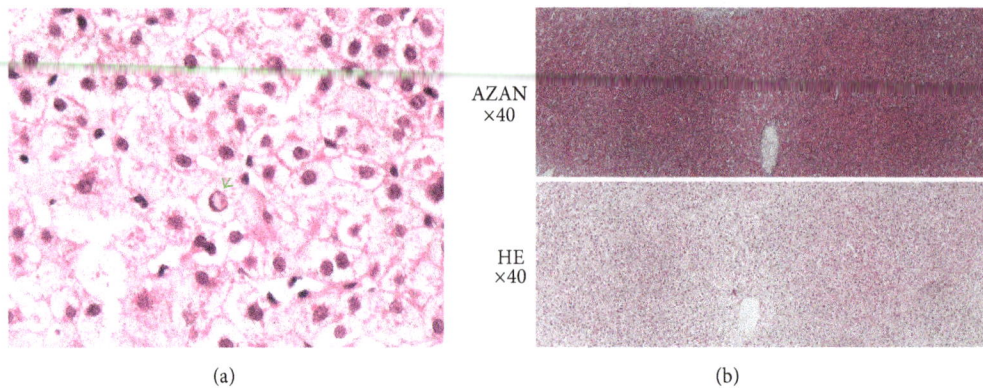

(a)   (b)

FIGURE 3: Findings of liver needle biopsy. (a) The arrow indicates a nuclear inclusion body. (b) Low magnification (×40) of a liver fragment with HE and AZAN staining.

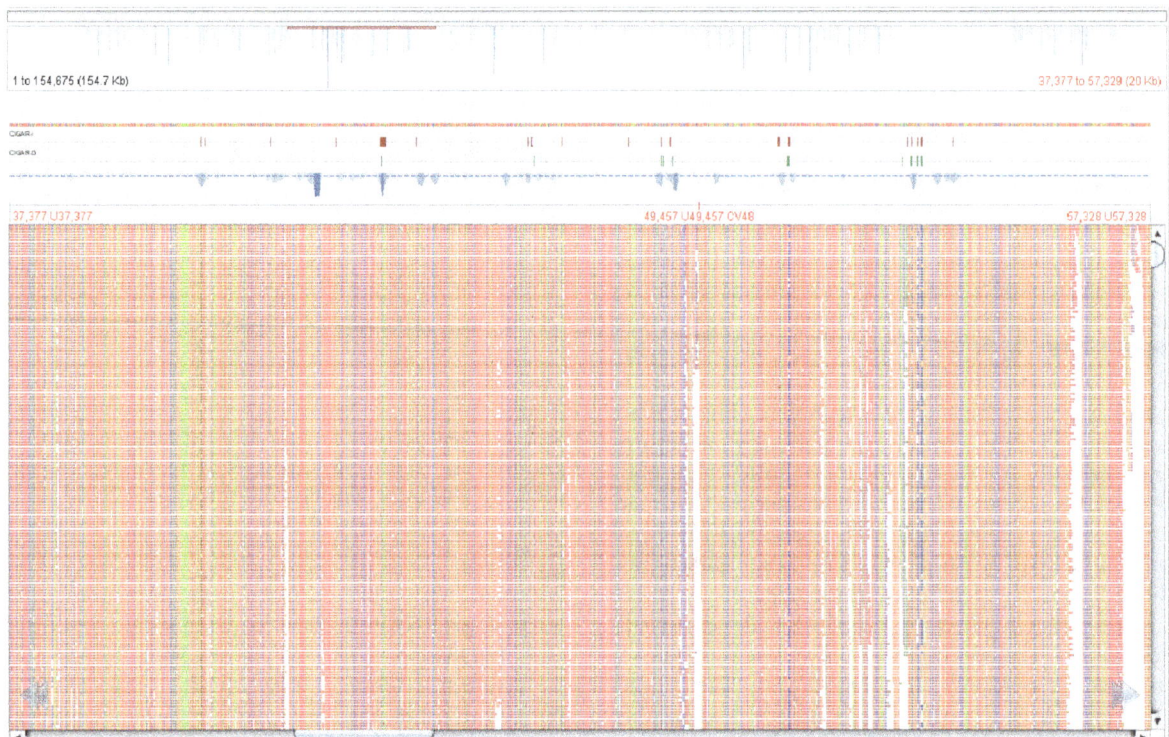

FIGURE 4: Alignment of patient serum RNA against human herpesvirus 2 reference genome. Reads were aligned using Bowtie2 and displayed using Tablet viewer [12].

human herpesvirus 2 reference genome, overlapping 80% of the 154,657 nt reference sequence with an average coverage depth of 768 and a maximum coverage depth of 6,991 (Figure 4).

2.3. Quantification of HSV-DNA. Based on the results of read mapping, real-time PCR was used to retrospectively quantify relative HSV-DNA levels in stored blood samples. DNA was extracted from 100 μL of serum (day 1 and day 2) and plasma (day 28) using SMI-TEST (Genome Science Laboratories, Tokyo, Japan) according to the manufacturer's instructions and dissolved in 20 μL of distilled water. Real-time PCR analysis was performed using the Mx300P System (Applied

Biosystems, Foster City, CA) according to the instructions provided by the manufacturer. We prepared 10 μL of Brilliant III Ultra-Fast SYBR Green QPCR Master Mix with Low ROX (Agilent Technologies, Santa Clara, CA), 100 nM of forward primer: TCAGCCCATCCTCCTTCGGCAGTA (target: Glycoprotein G, Nucleotide position: 138240–138262; derived from GenBank accession number Z86099), 100 nM of reverse primer: CGCGCGGTCCCAGATCGGCA (target: Glycoprotein G, Nucleotide position: 138398–138380), 2 μL of DNA, and 7.6 μL of distilled water. The cycling program was as follows: the sample was heated for 3 minutes at 95°C for denaturing, followed by a PCR cycling program consisting of 40 two-step cycles of 5 seconds at 95°C and 20 seconds at

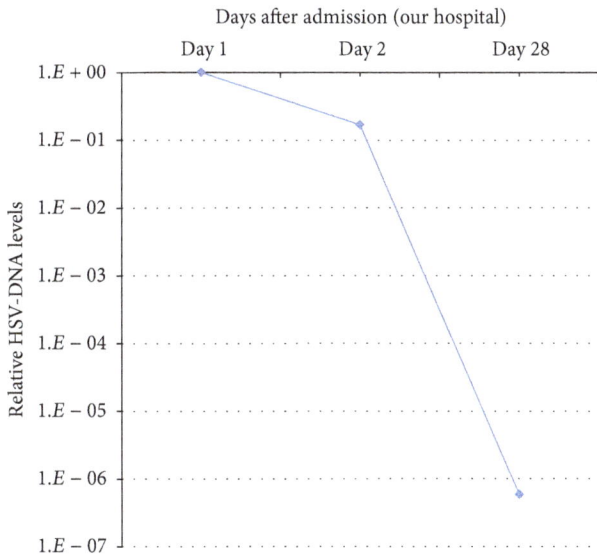

FIGURE 5: Relative HSV-DNA levels on days 1, 2, and 28. HSV-DNA levels decreased to lower than 10^{-6} from day 1 to day 28.

60°C. RT-PCR analysis confirmed the presence of HSV-DNA in the patient's blood samples at the time of admission and revealed that HSV-DNA levels had decreased by a factor of 10^{-6} between days 1 and 28 (Figure 5), shortly after which the patient was discharged. Acute HSV infection in this patient was also confirmed by a positive test for HSV-IgM antibody (8.6: normal range, <0.8) measured using stored serum samples.

3. Discussion

Although acute liver failure can result from several conditions, including viral hepatitis, drug-induced liver injury, and autoimmune hepatitis, in many cases the underlying cause cannot be conclusively determined. However, prognosis for this condition is poor, and failure to identify the cause may prevent selection of an effective treatment [15]. The findings presented here indicate that the patient had an undiagnosed acute HSV infection on admission to our hospital. Acute HSV infection in this patient was also confirmed by the presence of HSV-IgM antibody. HSV-2 is sexually transmitted, resulting in a lifelong, incurable infection and recurrent outbreaks of genital herpes. However, we can only speculate on when and how the patient was infected, and, considering that the patient was underage, it is unclear if she was unaware of the nature of the infection or perhaps reluctant to report it. We acknowledge this as a limitation of our study. Because HSV is an uncommon cause of ALF in nonimmunosuppressed and nonpregnant patients, the diagnosis of HSV infection was not considered during the acute phase in the case we presented. Although she was fortunately able to recover, diagnosis of HSV infection and antiviral treatment should have been initiated as soon as possible. Hence, the patient presented here was an instructive case that cautioned us to acknowledge the need to suspect HSV infection in patients with ALF even when the patient is neither pregnant nor immunosuppressed,

especially among patients who may be unwilling to self-report the condition.

HSV-associated hepatitis has been reported previously, but diagnosis of HSV hepatitis is complicated by the lack of specific clinical indications [13–15]. Early reports focused on HSV-related liver failure in neonates and children, and the patient described in the first report of HSV hepatitis in adults was a pregnant woman with several exacerbating factors, including hyperemesis gravidarum and treatment with tetracycline and stelazine [14]. In a more recent study of 5 cases of HSV-related ALF, 4 of the patients were immunosuppressed, and three of the patients were superinfected with HSV1 or HBV [15]. Three patients underwent liver transplantation. Two patients died within three days of admission, and the remaining patients died within a year after transplantation. Each of the patients presented with fever but without skin lesions, and HSV was not initially suspected. The most similar case is a recent report of HSV-associated ALF in an immunocompetent adult following a tongue piercing who presented with worsening fever and inflammation around the piercing site [13]. The patient died while in preparation for liver transplantation. HSV infection was detected during postmortem examination. These diverse cases have few features in common other than fever but together highlight the difficulty of diagnosis as well as the high mortality and rapid progression of HSV-associated ALF.

The case presented here also shows the potential for next generation sequencing technologies in diagnosis of cases of ALF of unclear etiology. Although the etiologies of many cases of ALF remain indeterminate, analysis of stored blood or tissue samples may retrospectively help to identify the cause, which may in turn help to improve diagnosis and treatment of ALF in future cases. In the simplest case, direct sequencing using PCR primers can be used to identify suspected viral pathogens. Next generation sequencing using mapping against a reference panel can also be used to identify suspected as well as unsuspected pathogens, and de novo assembly could be used to identify novel viruses following subtraction of host reads [18].

Accurate identification of the etiology using unbiased methods is important to establish and confirm an association between risk factors and clinical outcome. Early reports implicated viruses such as TTV and GBV-C as potential causes of hepatitis, but later studies have failed to identify an association between the presence of these viruses and acute hepatitis and ALF [19–21]. However, it remains possible that other viruses have yet to be identified. Retrospective sequence analysis will help to establish the role of these and other viruses in the etiology of ALF. Sequence data can also be mapped against the human genome and used to measure differential gene expression relative to healthy controls [22]. Microarrays could also be used for this purpose and compared against publically available expression data [23, 24]. Establishment of gene expression profiles from patients with ALF of known etiology might reveal useful biomarkers that could facilitate diagnosis and lead to more effective treatment.

While the sequencing and mapping approach described here is neither appropriate nor intended for diagnosis of patients in real time, given the urgency of decisions that must be made following admission as well as the costs and time required for sample preparation and analysis. However, the speed and affordability of next generation sequencing platforms is continuously improving, and systems such as the MinION Nanopore sequencer and its competitors are designed to support low-cost, real-time, long read benchtop sequencing of viral and plasmid genomes to rapidly identify viral pathogens or detect antibiotic resistance genes in clinical isolates [10, 11]. There is an urgent need for such systems to be able to respond effectively during outbreaks. By exchanging a measure of accuracy for a much faster turnaround time, cutting edge sequencing tools claim to achieve adequate sequencing results within 20 minutes with a laboratory prep time of only 10 minutes.

Even when sequencing results are already available, sequence identification using BLAST or mapping to a panel of reference genomes is a time-consuming and computationally demanding step, especially when the sample contains mainly human DNA or RNA. However, again by sacrificing accuracy for speed, kmer-based tools such as Taxonomer are able to perform rapid taxonomic profiling of reads using a web-based interface in real time [25]. The software begins classifying the reads while the raw fastq sequencing files are still uploading and can report a rough taxonomic classification down to genus or even species level within several minutes based on a random sample of reads. The combination of rapid sequencing methods with real-time classification methods sets the stage for a new era of informed diagnosis, although it is unclear when these methods will become routinely used in clinical practice.

Although the patient described here recovered without liver transplantation, the outcome might have been different, and had HSV infection been considered as a cause, effective antiviral treatment could have been started promptly. By reevaluating the etiology of unsolved ALF cases using next generation sequencing, we hope to identify overlooked causes in order to improve treatment for future patients. Next generation sequencing provides an unbiased method to detect agents not diagnosed at presentation and might also be useful in identifying unknown viruses.

Abbreviations

ALF: Acute liver failure
ALT: Alanine aminotransferase
AST: Aspartate aminotransferase
CT: Computed tomography
HSV: Herpes simplex virus
LT: Liver transplantation.

Disclosure

The funding body played no role in the design of the study, or in the collection, analysis, and interpretation of the data, or in the writing of the manuscript.

Authors' Contributions

Atsushi Ono and C. Nelson Hayes equally contributed to this work.

Acknowledgments

The authors thank Emi Nishio and Akemi Sata for clerical assistance. Computation time was provided by Supercomputing Services, Human Genome Center, Institute of Medical Science, University of Tokyo. This study was funded in part by the Research Program on Hepatitis from the Japan Agency for Medical Research and Development, AMED (Grant no. 15fk0210001h0002).

References

[1] W. M. Lee, "Acute liver failure," *Seminars in Respiratory and Critical Care Medicine*, vol. 33, no. 1, pp. 36–45, 2012.

[2] C. Trey and C. S. Davidson, "The management of fulminant hepatic failure," *Progress in Liver Diseases*, vol. 3, pp. 282–298, 1970.

[3] W. M. Lee, R. H. Squires Jr., S. L. Nyberg, E. Doo, and J. H. Hoofnagle, "Acute liver failure: summary of a workshop," *Hepatology*, vol. 47, no. 4, pp. 1401–1415, 2008.

[4] W. M. Lee and E. Seremba, "Etiologies of acute liver failure," *Current Opinion in Critical Care*, vol. 14, no. 2, pp. 198–201, 2008.

[5] K. Sugawara, N. Nakayama, and S. Mochida, "Acute liver failure in Japan: Definition, classification, and prediction of the outcome," *Journal of Gastroenterology*, vol. 47, no. 8, pp. 849–861, 2012.

[6] C. Bihari, A. Rastogi, P. Saxena et al., "Parvovirus B19 associated hepatitis," *Hepatitis Research and Treatment*, vol. 2013, Article ID 472027, 9 pages, 2013.

[7] Y. Maneerat, P. Wilairatana, E. Pongponratn et al., "Herpes simplex virus type-2, cytomegalovirus and Epstein-Barr virus infection in acute non A to E hepatitis Thai patients," *Asian Pacific Journal of Allergy and Immunology*, vol. 15, no. 3, pp. 147–151, 1997.

[8] S. K. Wollersheim, R. M. Humphries, J. D. Cherry, and P. Krogstad, "Serological misdiagnosis of acute liver failure associated with echovirus 25 due to immunological similarities to hepatitis a virus and prozone effect," *Journal of Clinical Microbiology*, vol. 53, no. 1, pp. 309-310, 2015.

[9] A. Sagir, O. Kirschberg, T. Heintges, A. Erhardt, and D. Häussinger, "SEN virus infection," *Reviews in Medical Virology*, vol. 14, no. 3, pp. 141–148, 2004.

[10] J. Wang, Y. H. Ke, Y. Zhang et al., "Rapid And Accurate Sequencing of Enterovirus Genomes Using Minion Nanopore Sequencer," *Biomedical and Environmental Sciences*, vol. 30, pp. 718–726, 2017.

[11] J. K. Lemon, P. P. Khil, K. M. Frank, J. P. Dekker, and A. Mellmann, "Rapid nanopore sequencing of plasmids and resistance gene detection in clinical isolates," *Journal of Clinical Microbiology*, vol. 55, no. 12, pp. 3530–3543, 2017.

[12] I. Milne, G. Stephen, M. Bayer et al., "Using tablet for visual exploration of second-generation sequencing data," *Briefings in Bioinformatics*, vol. 14, no. 2, Article ID bbs012, pp. 193–202, 2013.

[13] S. E. Lakhan and L. Harle, "Fatal fulminant herpes simplex hepatitis secondary to tongue piercing in an immunocompetent adult: A case report," *Journal of Medical Case Reports*, vol. 2, article no. 356, 2008.

[14] T. H. Flewett, R. G. Parker, and W. M. Philip, "Acute hepatitis due to *Herpes simplex* virus in an adult," *Journal of Clinical Pathology*, vol. 22, no. 1, pp. 60–66, 1969.

[15] P. Ichai, A. M. Roque Afonso, M. Sebagh et al., "Herpes simplex virus-associated acute liver failure: A difficult diagnosis with a poor prognosis," *Liver Transplantation*, vol. 11, no. 12, pp. 1550–1555, 2005.

[16] S. Mochida, Y. Takikawa, N. Nakayama et al., "Classification of the etiologies of acute liver failure in japan: A report by the intractable hepato-biliary diseases study group of japan," *Hepatology Research*, vol. 44, no. 4, pp. 365–367, 2014.

[17] B. Langmead and S. L. Salzberg, "Fast gapped-read alignment with Bowtie 2," *Nature Methods*, vol. 9, no. 4, pp. 357–359, 2012.

[18] Z. Chang, G. Li, J. Liu et al., "Bridger: A new framework for de novo transcriptome assembly using RNA-seq data," *Genome Biology*, vol. 16, no. 1, article no. 30, 2015.

[19] A. C. Lyra, J. R. R. Pinho, L. K. Silva et al., "HEV, TTV and GBV-C/HGV markers in patients with acute viral hepatitis," *Brazilian Journal of Medical and Biological Research*, vol. 38, no. 5, pp. 767–775, 2005.

[20] H. J. Alter, "The cloning and clinical implications of HGV and HGBV-C," *The New England Journal of Medicine*, vol. 334, no. 23, pp. 1536-1537, 1996.

[21] R. Tuveri, F. Jaffredo, F. Lunel et al., "Impact of TT virus infection in acute and chronic, viral- and non viral- related liver diseases," *Journal of Hepatology*, vol. 33, no. 1, pp. 121–127, 2000.

[22] C. Trapnell, A. Roberts, L. Goff et al., "Differential gene and transcript expression analysis of RNA-seq experiments with TopHat and Cufflinks," *Nature Protocols*, vol. 7, no. 3, pp. 562–578, 2012.

[23] A. Naik, A. Goel, V. Agrawal et al., "Changes in gene expression in liver tissue from patients with fulminant hepatitis e," *World Journal of Gastroenterology*, vol. 21, no. 26, pp. 8032–8042, 2015.

[24] R. M. Rodrigues, O. Govaere, T. Roskams, T. Vanhaecke, V. Rogiers, and J. De Kock, "Gene expression data from acetaminophen-induced toxicity in human hepatic in vitro systems and clinical liver samples," *Data in Brief*, vol. 7, pp. 1052–1057, 2016.

[25] S. Flygare, K. Simmon, C. Miller et al., "Taxonomer: An interactive metagenomics analysis portal for universal pathogen detection and host mRNA expression profiling," *Genome Biology*, vol. 17, no. 1, article no. 111, 2016.

28

Hepatotoxicity due to Clindamycin in Combination with Acetaminophen in a 62-Year-Old African American Female: A Case Report and Review of the Literature

Jerome Okudo[1] and Nwabundo Anusim[2]

[1]School of Public Health, University of Texas, 1200 Pressler Street, Houston, TX 77030, USA
[2]Department of Medicine, Saint Joseph Regional Medical Center, 5215 Holy Cross Parkway, Mishawaka, IN 46545, USA

Correspondence should be addressed to Jerome Okudo; jeromeokudo@yahoo.com

Academic Editor: Fumio Imazeki

Clindamycin is a bacteriostatic lincosamide antibiotic with a broad spectrum. Side effects include nausea, vomiting, diarrhea, and metallic taste; however, hepatotoxicity is rare. The incidence is unknown. It is characterized by increases in aspartate and alanine transaminases. There may be no symptoms and the treatment is to stop the administration of clindamycin. We have described a 62-year-old African American female medicated with acetaminophen and clindamycin who had initially presented to the dental clinic for the evaluation of gum pain following tooth extraction. She had significantly increased levels of liver transaminases, which trended downwards on quitting the medication.

1. Introduction

Clindamycin is a common bacteriostatic antibiotic with wide coverage against several organisms [1–3]. It is useful in the treatment of oral infections and is quickly distributed in the body following oral administration. It is metabolized and excreted by the liver.

While clindamycin has many side effects, hepatotoxicity is a rare culprit in liver damage [4, 5]. There is limited medical literature supporting the role of clindamycin in liver damage even though apoptosis plays a role. Damage from clindamycin causes significant increases in both aspartate transaminase and alanine transaminase and liver biopsy may demonstrate damage to the portal system, which may show reversal to baseline when clindamycin administration is stopped [4, 5]. We have discussed a patient who received oral clindamycin for a dental infection and subsequently developed clindamycin hepatotoxicity.

2. Case Report

A 62-year-old African American female with a history of tobacco use, alcohol use, hypertension, and hyperlipidemia presented to the hospital with severe pains in her gum nine days following a tooth extraction at sites 19 and 30. She self-medicated with several alternated tablets of 750 mg acetaminophen every six hours and ibuprofen 400 mg prn but her gum pain was unrelenting. In the interim, she saw her primary care physician who prescribed 450 mg 6 hourly clindamycin for ten days for a possible dental infection. In spite of her compliance to clindamycin, after five days of treatment, her gum pain persisted and was severe. It became evident that she would require hospitalization. At presentation at the emergency department, physical examination was unremarkable; the maxillofacial surgeon made an assessment of alveolar osteitis and chlorhexidine mouthwash was started for the patient. Upon initial evaluation of the laboratory results in the emergency department, it was found that the patient had the following results: alanine aminotransferase (ALT) was 423 IU/L (normal range 0–40); aspartate aminotransferase (AST) was 338 IU/L (normal range 5–40); her total bilirubin and INR levels were within reference ranges, gamma-glutamyl transpeptidase (GGT) was 179 IU/L (normal range of 10–64); and alkaline phosphatase (ALP) was 321 IU/L (normal range 40–100). Her acetaminophen level was 31 mcg/mL and alcohol level was 7 mg/dL. At this time, there was suspicion of acetaminophen poisoning and poison control was notified and she was started on acetylcysteine 21-hour dose regimen; this was extended after 48 hours per protocol. On the 7th day on oral clindamycin, there was suspicion of clindamycin toxicity as indicated by her latest ALT (1579) and AST (1512) results which had trended upwards; additional history was sought from the patient. There was no fever, chills, fatigue, anorexia, weakness, nausea, abdominal pain, dark-colored urine, jaundice, pruritus, lymphadenopathy, or rash. There was neither history of chronic liver disease nor hypersensitivity features in the patient. There were also no hypersensitivity features in the patient. Her other blood tests included glucose, cholesterol, triglycerides, protein, albumin, uric acid, blood urea nitrogen (BUN), and serum creatinine and they were determined to be within normal ranges. Hepatitis A antibody IgM, B core IgM, surface antigen, hepatitis C, HIV, cytomegalovirus, Epstein Barr virus, and antinuclear antibody screen (ANA) were negative. We did not test hepatitis E virus in this patient; however, the patient had not recently traveled to any regions in Africa, Asia, or Central America where the virus is well known. A review of the patient by the gastroenterology team was performed and a Doppler of the hepatic vein, hepatitis panel (already performed), and a liver ultrasound scan were ordered to rule out Budd-Chiari syndrome, acute hepatitis, and biliary obstruction; however, all tests were negative. A liver biopsy was not performed for financial reasons. During this time, ALT and AST values were monitored continuously with very high values. By day 9 on clindamycin, the highest values of ALT (1927) and AST (1812) were gotten in the patient and it was suggested that clindamycin be discontinued, and clindamycin was therefore discontinued on day 10. By the third week, the values of ALT and AST began to trend downwards; ALT (976) and AST (878) were the latest results. During the 4th week, her values had improved to ALT (822) and AST (676). She is being followed up in the clinic on several clinic visits as outpatient until her results return to normal.

3. Discussion

Drug-induced liver injury (DILI) is very common and has been reported as being responsible for drug withdrawal from the market. It has been implicated in liver failure. It is imperative to make a clear distinction between DILI caused by overdose and that caused by administration of drug, that is, idiosyncratic DILI. It is also imperative to consider the effect of two main drug categories, one that can lead to severe injury and another that has a low likelihood of causing severe liver damage. To ensure a proper classification of DILI, DILI criteria have long been made available in the medical literature. DILI criteria and classification (adapted from Aithal et al. 2011) will be used in this patient [9–12]. The medical literature has suggested that there should be minimal elements for reporting drug-induced liver injury. Though this is a long list, our case report met more than 90% of the criteria and has discussed these elements in the case reports. They include the demographics such as sex and age of the patient. Other criteria are drugs and their respective doses, indication, and disease for which the medication was used

and other comorbid or concurrent conditions or pertinent past medical history in the patient such as previous drug reactions and liver disease, history of alcohol use, time of onset of event, symptoms, pertinent liver symptoms and signs, detailed medication history prior to the current culprit medication, abnormal laboratory tests and dates reported and baseline liver tests, exclusion of hepatitis by a panel, other liver tests with their course, imaging studies, liver histology, and rechallenge [9–12]. Of all these, the last two were not performed in this patient for financial reasons.

In meeting the DILI criteria, seven major criteria were considered and they include the following: (i) clinical chemistry criteria for drug-induced liver injury (DILI) (two criteria were met even though one criterion is required out of three criteria; they include more than or equal to fivefold elevation above the upper limit of normal for alanine aminotransferase (ALT) and more than or equal to threefold elevation in ALT concentration and simultaneous elevation of bilirubin concentration exceeding 2x ULN). (ii) clinical pattern of drug-induced liver injury (DILI) which was hepatocellular based on the formula (it is important to bear in mind that R ratios of >5 have a high likelihood to be hepatocellular, <2 a cholestatic pattern, and between 2 and 5 a mixed pattern of enzymes. If the ALT value is determined to be greater than twice the upper limit of the normal range (ULN) and the alkaline phosphatase is normal, the pattern should be considered hepatocellular and R ratio need not be calculated. Also, if the alkaline phosphatase value is more than twice ULN but the ALT is normal, the pattern should be considered cholestatic, and R ratio may not be calculated. In the RUCAM system, cases determined to be mixed are given scores as if they were cholestatic [9–12]), (iii) DILI severity index which we inferred to be moderate because of the elevated ALT/ALP concentration reaching criteria for DILI and bilirubin concentration ≥2x ULN, (iv) DILI causality assessment which was computed for clindamycin and acetaminophen, respectively, (scores of 10 and 9 were computed, respectively, using the Roussel Uclaf Causality Assessment Method (RUCAM) scale), (v) persistent and chronic drug-induced liver injury (DILI) based on a timeframe beyond three months' follow-up for which the liver transaminases had returned to normal, (vi) drug-associated chronic liver disease (this patient did not display any evidence of chronic liver disease, and for financial reasons a liver biopsy was not performed), and (vii) drug-induced autoimmune hepatitis (ALH). To determine drug induced autoimmune hepatitis, a scoring system using a simplified set of diagnostic criteria will prove useful. A score of >6 is obtainable if a liver biopsy is performed for histological evaluation of the liver. In addition, assessment of multiple autoantibodies (antinuclear antibody, smooth muscle cell antibody, liver-kidney microsomal antibodies, and soluble liver/liver-pancreas antibodies), quantitative serum-globulins, and exclusion of viral hepatitis are also required. However, histological evaluation of the liver was not performed due to financial difficulties of the patient.

Many drugs have been known to cause liver toxicity and clindamycin is a rare one [7, 13–15]. Very few cases of liver toxicity caused by clindamycin administration have been reported (Table 1). The pharmacokinetics of clindamycin is

TABLE 1: Cases of clindamycin hepatotoxicity in adults searched on PubMed till date.

Author	Year	Age	Sex	Reason for taking clindamycin	Presentation	Biopsy	Liver enzymes (ALT, AST, ALP)	Trend of liver enzymes	Evolution of liver injury after cessation of clindamycin	Treatment
[5]	1977	57	M	Endocarditis	N/A	H	I	DW	Two patients had hepatotoxicity which resolved rapidly after clindamycin was stopped	CS
[4]	1974	18	M	Endocarditis and pulmonary abscesses	N/A	HC/C	I	DW	Repeat liver biopsy after 12 days of stopping clindamycin showed significant resolution of SGOT level; SGOT returned to normal in 30 days	CS
[2]	1994	67	M	Skin abscess	Jaundice	C	I	DW	Persistence of duct paucity	CS
[3]	2007	42	F	Dental infection	Jaundice, pruritus	NP	I	DW	LFTs returned to normal after 8 weeks	CS
[1]	2009	52	F	Cerebral abscess	N/A	NP	I	DW	Complete resolution	CS
[6]	2009	48	F	Bronchial infection	Jaundice, pruritus	C	I	DW	Stevens Johnson Syndrome and intrahepatic cholestasis simultaneously	CS
[7]	2013	73	M	Pneumonia	Jaundice	NP	I	DW	Developed liver failure	CS
[8]	2015	75	F	Urinary tract infection	Jaundice	C	I	DW	At 4 weeks' follow-up, biochemical tests returned to baseline normal values	CS
Present case report	2016	62	F	Dental infection	Accidental finding	NP	I	DW	Patients LFTs gradually returned to normal; patient is being followed up in the clinic	CS

H: hepatocellular, C: cholestasis, CS: clindamycin stopped, NP: not performed, DW: downward trend, and I: increased.

well studied. Oral administration of clindamycin is absorbed almost completely and rapidly so that peak plasma concentration is attained within 45 minutes after it has been orally administered. Absorption is not affected by food. It is well prescribed and oral administration has a high bioavailability. It is also widely distributed in body fluids and tissues. While it is known to diffuse across the placenta, it is not known to diffuse across a healthy blood brain barrier. Majority of clindamycin in the circulation is bound to plasma proteins. It is distributed highly intracellular due to the lipophilic properties. The intracellular concentrations are higher than the extracellular concentrations. It is metabolized in the liver to active metabolites, which include N-dimethyl and sulphoxide, and inactive metabolites and about 4% in the feces. The half-life is about two and a half hours in children and three hours in adults. It is excreted as biologically active and biologically inactive metabolites in feces, urine, and bile. 10% of the drug is excreted in the urine as active drug and 4% in the feces and the rest is excreted as inactive metabolites. It is important to consider special populations such as the elderly and patients with renal and hepatic disease. The half-life, volume of distribution, clearance, and absorption of the drug are not altered by increased age. However, for patients with renal dysfunction, elimination half-life is prolonged. If renal impairment is mild to moderate, there is no reason to reduce the dosage of the medication. In patients who have moderate to severe hepatic impairment, the half-life is also prolonged [16]. Clindamycin is a lincosamide antibiotic known to inhibit bacterial protein synthesis by binding to the 50S subunit of the ribosome. It is known to be active against Gram-positive aerobes and anaerobes, Gram-negative anaerobes.

Even though hepatotoxicity is not a well-known side effect, it causes hepatotoxicity in two forms: transient serum aminotransferase elevations usually occurring after several days of high intravenous doses and an acute idiosyncratic liver injury that starts within 1 to 3 weeks of therapy and is usually mild and self-limited [5, 7, 8, 15]. Several case reports and reviews have been reported on drug related liver injury for which 176 cases were identified and 39 were due to antimicrobial agents but none was related to clindamycin explaining how rarely studied this entity is [6, 13–15, 17].

An ultrasound of the liver is important to rule out biliary obstruction [1–3]. This patient self-medicated with acetaminophen for a long period of time and also received clindamycin and both medications are implicated in increased levels of transaminases. To differentiate the liver damage by acetaminophen and clindamycin, clindamycin would cause an increase in both alkaline phosphatase and alanine transaminase described as mixed; however, acetaminophen would cause an increase in alanine transaminase alone [5, 7]. In addition, this patient received n acetyl cysteine for acetaminophen poisoning but her liver enzymes continued to rise so acetaminophen was not the culprit. While a liver biopsy is important in evaluation, it was not performed in this patient for financial reasons. The following are the likely findings on liver biopsy: significant cholestasis, inflamed portal system, bile duct injury ductopenia, centrilobular, and portal cholestatic hepatitis, without fibrosis or necrosis [3]. Treatment of this condition is to stop clindamycin immediately [1–6]. Symptom resolution, transaminases returning back to baseline on quitting clindamycin, timeline between clindamycin administration and elevation of transaminases, and no other demonstrable causes for rise in liver enzymes are the unique features of this case.

4. Conclusion

We reported a case of clindamycin-induced hepatotoxicity, which was an incidental finding. A significant elevation in liver enzymes, which improves when clindamycin is stopped, may aid in the diagnosis of clindamycin-induced hepatotoxicity. The type of injury in this patient was hepatocellular; however, this may vary from one person to another. It is important to look out for patients who take clindamycin because of the potential of more severe presentation of hepatotoxicity. It is important to carefully evaluate patients to make an accurate diagnosis. When making clinical decisions, anchoring is likely. The importance of precise decision making cannot be overemphasized [18].

References

[1] S. Senanayake, "Possible acute hepatotoxicity from oral clindamycin," *Australian Prescriber*, vol. 32, article 140, 2009.

[2] I. Altraif, L. Lilly, I. R. Wanless, and J. Heathcote, "Cholestatic liver disease with ductopenia (vanishing bile duct syndrome) after administration of clindamycin and trimethoprim-sulfamethoxazole," *The American Journal of Gastroenterology*, vol. 89, no. 8, pp. 1230–1234, 1994.

[3] C. Aygün, O. Kocaman, Y. Gürbüz, Ö. Şentürk, and S. Hülagü, "Clindamycin-induced acute cholestatic hepatitis," *World Journal of Gastroenterology*, vol. 13, no. 40, pp. 5408–5410, 2007.

[4] M. Elmore, J. P. Rissing, L. Rink, and G. F. Brooks, "Clindamycin-associated hepatotoxicity," *The American Journal of Medicine*, vol. 57, no. 4, pp. 627–630, 1974.

[5] D. R. Hinthorn, L. H. Baker, D. A. Romig, D. W. Voth, and C. Liu, "Endocarditis treated with clindamycin: relapse and liver dysfunction," *Southern Medical Journal*, vol. 70, no. 7, pp. 823–826, 1977.

[6] J. E. Sahagún Flores, J. A. Soto Ortiz, C. E. Tovar Méndez, E. C. Cárdenas Ochoa, and G. Hernández Flores, "Stevens-Johnson syndrome with intrahepatic cholestasis induced by clindamycin or chlorpheniramine," *Dermatology Online Journal*, vol. 15, no. 5, article 12, 2009.

[7] M. Z. Bawany, B. Bhutto, W. I. Youssef, A. Nawras, and T. Sodeman, "Acute liver failure: an uncommon complication of commonly used medication," *American Journal of Therapeutics*, vol. 20, no. 5, pp. 566–568, 2013.

[8] H. Moole, Z. Ahmed, N. Saxena, S. R. Puli, and S. Dhillon, "Oral clindamycin causing acute cholestatic hepatitis without ductopenia: a brief review of idiosyncratic drug-induced liver injury and a case report," *Journal of Community Hospital Internal Medicine Perspective*, vol. 5, article 28746, pp. 1–5, 2015.

[9] G. P. Aithal, P. B. Watkins, R. J. Andrade et al., "Case definition and phenotype standardization in drug-induced liver injury," *Clinical Pharmacology and Therapeutics*, vol. 89, no. 6, pp. 806–815, 2011.

[10] E. S. Björnsson and J. H. Hoofnagle, "Categorization of drugs implicated in causing liver injury: critical assessment based on published case reports," *Hepatology*, vol. 63, no. 2, pp. 590–603, 2016.

[11] V. K. Agarwal, J. G. McHutchison, J. H. Hoofnagle, and Drug-Induced Liver Injury Network (DILIN), "Important elements for the diagnosis of drug-induced liver injury," *Clinical Gastroenterology and Hepatology*, vol. 8, no. 5, pp. 463–470, 2010.

[12] R. J. Fontana, L. B. Seeff, R. J. Andrade et al., "Standardization of nomenclature and causality assessment in drug-induced liver injury: summary of a clinical research workshop," *Hepatology*, vol. 52, no. 2, pp. 730–742, 2010.

[13] N. Hernández, F. Bessone, A. Sánchez et al., "Profile of idiosyncratic drug induced liver injury in Latin America: an analysis of published reports," *Annals of Hepatology*, vol. 13, no. 2, pp. 231–239, 2014.

[14] M. B. De Valle, V. Av Klinteberg, N. Alem, R. Olsson, and E. Björnsson, "Drug-induced liver injury in a Swedish University hospital out-patient hepatology clinic," *Alimentary Pharmacology and Therapeutics*, vol. 24, no. 8, pp. 1187–1195, 2006.

[15] J. M. Leitner, W. Graninger, and F. Thalhammer, "Hepatotoxicity of antibacterials: pathomechanisms and clinical," *Infection*, vol. 38, no. 1, pp. 3–11, 2010.

[16] M. Smieja, "Current indications for the use of clindamycin: a critical review," *Canadian Journal of Infectious Diseases*, vol. 9, no. 1, pp. 22–28, 1998.

[17] C. Y. Chang and T. D. Schiano, "Review article: drug hepatotoxicity," *Alimentary Pharmacology and Therapeutics*, vol. 25, no. 10, pp. 1135–1151, 2007.

[18] T. Ajayi and J. Okudo, "Cardiac arrest and gastrointestinal bleeding: a case of medical heuristics," *Case Reports in Medicine*, vol. 2016, Article ID 9621390, 4 pages, 2016.

29

Fulminant Hepatic Failure in a Patient with Crohn's Disease on Infliximab Possibly Related to Reactivation of Herpes Simplex Virus 2 Infection

Gary Golds[1] and Lawrence Worobetz[2]

[1]Department of Medicine, University of Saskatchewan, 103 Hospital Drive, Saskatoon, SK, Canada S7N 0W8
[2]Division of Gastroenterology, Department of Medicine, University of Saskatchewan, 103 Hospital Drive, Saskatoon, SK, Canada S7N 0W8

Correspondence should be addressed to Gary Golds; gbg350@mail.usask.ca

Academic Editor: Sandeep Mukherjee

HSV hepatitis is a rare but often fatal cause of liver failure which tends to affect immunocompromised individuals. Early treatment with Acyclovir has been shown to reduce mortality in HSV hepatitis making recognition of the condition critically important. Here, we present a case of HSV hepatitis in a young woman with Crohn's disease on Prednisone, Azathioprine, and Infliximab. We discuss the clinical presentation of HSV hepatitis as well as the possible causes of hepatitis in a patient on these medications. This case helps demonstrate the importance of early clinical suspicion for HSV in undifferentiated fulminate liver failure. It is also the first reported case of HSV hepatitis in a patient on Infliximab, raising the possibility of HSV reactivation in patients on Infliximab.

1. Introduction

Herpes simplex virus (HSV) is a rare but often fatal cause of acute liver failure which generally affects immunosuppressed individuals and pregnant women in the third trimester [1]. Mortality rates for HSV hepatitis are high, but early intervention with Acyclovir appears to greatly reduce morality. As such, early clinical recognition of HSV hepatitis can be potentially life-saving. Many patients with inflammatory bowel disease (IBD) utilize immunomodulators and biologic therapies to help control their disease. It has long been known that these agents, particularly the tumor necrosis factor-alpha (TNFα) inhibitors such as Infliximab, put patients at increased risk for opportunistic infections and reactivation of latent infections such as tuberculosis. Here we report a case of HSV-2 reactivation causing fulminant liver failure in a patient with IBD recently started on Infliximab.

2. Case Presentation

A 33-year-old female with Crohn's disease presented with a two-day history of subjective fevers and chills and right upper quadrant pain. Her past medical history included endometriosis, cholecystectomy, previous liver abscess, and Crohn's disease. Her medications were venlafaxine, norgestimate/ethinylestradiol contraceptive pill, Azathioprine 100 mg daily, Infliximab, and Prednisone. The Infliximab was started 5 months prior to presentation at a dose of 300 mg every four weeks with the most recent dose 9 days prior to symptom onset. Prednisone was started two weeks priorly for Crohn's flare and was being tapered at 5 mg per week with a dose of 40 mg daily at the time of admission. The patient had no known drug allergies and no family history of autoimmune disease or liver disease.

The patient presented to her local hospital on her second day of symptoms. Her temperature was 38.9°C for which she received a dose of acetaminophen. Initial investigations revealed elevated ALT and AST of 2210 U/L and 2935 U/L, respectively. She was then transferred to the care of the Gastroenterology Team at Royal University Hospital for further assessment.

Regarding her history, she denied any medication changes, over the counter medication use, or intentional ingestions. There were no new food exposures, sick contacts, intravenous drug use, new sexual partners, or recent alcohol use. She denied pruritus, jaundice, change in mental status, nausea or vomiting, rashes, inflamed joints, or eye changes. Her bowel movements were once daily with no blood or mucous or melena and she had no abdominal cramping. She did report a two-day history of white oral plaques and odynophagia without dysphagia. She had travelled to the Dominican Republic three months priorly and felt well during and after the trip.

On exam, vital signs were within normal limits including a temperature of 36.5°C. Cardiovascular and respiratory exam were unremarkable except for signs of mild dehydration. Abdomen was nonprotuberant with bowel sounds present. There was tenderness to palpation in the right upper quadrant with voluntary guarding. The liver edge was palpable just below the costal margin and was smooth and nontender. Traube's space was resonant suggesting no splenomegaly. There were no stigmata of chronic liver disease, and the patient did not exhibit asterixis. In the mouth there were multiple small nonvesicular white plaques with surrounding erythema.

Laboratory investigations showed ALT 2309 U/L, AST 3481 U/L, AP 80 U/L, GGT 50 U/L, Total Bilirubin 6 μmol/L, Albumin 28 g/L, and INR 1.3. White blood cells were normal at $5.96 \times 10e9$/L with a normal differential except for mildly diminished monocyte count of $0.18 \times 10e9$/L. Hemoglobin was normal but platelets were low at $111 \times 10e9$/L. Serum acetaminophen level was positive at 20 μmol/L, but based on the modified Rumack-Matthew nomogram the patient did not meet criteria for N-acetylcysteine administration. The patient was admitted to hospital for further investigations and was started on nystatin oral suspension for suspected oral candidiasis. On postadmission day (PAD) 1 the patient's ALT and AST continued to rise as did her INR and bilirubin (Figure 1). Abdominal ultrasound with Doppler was normal with no evidence of Budd-Chiari syndrome. Infectious workups for EBV, CMV, hepatitis C, and hepatitis B were all negative, but hepatitis A IgG was positive with IgM pending. Investigations for autoimmune hepatitis and Wilson's disease were also still pending. Based upon these initial results it was thought that the patient had either an acute viral or autoimmune hepatitis.

On PAD 2 the patient developed tachycardia and her platelets continued to decline. There was laboratory evidence of disseminated intravascular coagulation (DIC) with decreased fibrinogen, elevated D-dimer, haptoglobin, and LDH. Hematology was consulted and they confirmed the diagnosis of DIC. The patient was started on a two-day course of intravenous immune globulin and given fresh frozen plasma and cryoprecipitate. Platelet transfusion was recommended but withheld due to lack of Rh− platelets being available. Hepatitis A IgM also came back negative and the patient was started on Solumedrol 40 mg IV every 8 hours for presumed autoimmune hepatitis. Azathioprine was also stopped given the possibility for drug induced hepatotoxicity.

On PAD 3 the ANA titre came back positive at 1 : 160 which further suggested autoimmune hepatitis, and as such IV steroids were continued. The liver transplant team was

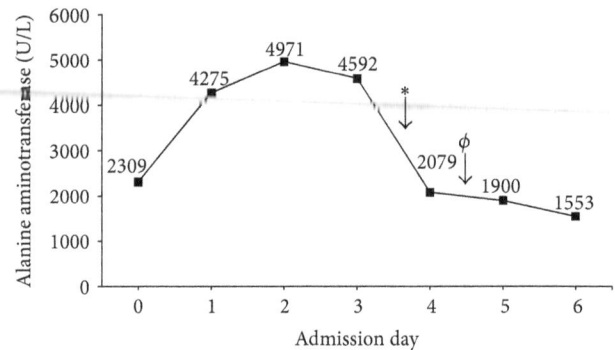

FIGURE 1: Alanine aminotransferase (ALT) levels during hospital admission in relation to medical therapy. Solumedrol initiation is denoted by ∗ while initiation of Acyclovir is indicated by φ.

notified of the patient and plans for liver biopsy were made, but due to ongoing severe coagulopathy and clinically significant bleeding, the biopsy was delayed for fear of significant postprocedure bleeding. On PAD 4 the patient developed spontaneous hematemesis prompting IV pantoprazole infusion, ICU admission, and emergent gastroscopy. This demonstrated a normal stomach and duodenum but diffuse esophagitis with mucosal sloughing suspicious for an infectious process. Biopsies of the esophagus were taken and the infectious disease team was consulted. Subsequently, multiple erosive lesions on the vulva which appeared herpetiform in nature were discovered. The patient was then started on Acyclovir 300 mg IV every 8 hours for a suspected disseminated HSV infection and the Solumedrol was stopped. Due to the patient's travel history, investigations for potentially liver toxic pathogens endemic to the Dominican Republic (hepatitis E, yellow fever virus, dengue virus, chikungunya virus, and *Leptospira*) were also done. These all eventually came back negative.

The next day, the patient's clinical status further declined with decreasing level of consciousness necessitating intubation. Her change in mental status was thought to be from hepatic encephalopathy and she was given lactulose via nasogastric tube. She was started on meropenem in case of concomitant bacteria infection. The patient then became anuric and went into respiratory failure and after aggressive resuscitation attempts the patient passed away. An autopsy was declined by the patient's family.

The results of the esophageal biopsy came back positive for fungal hyphae as well as HSV-2. Swabs from the vulvar lesions were positive for HSV-2 and serum PCR was also positive for HSV-2 but negative for varicella. Given this clinical picture, the patient was determined to have died from fulminant HSV-2 hepatitis with concomitant DIC and multiorgan failure. The fact that the patient had HSV-2 IgG suggests this was likely a reactivation of a previous HSV-2 infection.

3. Discussion

HSV hepatitis is a rare but often fatal cause of acute liver failure. It likely accounts for less than 1% of all cases of acute liver failure [2], but given its mortality rates of up to 74% [1], it is an important diagnosis to consider in any patient presenting with acute liver failure of unknown origin. HSV hepatitis primarily affects immunosuppressed individuals and pregnant females in their third trimester [1, 3]; however there have been many reported cases of immunocompetent individuals developing HSV hepatitis [4–11]. Patients with HSV hepatitis most commonly present with fever, thrombocytopenia, coagulopathy, and encephalopathy [1]. Cutaneous manifestations of the virus are present in less than half of all cases [1], and most diagnoses are made on autopsy [1]. Even with treatment using Acyclovir, mortality rates of HSV hepatitis are still as high as 51% [1]. Additionally, there is evidence that a delay in administration of Acyclovir is associated with increased mortality rates [12]. The significantly reduced mortality of HSV hepatitis with Acyclovir treatment, as well as its relatively safe drug profile [13, 14], has prompted some clinicians to recommend empiric Acyclovir therapy in any patient presenting with hepatitis who is at risk of HSV infection [15, 16].

The clinical features in our case report are very similar to what has been described for HSV hepatitis in the literature. Given these similarities in presentation, the positive serum PCR, and esophageal biopsy for HSV-2 and previous HSV IgG, the most likely cause of hepatitis in our case is HSV-2 reactivation. Other potential causes of hepatitis to consider in our patient include autoimmune or drug induced causes. In our case, while the patient's serum ANA titre was significant at 1 : 160, the lack of clinical improvement with pulse steroids as well as negative antismooth muscle antibody assay and nonelevated IgG makes autoimmune hepatitis unlikely in our patient. Our patient was on both Infliximab and Azathioprine, two medications known to cause drug induced liver injury. In the case of Azathioprine, drug induced hepatotoxicity can occur over a broad range of time frame and is generally associated with drug initiation or dose changes [17]. In our case, however, there had been no recent changes in Azathioprine and the drug was also discontinued without an improvement in the patient's condition. Therefore, it is unlikely that Azathioprine was the cause of our patient's fulminant liver failure. The anti-TNFα agents, primarily Infliximab, have also been reported to cause drug induced liver injury [18]. However, most of these cases only had mild elevation of liver enzymes, occurring months after initiation of the anti-TNFα agent [18, 19]. Our patient on the other hand had dramatic elevations in her liver enzymes. Interestingly there have been case reports of ANA positive hepatitis following Infliximab infusions which suggest the possible induction of autoimmune hepatitis by Infliximab [20]. However, given the lack of ANA titres prior to Infliximab administration in many of the patients, it is hard to determine whether development of autoimmune hepatitis was associated with Infliximab administration or merely coincidental. Similarly in our case, our patient had a positive ANA titre with an unknown titre prior to hospitalization.

While HSV hepatitis has not previously been reported in a patient on Infliximab, it is well known that the use of TNFα inhibitors can lead to reactivation of latent infections [21]. In terms of viral infections, hepatitis B (HBV) and hepatitis C

(HCV) are the best studied in patients on TNFα inhibitors [22]. Overall, HBV reactivation is much more common [23, 24] and this is thought to be due to the required involvement of TNFα in the host immune response to HBV infection [25, 26]. Similarly, the role of TNFα in host defense mechanisms against the herpes simplex virus is thought to be important and likely involves macrophage activation and immune cell signalling [27]. Mouse models have demonstrated that TNFα depletion leads to rapid reactivation of HSV-1 infections and TNFα knockout mice are more susceptible to primary HSV-1 infection and had higher subsequent rates of mortality [28]. Following from this, it would not be unexpected for patients on TNFα inhibitors to have increased rates of viral herpes infections. Indeed, there are a large number of reports of herpes zoster infections in patients on Infliximab as well as case reports of HSV-1 encephalitis, necrotizing tonsillitis, and diffuse cutaneous infection in patients treated with Infliximab [29–32]. Therefore, it would not be unreasonable to believe that HSV reactivation could cause viral hepatitis in a patient on a TNFα inhibitor.

In conclusion, we have presented a case of acute hepatitis from HSV-2 reactivation leading to thrombocytopenia, coagulopathy, multiorgan failure, and death despite IV Acyclovir treatment. The patient had recently started taking Infliximab and this is the first case to our knowledge of HSV hepatitis in a patient on this medication [1, 21, 33]. This case raises the possibility of Infliximab causing HSV-2 reactivation in patients leading to hepatitis. It also further emphasizes the need to have a high clinical suspicion for HSV hepatitis in any patient presenting with acute hepatitis who is immunosuppressed as early Acyclovir administration has been demonstrated to significantly reduce mortality [1, 12]. Due to this reduced mortality, the challenge of diagnosing HSV hepatitis, and the relatively safe drug profile of Acyclovir [16], we recommend that any patient who is immunosuppressed and presenting with hepatitis of unknown origin should be started on empiric Acyclovir therapy.

References

[1] J. P. Norvell, A. T. Blei, B. D. Jovanovic, and J. Levitsky, "Herpes simplex virus hepatitis: an analysis of the published literature and institutional cases," *Liver Transplantation*, vol. 13, no. 10, pp. 1428–1434, 2007.

[2] F. V. Schiødt, T. J. Davern, A. O. Shakil, B. McGuire, G. Samuel, and W. M. Lee, "Viral hepatitis-related acute liver failure," *American Journal of Gastroenterology*, vol. 98, no. 2, pp. 448–453, 2003.

[3] S. Sharma and M. Mosunjac, "Herpes simplex hepatitis in adults: a search for muco-cutaneous clues," *Journal of Clinical Gastroenterology*, vol. 38, no. 8, pp. 697–704, 2004.

[4] G. Biancofiore, M. Bisà, L. M. Bindi et al., "Liver transplantation due to Herpes Simplex virus-related sepsis causing massive

hepatic necrosis after thoracoscopic thymectomy," *Minerva Anestesiologica*, vol. 73, no. 5, pp. 319–322, 2007.

[5] G. Boivin, B. Malette, and N. Goyette, "Disseminated herpes simplex virus type 1 primary infection in a healthy individual," *Canadian Journal of Infectious Diseases and Medical Microbiology*, vol. 20, no. 4, pp. 122–125, 2009.

[6] A. Chaillon, N. Schnepf, M. Jonas et al., "Case report: benefits of quantitative polymerase chain reaction in the clinical management of herpes simplex virus 1 infection with prominent hepatitis and unusual secondary progression," *Journal of Medical Virology*, vol. 84, no. 3, pp. 457–461, 2012.

[7] L. Czakó, M. Dobra, V. Terzin, L. Tiszlavicz, and T. Wittmann, "Sepsis and hepatitis together with herpes simplex esophagitis in an immunocompetent adult," *Digestive Endoscopy*, vol. 25, no. 2, pp. 197–199, 2013.

[8] T. Czartoski, C. Liu, D. M. Koelle, S. Schmechel, A. Kalus, and A. Wald, "Fulminant, acyclovir-resistant, herpes simplex virus type 2 hepatitis in an immunocompetent woman," *Journal of Clinical Microbiology*, vol. 44, no. 4, pp. 1584–1586, 2006.

[9] M. Glas, S. Smola, T. Pfuhl et al., "Fatal multiorgan failure associated with disseminated herpes simplex virus-1 infection: a case report," *Case Reports in Critical Care*, vol. 2012, Article ID 359360, 4 pages, 2012.

[10] A. Peppercorn, L. Veit, C. Sigel, D. J. Weber, S. Jones, and B. A. Cairns, "Overwhelming disseminated herpes simplex virus type 2 infection in a patient with severe burn injury: case report and literature review," *Journal of Burn Care and Research*, vol. 31, no. 3, pp. 492–498, 2010.

[11] L. Wind, M. V. van Herwaarden, F. Sebens, and M. Gerding, "Severe hepatitis with coagulopathy due to HSV-1 in an immunocompetent man," *Netherlands Journal of Medicine*, vol. 70, no. 5, pp. 227–229, 2012.

[12] M. Montalbano, G. I. Slapak-Green, and G. W. Neff, "Fulminant hepatic failure from herpes simplex virus: post liver transplantation acyclovir therapy and literature review," *Transplantation Proceedings*, vol. 37, no. 10, pp. 4393–4396, 2005.

[13] M. D. Moomaw, P. Cornea, R. C. Rathbun, and K. A. Wendel, "Review of antiviral therapy for herpes labialis, genital herpes and herpes zoster," *Expert Review of Anti-Infective Therapy*, vol. 1, no. 2, pp. 283–295, 2003.

[14] S. K. Tyring, D. Baker, and W. Snowden, "Valacyclovir for herpes simplex virus infection: long-term safety and sustained efficacy after 20 years' experience with acyclovir," *Journal of Infectious Diseases*, vol. 186, supplement 1, pp. S40–S46, 2002.

[15] U. Navaneethan, E. Lancaster, P. G. Venkatesh, J. Wang, and G. W. Neff, "Herpes simplex virus hepatitis-it's high time we consider empiric treatment," *Journal of Gastrointestinal and Liver Diseases*, vol. 20, no. 1, pp. 93–96, 2011.

[16] C. Riediger, P. Sauer, E. Matevossian, M. W. Müller, P. Büchler, and H. Friess, "Herpes simplex virus sepsis and acute liver failure," *Clinical Transplantation*, vol. 23, supplement 21, pp. 37–41, 2009.

[17] G. P. Aithal, "Hepatotoxicity related to antirheumatic drugs," *Nature Reviews Rheumatology*, vol. 7, no. 3, pp. 139–150, 2011.

[18] E. Shelton, K. Chaudrey, J. Sauk et al., "New onset idiosyncratic liver enzyme elevations with biological therapy in inflammatory bowel disease," *Alimentary Pharmacology and Therapeutics*, vol. 41, no. 10, pp. 972–979, 2015.

[19] I. Parisi, J. O'Beirne, R. E. Rossi et al., "Elevated liver enzymes in inflammatory bowel disease," *European Journal of Gastroenterology & Hepatology*, vol. 28, no. 7, pp. 786–791, 2016.

[20] F. Colina, A. Molero, B. Casís, and P. Martínez-Montiel, "Infliximab-related hepatitis: a case study and literature review," *Digestive Diseases and Sciences*, vol. 58, no. 11, pp. 3362–3367, 2013.

[21] G. Murdaca, F. Spanò, M. Contatore et al., "Infection risk associated with anti-TNF-γ agents: a review," *Expert Opinion on Drug Safety*, vol. 14, no. 4, pp. 571–582, 2015.

[22] F. Atzeni, A. Batticciotto, I. F. Masala, R. Talotta, M. Benucci, and P. Sarzi-Puttini, "Infections and biological therapy in patients with rheumatic diseases," *The Israel Medical Association Journal*, vol. 18, no. 3-4, pp. 164–167, 2016.

[23] A. M. G. Brunasso, M. Puntoni, A. Gulia, and C. Massone, "Safety of anti-tumour necrosis factor agents in patients with chronic hepatitis C infection: a systematic review," *Rheumatology*, vol. 50, no. 9, pp. 1700–1711, 2011.

[24] M. Viganò, G. Serra, G. Casella, G. Grossi, and P. Lampertico, "Reactivation of hepatitis B virus during targeted therapies for cancer and immune-mediated disorders," *Expert Opinion on Biological Therapy*, vol. 16, no. 7, pp. 917–926, 2016.

[25] H.-T. Tzeng, H.-F. Tsai, I.-T. Chyuan et al., "Tumor necrosis factor-alpha induced by hepatitis B virus core mediating the immune response for hepatitis B viral clearance in mice model," *PLoS ONE*, vol. 9, no. 7, article e103008, 2014.

[26] J. Chang, T. M. Block, and J.-T. Guo, "The innate immune response to hepatitis B virus infection: implications for pathogenesis and therapy," *Antiviral Research*, vol. 96, no. 3, pp. 405–413, 2012.

[27] S. Ellermann-Eriksen, "Macrophages and cytokines in the early defence against herpes simplex virus," *Virology Journal*, vol. 2, p. 59, 2005.

[28] H. Minagawa, K. Kashimoto, and Y. Yanagi, "Absence of tumour necrosis factor facilitates primary and recurrent herpes simplex virus-1 infections," *Journal of General Virology*, vol. 85, no. 2, pp. 343–347, 2004.

[29] J. Segan, M. P. Staples, L. March, M. Lassere, E. F. Chakravarty, and R. Buchbinder, "Risk factors for herpes zoster in rheumatoid arthritis patients: the role of tumour necrosis factor-α inhibitors," *Internal Medicine Journal*, vol. 45, no. 3, pp. 310–318, 2015.

[30] E. A. Justice, S. Y. Khan, S. Logan, and P. Jobanputra, "Disseminated cutaneous herpes simplex virus-1 in a woman with rheumatoid arthritis receiving infliximab: a case report," *Journal of Medical Case Reports*, vol. 2, article 282, 2008.

[31] R. D. Bradford, A. C. Pettit, P. W. Wright et al., "Herpes simplex encephalitis during treatment with tumor necrosis factor-α inhibitors," *Clinical Infectious Diseases*, vol. 49, no. 6, pp. 924–927, 2009.

[32] L. Jansen, X. G. Vos, and M. Löwenberg, "Herpes simplex induced necrotizing tonsillitis in an immunocompromised patient with ulcerative colitis," *World Journal of Clinical Cases*, vol. 4, no. 2, pp. 60–62, 2016.

[33] R. M. Nanau, L. B. Cohen, and M. G. Neuman, "Risk of infections of biological therapies with accent on inflammatory bowel disease," *Journal of Pharmacy and Pharmaceutical Sciences*, vol. 17, no. 4, pp. 485–528, 2014.

30

Diphenhydramine as a Cause of Drug-Induced Liver Injury

Yunseok Namn,[1] **Yecheskel Schneider,**[1] **Isabelle H. Cui,**[2] **and Arun Jesudian**[1]

[1]*Department of Gastroenterology and Hepatology, Weill Cornell Medical College, New York Presbyterian Hospital, New York, NY, USA*
[2]*Department of Pathology, Weill Cornell Medical College, New York Presbyterian Hospital, New York, NY, USA*

Correspondence should be addressed to Yunseok Namn; yun9007@nyp.org

Academic Editor: Melanie Deutsch

Drug-induced liver injury (DILI) is the most common cause of acute liver failure in the Unites States and accounts for 10% of acute hepatitis cases. We report the only known case of diphenhydramine-induced acute liver injury in the absence of concomitant medications. A 28-year-old man with history of 13/14-chromosomal translocation presented with fevers, vomiting, and jaundice. Aspartate-aminotransferase and alanine-aminotransferase levels peaked above 20,000 IU/L and 5,000 IU/L, respectively. He developed coagulopathy but without altered mental status. Patient reported taking up to 400 mg diphenhydramine nightly, without concomitant acetaminophen, for insomnia. He denied taking other medications, supplements, antibiotics, and herbals. A thorough workup of liver injury ruled out viral hepatitis (including A, B, C, and E), autoimmune, toxic, ischemic, and metabolic etiologies including Wilson's disease. A liver biopsy was consistent with DILI without evidence of iron or copper deposition. Diphenhydramine was determined to be the likely culprit. This is the first reported case of diphenhydramine-induced liver injury without concomitant use of acetaminophen.

1. Introduction

Drug-induced liver injury (DILI) is the most common cause of acute liver failure in the Unites States, accounting for nearly 50% of cases and 10% of acute hepatitis cases [1–3]. Other etiologies of acute liver injury include viral, autoimmune, metabolic, and ischemic etiologies. When acute liver injury progresses to fulminant hepatic failure, it is associated with high mortality [4, 5]. Therefore, prompt recognition of the underlying etiology and initiation of treatment are of paramount importance. Medications such as acetaminophen, antiepileptics, and antibiotics are well known causes of DILI; however, thousands of drugs, herbs, and toxins can cause idiosyncratic liver injury. We report the first case of diphenhydramine-induced liver injury without concomitant use of acetaminophen.

2. Case

A 28-year-old man with history of chromosomal translocation 13/14 and no prior liver disease presented to the hospital with complaint of fevers, nonbloody emesis, and dark urine. History revealed ingestion of diphenhydramine 400 mg nightly, taken for insomnia, over the previous 4 months; the medication was inspected in the hospital and confirmed not to contain acetaminophen. He denied use of herbal compounds, supplements, teas, and any other medication. The patient endorsed rare alcohol consumption and rare intranasal cocaine use in the distant past. Family history was notable for possible statin-induced liver disease and hereditary angioedema.

Vital signs on presentation were within normal limits. Physical exam revealed icteric conjunctiva, a 15 cm liver palpable 3 cm below the right costal margin, nonpalpable spleen, normal mentation, and neurologic exam without asterixis. Initial laboratory studies revealed aspartate aminotransferase (AST) 10,425 IU/L, alanine aminotransferase (ALT) 2,471 IU/L, alkaline phosphatase (ALP) 65 IU/L, total bilirubin 2.7 mg/dL (direct 1.4 mg/dL), INR 2.6, and a hemoglobin level of 12.7 g/dL; the remainder of the laboratory studies were normal, including creatinine, blood glucose, and lactate. Hepatology and toxicology consultations were requested, and empiric intravenous N-acetylcysteine (NAC) was initiated. By day two, his transaminases and coagulopathy worsened,

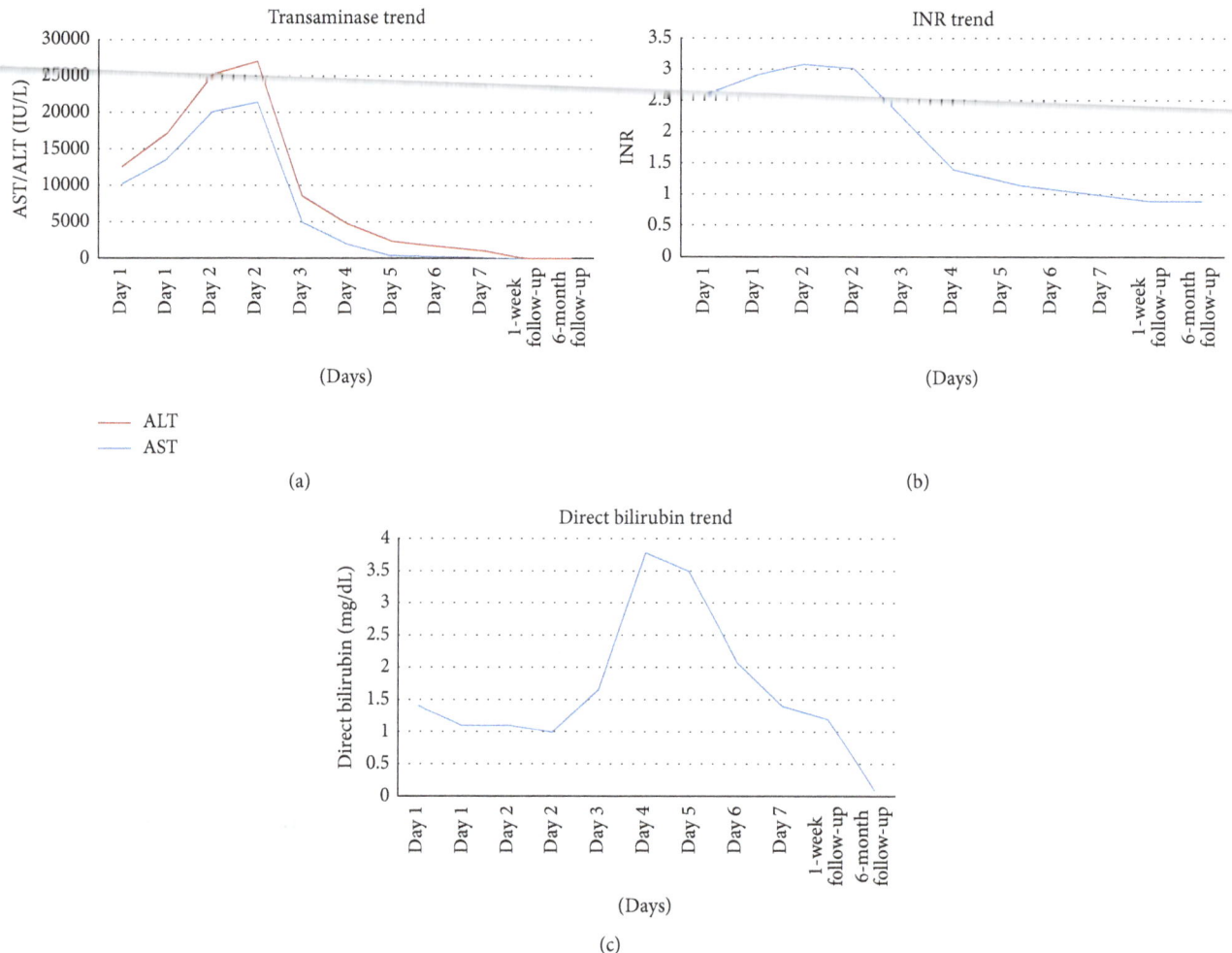

FIGURE 1: Linear graphs representing the trend of transaminases, INR, and direct bilirubin throughout patient's hospital course and outpatient follow-up.

with AST 20,176 IU/L, ALT 5,076 IU/L, and INR 3.1 (Figures 1(a), 1(b), and 1(c)). The patient did not exhibit signs of hepatic encephalopathy, but was transferred to the intensive care unit for closer monitoring. By the third day of NAC treatment, transaminases started to improve. A complete evaluation for causes of acute liver injury, including viral hepatitis (hepatitis A, B, C, and E), workup for other viruses (including EBV, CMV, HHV-6, and HIV), autoimmune workup (ANA, ASMA, AMA, A1AT, IgG, and LTK Ab), metabolic testing (ceruloplasmin, 24-hour urine copper, ophthalmologic examination for Keyser-Fleischer rings, MRI brain to evaluate for lenticular degeneration, and iron studies), urine toxicology, and SPEP/UPEP, was all normal and did not reveal an alternative etiology of the patient's acute liver injury. Abdominal ultrasound demonstrated a 17.4 cm liver with smooth contour and normal echogenicity with patent hepatic and portal vasculature. He underwent a transjugular biopsy which revealed centrilobular and bridging necrosis accompanied by portal and lobular inflammation, favoring drug-induced liver injury (Figures 2(a) and 2(b)). Rhodanine stain for copper and quantitative copper analysis were both negative, ruling out Wilson's disease. Iron staining was not

consistent with hemochromatosis. The patient ultimately recovered completely from acute liver injury and was discharged home. Upon the 6-month outpatient follow-up, patient was asymptomatic and reported feeling well, and repeat liver function tests did not show any evidence of liver injury.

3. Discussion

Acute liver injury can be attributed to a wide array of causes, with viral and drug etiologies being the most common in adults. In the United States, acetaminophen toxicity and idiosyncratic drugs reaction are the leading causes of acute liver failure while viral hepatitis is the leading cause in Asia and Europe [4, 5].

Drug-induced liver injury remains one of the most challenging diagnoses to make but must be considered in the differential diagnosis of any liver injury [6, 7]. Patients should undergo careful evaluation to exclude other causes of liver disease, including viral hepatitides (hepatitis A, B, C, and E), EBV, CMV, HHV-6, autoimmune hepatitis, and Wilson's disease if age is less than 40 [8, 9]. Offending agents

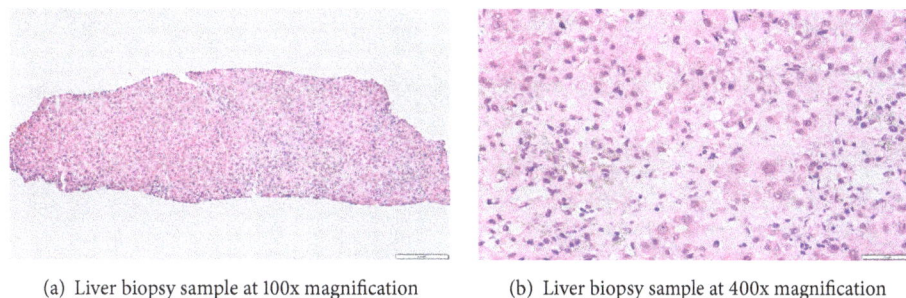

(a) Liver biopsy sample at 100x magnification

(b) Liver biopsy sample at 400x magnification

FIGURE 2: On Hematoxylin and Eosin stain (100x and 400x), there is centrilobular and bridging necrosis accompanied by portal and lobular inflammation including eosinophils and plasma cells. There is evidence of cholestasis and bile duct injury is noted in some portal tracts. Hepatocellular injury, that is, hepatocyte ballooning degeneration, is also present. Fibrosis is absent on Trichrome staining. There is no evidence of steatosis, glycogenic nuclei, Mallory's hyaline, or copper deposition. Overall, these findings favor a diagnosis of drug-induced liver injury.

can include prescription and over-the-counter medications, such as antibiotics (nitrofurantoin, isoniazid, and trimethoprim/sulfamethoxazole), immunomodulatory agents (such as infliximab), analgesics (especially those that contain acetaminophen), antineoplastic agents, antiepileptics, and statins [10, 11]. Additionally, DILI can result from herbal ingestions or dietary supplements [12, 13]. Manifestations of liver injury can range from asymptomatic transaminase elevation and/or jaundice (depending on a hepatocellular or cholestatic pattern of injury, resp.) to development of acute liver failure marked by encephalopathy and synthetic dysfunction [13, 14].

Drug-induced liver injury can be divided into two classes of medication-related hepatotoxicity: intrinsic and idiosyncratic. The former, which includes acetaminophen, is often dose-dependent with predictable liver injury at hepatotoxic doses [11, 15]. Idiosyncratic DILI is not dose-dependent and thus is harder to predict. It is thought to mainly affect individuals with underlying susceptibility or predisposition and therefore, may have variable latency [11, 16].

In the presented case, multiple etiologies for the liver injury were considered and excluded. The liver biopsy was consistent with DILI and after ascertainment of an exhaustive mediation history diphenhydramine was identified as the only possible culprit. Although there are reports of diphenhydramine and acetaminophen causing liver injury when ingested together, there are no prior cases in the literature of diphenhydramine alone causing DILI. Although considered to have minimal to no hepatotoxic effects, this case suggests that diphenhydramine may be hepatotoxic at high doses with chronic use (as the patient had been taking at least 400 mg per day for over four months). It has been reported that compounds with more than 50% hepatic metabolism given at doses higher than 50 mg/day were at highest risk of hepatotoxicity [13, 17]. Diphenhydramine undergoes extensive first-pass metabolism, whereby 50–60% of ingested medication is metabolized by the liver before reaching the systemic circulation. Nearly all the available drug is metabolized by the liver within 24–48 hours, thus increasing risk for liver injury. It is unclear if a predisposition for hepatotoxicity was present in this patient given his history

of a balanced chromosomal translocation. However, certain genetic predispositions have been noted to play a role in risk for DILI. For example, the HLA-1 and HLA-II genotypes have been shown to confer an increased susceptibility to DILI for patients taking amoxicillin-clavulanate [7, 17, 18].

In summary, we present a case of diphenhydramine-induced liver injury, without the concomitant use of acetaminophen. Although not previously thought to cause liver injury, this case highlights that any medication metabolized by the liver has potential to lead to liver injury when ingested at high enough doses and for long enough duration in susceptible individuals.

Authors' Contributions

Yunseok Namn is the main author of manuscript and article guarantor; Yecheskel Schneider is the 2nd author of manuscript; Isabelle H. Cui attained and analyzed the histological slide; Arun Jesudian is the advisor.

References

[1] H. J. Zimmerman, "Drug-induced liver disease," *Clinical Liver Disease*, vol. 4, no. 1, pp. 73–96, 2000.

[2] G. Ostapowicz, "Results of a prospective study of acute liver failure at 17 tertiary care centers in the United States," *Annals of Internal Medicine*, vol. 137, no. 12, pp. 947–954, 2002.

[3] A. M. Larson, J. Polson, R. J. Fontana et al., "Acetaminophen-induced acute liver failure: results of a United States multicenter, prospective study," *Hepatology*, vol. 42, no. 6, pp. 1364–1372, 2005.

[4] D. Gotthardt, C. Riediger, K. H. Weiss et al., "Fulminant hepatic failure: etiology and indications for liver transplantation,"

Nephrology Dialysis Transplantation, vol. 22, supplement 8, pp. viii5–viii8, 2007.

[5] C. Stephens, R. J. Andrade, and M. I. Lucena, "Mechanisms of drug-induced liver injury," *Current Opinion in Allergy and Clinical Immunology*, vol. 14, no. 4, pp. 286–292, 2014.

[6] R. Marudanayagam, V. Shanmugam, B. Gunson et al., "Aetiology and outcome of acute liver failure," *HPB: The Official Journal of the International Hepato Pancreato Biliary Association*, vol. 11, no. 5, pp. 429–434, 2009.

[7] M. Ghabril, N. Chalasani, and E. Björnsson, "Drug-induced liver injury: a clinical update," *Current Opinion in Gastroenterology*, vol. 26, no. 3, pp. 222–226, 2010.

[8] M. D. Leise, J. J. Poterucha, and J. A. Talwalkar, "Drug-induced liver injury," *Mayo Clinic Proceedings*, vol. 89, no. 1, pp. 95–106, 2014.

[9] N. Kaplowitz, "Drug-induced liver injury," *Clinical Infectious Diseases*, vol. 38, no. 2, pp. S44–S48, 2004.

[10] P. Sarges, J. M. Steinberg, and J. H. Lewis, "Drug-induced liver injury: highlights from a review of the 2015 literature," *Drug Safety*, vol. 39, no. 9, pp. 801–821, 2016.

[11] R. A. Roth and P. E. Ganey, "Intrinsic versus idiosyncratic drug-induced hepatotoxicity—two villains or one?" *Journal of Pharmacology and Experimental Therapeutics*, vol. 332, no. 3, pp. 692–697, 2010.

[12] A. Reuben, D. G. Koch, and W. M. Lee, "Drug-induced acute liver failure: results of a U.S. multicenter, prospective study," *Hepatology*, vol. 52, no. 6, pp. 2065–2076, 2010.

[13] C. Lammert, S. Einarsson, C. Saha, A. Niklasson, E. Bjornsson, and N. Chalasani, "Relationship between daily dose of oral medications and idiosyncratic drug-induced liver injury: search for signals," *Hepatology*, vol. 47, no. 6, pp. 2003–2009, 2008.

[14] R. Marudanayagam, V. Shanmugam, B. Gunson et al., "Aetiology and outcome of acute liver failure," *HPB*, vol. 11, no. 5, pp. 429–434, 2009.

[15] N. Chalasani, H. L. Bonkovsky, R. Fontana et al., "Features and outcomes of 899 patients with drug-induced liver injury: the DILIN prospective study," *Gastroenterology*, vol. 148, no. 7, pp. 1340–1352.e7, 2015.

[16] S. R. Knowles, J. Uetrecht, and N. H. Shear, "Idiosyncratic drug reactions: the reactive metabolite syndromes," *The Lancet*, vol. 356, no. 9241, pp. 1587–1591, 2000.

[17] B. Fromenty, "Drug-induced liver injury in obesity," *Journal of Hepatology*, vol. 58, no. 4, pp. 824–826, 2013.

[18] N. Chalasani, H. L. Bonkovsky, R. Fontana et al., "Features and outcomes of 899 patients with drug-induced liver injury: the DILIN prospective study," *Gastroenterology*, vol. 148, no. 7, pp. 1340.e7–1352.e7, 2015.

31

Tubulocystic Carcinoma of the Bile Duct

Masahiro Takeuchi ⓘ,[1] **Yoshitaka Sakamoto,**[2] **Hirotsugu Noguchi,**[3]
Sohsuke Yamada,[4] **and Keiji Hirata**[1]

[1]*Department of Surgery 1, School of Medicine, University of Occupational and Environmental Health, 1-1 Iseigaoka,*
Yahatanishi-ku, Kitakyushu-shi, Fukuoka 807-0804, Japan
[2]*Department of Surgery, Moji Medical Center, 3-1 Higashiminatomachi, Moji-ku, Kitakyushu-shi, Fukuoka 801-8502, Japan*
[3]*Department of Pathology, School of Medicine, University of Occupational and Environmental Health, 1-1 Iseigaoka,*
Yahatanishi-ku, Kitakyushu-shi, Fukuoka 807-0804, Japan
[4]*Department of Pathology and Laboratory Medicine, Kanazawa Medical University, 1-1 Uchinada, Ishikawa 920-0293, Japan*

Correspondence should be addressed to Masahiro Takeuchi; masahiro99@med.uoeh-u.ac.jp

Academic Editor: Ned Snyder

Tubulocystic carcinoma of the bile duct is extremely rare and has not been reported in the literature. We reported a case of cystic neoplasm of the liver with distinct histopathological features that could not be clearly classified as of either mucinous or intraductal papillary neoplasm. A 68-year-old Japanese patient had a multicystic biliary tumor within the liver. This tumor was detected on follow-up of polymyalgia rheumatica. The exophytic, multicystic, 35 × 50 mm mass was composed of complex tubulocystic structures. We initially suspected cystadenocarcinoma of the liver and performed radical operation. However, pathology ultimately showed it to be very rare tubulocystic carcinoma that derived from the bile duct. We reviewed the literature and describe the process of our differential diagnosis.

1. Introduction

Tubulocystic carcinoma is one of subtypes of kidney cancer, but it is a rare structure in kidney cancer [1]. On the other hand, intrahepatic bile duct carcinoma is a malignant tumor that develops from the intrahepatic bile duct epithelium, including the glands [2, 3]. Intrahepatic cholangiocarcinoma is the second most common type of hepatocellular carcinoma in primary malignant liver tumors. Many clinicopathologic studies on hepatocellular carcinoma have been published, but intrahepatic bile duct carcinoma remains unstudied in many respects, including its pathology form. We herein report that cystic tumor of biliary tract with feature mimicking a subtype of renal carcinoma.

2. Case Report

A 68-year-old man was referred to our department for the evaluation and treatment of a liver mass detected on inspections that were performed due to poor control of polymyalgia rheumatica. Abdominal ultrasound (US) and computed tomography (CT) revealed a solid 3.0 cm mass, which was suspected to be cystadenocarcinoma, in the right liver lobe (Couinaud segment 8). The patient was asymptomatic and had no remarkable medical history, including liver disease. He was not a habitual drinker or a smoker. A general examination that included the abdomen showed no particular findings. The laboratory data (complete blood count, chemistry, urinalysis, tumor markers, and coagulation) showed an elevated white blood cell count (11000/μl) and CRP level (10.83 mg/dl). AFP, CEA, CA19-9, PSA, and PIVKA-II values were all within normal limits.

US showed an isoechoic nodule of 30 × 35 mm with hypoechoic areas in segment 8 of the liver (Figure 1). CT showed a tumor that was slowly enhanced from the early phase to the parallel phase (Figure 2).

Furthermore, drip-infusion-cholecystocholangiography-CT (DIC-CT) showed that there was no traffic between the tumor and the bile duct (data not shown).

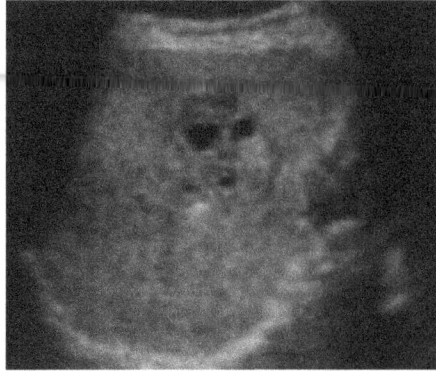

FIGURE 1: Ultrasonography (US) images. US showed an isoechoic nodule with small hypoechoic areas in segment 8 of the liver.

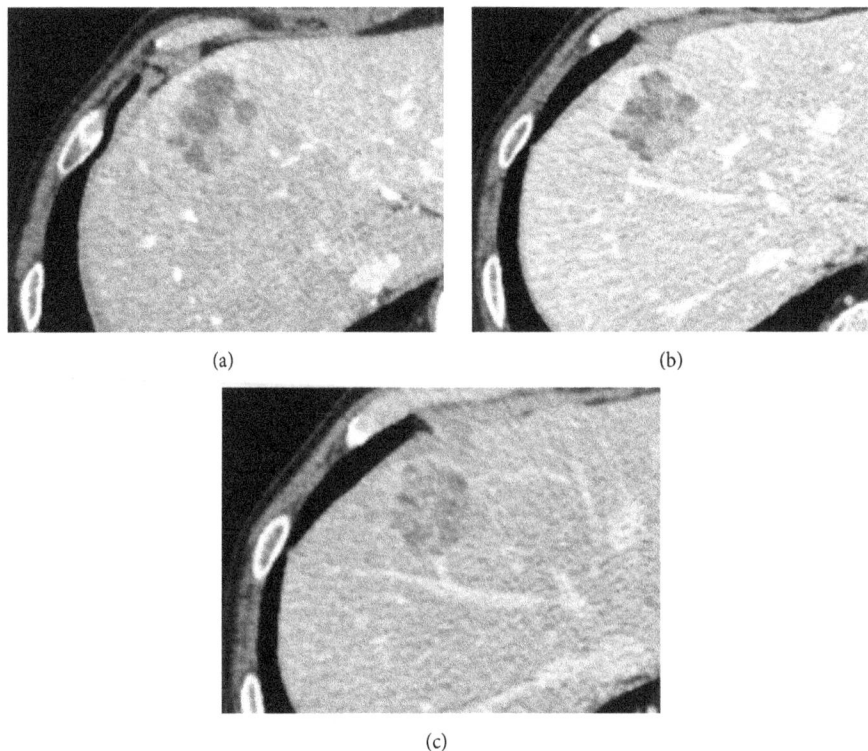

(a)

(b)

(c)

FIGURE 2: Images of contrast abdominal computed tomography (CT). CT showed that the tumor was slowly enhanced from the early phase to the parallel phase. (a) Early phase. (b) Delayed phase. (c) Parallel phase.

Magnetic resonance imaging (MRI) using Gd-EOB-DTPA contrast agent revealed a tumor with a high signal on T2-weighted imaging and a low signal on T1-weighted imaging accompanied by an enhancement effect on the cyst wall, and a bulkhead was found. Diffusion-weighted imaging revealed markedly high intensity (Figure 3). The patient had poor control of polymyalgia rheumatica and did not have a lesion other than on the liver, so the clinical decision was made to resect the mass for a diagnosis and treatment.

Surgical resection of the anterior segment of the right hepatic lobe showed a 35 × 50 mm mass on the hepatic capsule. Tumor cleft was a mass with cystic structure in solid part (Swiss cheese-like); there was no necrosis inside (Figure 4).

3. Pathology

Histopathologically, when viewed at high-power magnification, tubular and tubulocystic structures were conspicuous, and these tubules/cysts were separated by thin fibrous stroma without any evidence of desmoplastic reaction. The tumor cells had large nucleoli and eosinophilic or amphotropic cytoplasm with mildly cellular variety, showing a cuboidal to flattened shape lining the tubules and microcysts (Figure 5). Immunohistochemically, these atypical epithelial cells were positive for CD10, cellular adhesion molecule (CAM) 5.2 (low-molecular cytokeratin), and vimentin, suggesting a biliary epithelial nature, and were occasionally positive for

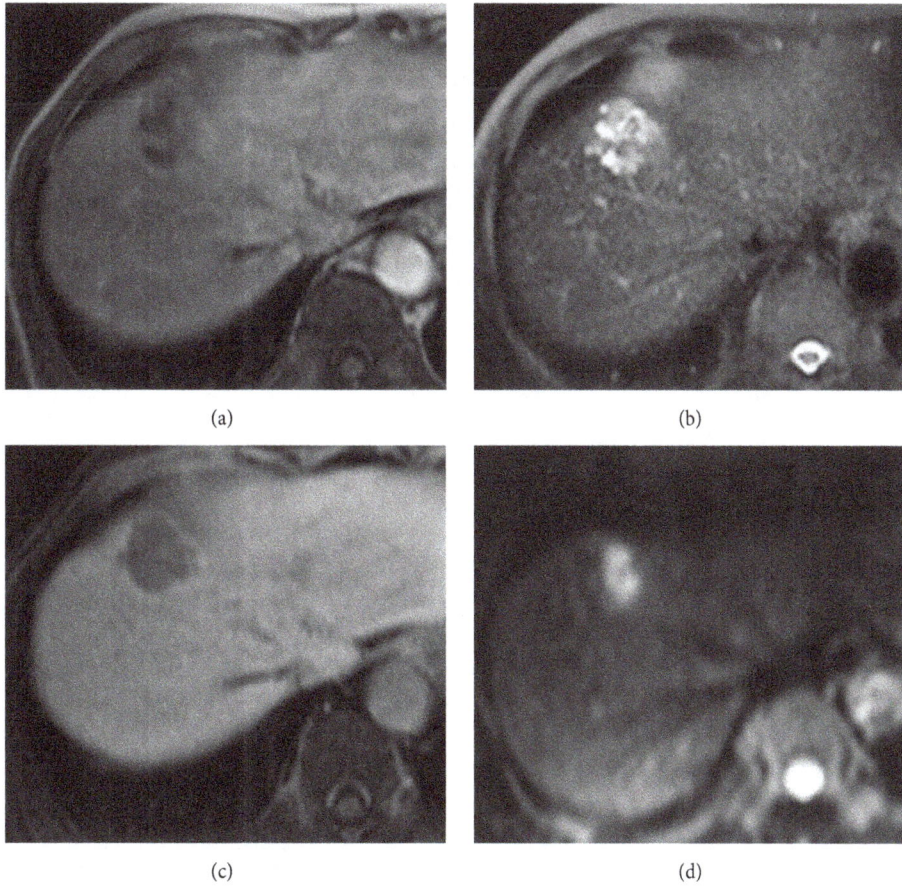

(a)

(b)

(c)

(d)

FIGURE 3: (a) T1-weighted magnetic resonance (MR) images showed the tumor with low intensity with lobulated borders. (b) The T2-weighted MR image shows the low signal portion indicating the cyst wall or bulkhead inside the high signal region. (c) In the hepatobiliary phase, the tumor showed low intensity. (d) On diffusion-weighted images, markedly high intensity was noted.

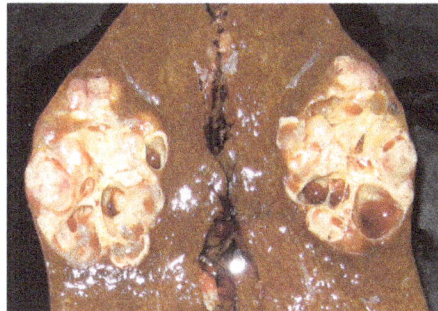

FIGURE 4: Resected specimen. The mass measured 35 × 50 mm and was located on the hepatic capsule.

cytokeratin (CK) 7 (Figure 6). However, cytokeratin (clone: AE1AE3), β-catenin, progesterone receptor (PgR), thyroid transcription factor- (TTF-) 1, synaptophysin, thyroglobulin, surfactant apoprotein (SPA), epithelial-CMA (EpCAM), MUC5AC (a mucinous-associated protein), neural cell-CAM (NCAM), human melanin black (HMB) 45, and CD20 were negative (Figures 7(a) and 7(b)). On staining of hepatocytes (Figure 7(c)), alpha-fetoprotein (AFP), glypican-3, and arginase-1 were negative. In the tumor region, these carcinoma cells were specifically positive for p53 (Figure 7(d)).

Based on these findings, we made a conclusive diagnosis of tubulocystic carcinoma of the bile duct. The patient was well with no recurrence of the tumor in the liver at four-year follow-up after surgery.

4. Discussion

Most common biliary cystic tumors are of two types: biliary cystadenomas and adenocarcinoma. These are classified as either mucinous cystic neoplasm (MCN) or intraductal

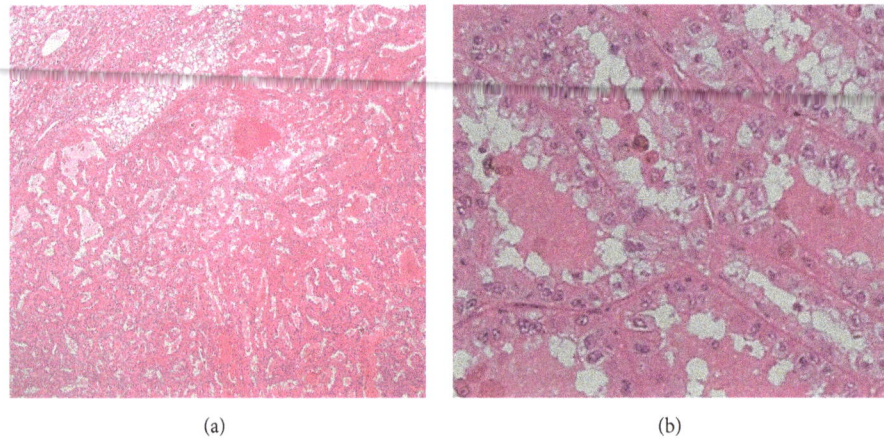

(a)　　　　　　　　　　　　　(b)

Figure 5: (a) The tumor comprised tubulocystic structured lesions (H&E). (b) Tumor cells have cell mutation with large nucleoli and eosinophilic cytoplasm, cubic and flat, forming small glands.

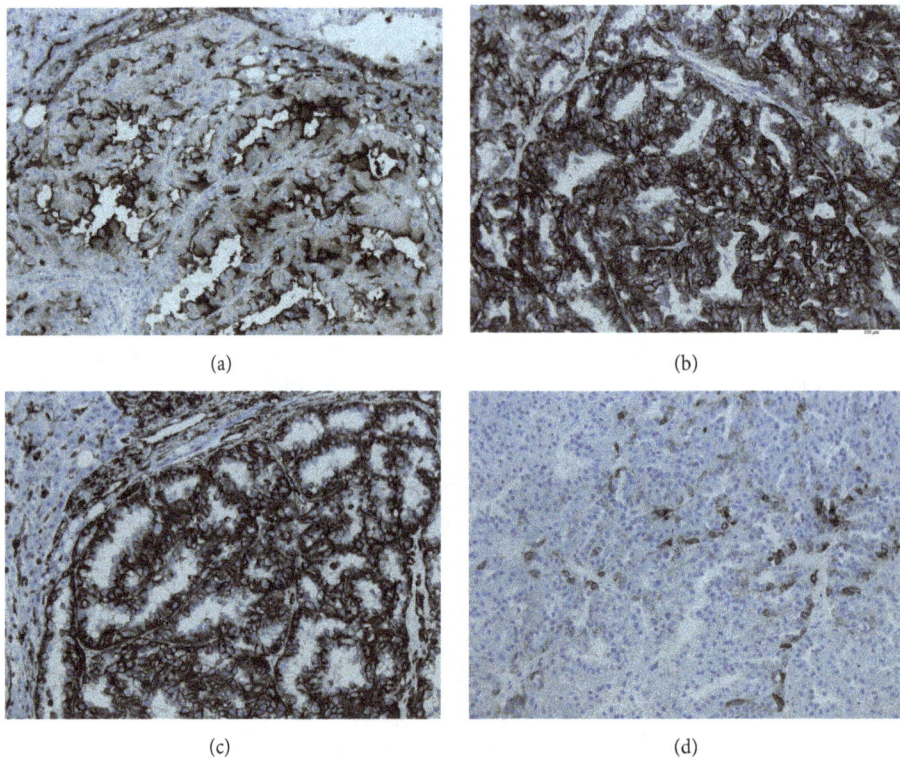

(a)　　　　　　　　　　　　　(b)

(c)　　　　　　　　　　　　　(d)

Figure 6: (a) CD10 positivity in the tumor cells. (b) CAM5.2 positivity in the tumor cells. (c) Vimentin positivity in the tumor cells. (d) CK7 being occasionally positive.

papillary neoplasm of bile duct (IPN-B) depending on the presence of ovarian stroma and bile duct communication (BDC), respectively [4].

Tubulocystic carcinoma (TCC) of the kidney is an exceedingly rare, recently recognized subtype of renal cell carcinoma and considered in differential diagnosis of cystic renal neoplasms. Diagnosis is based on distinct histological features combined with immune histochemical features. This case had histological and pathological features of tubulocystic carcinoma of the kidney. Only six cases of tubulocystic carcinoma that derived from the bile duct have been reported

as subtype of the collecting duct carcinoma of the kidney in abstracts of the 102nd United States and Canadian Academy of Pathology (USCAP) annual meeting in 2013, and the details of the entity are unknown. Masson originally described tubulocystic carcinoma with Bellinian epithelioma as a tumor of the collecting ducts of Bellini in the kidney [5]. Therefore, an evolving concept of collecting duct carcinomas was proposed, and low-grade collecting duct carcinoma at the beginning of the spectrum corresponds to the current concept of tubulocystic carcinoma. Supportive findings include the expression of proximal convoluted tubule markers

(a)

(b)

(c)

(d)

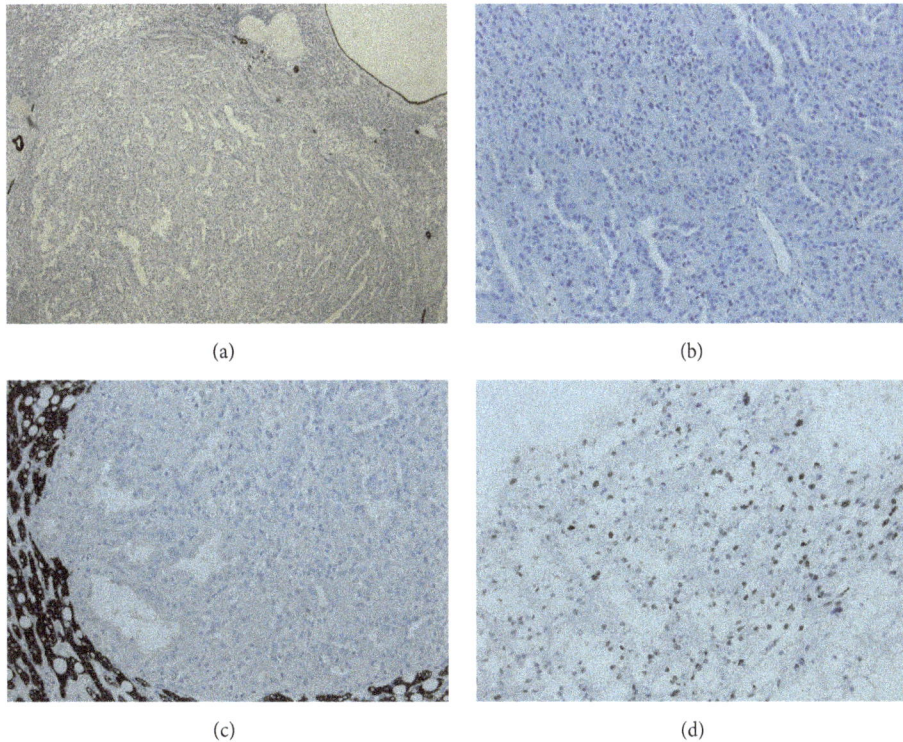

FIGURE 7: (a) AE1AE3 negativity in the tumor. (b) CD20 negativity in the tumor. (c) Hepatocyte negativity in the tumor. (d) p53 positivity in the tumor.

(CD10 and alpha-methylacyl-CoA racemase; AMACR), distal nephron proteins (parvalbumin, high-molecular-weight CK, and CD19) [1, 6], and the detection of intercalated cells and cells similar to those in the proximal tubule using electron microscopy [1, 7, 8]. In addition, Osunkoya et al. [8] reported that all tubulocystic carcinomas were strongly positive for the proximal convoluted tubule markers CD10, vimentin, and AMACR. Tubulocystic carcinoma exhibits a histopathological image that suggests a poor proliferative response from its cell heterotypes and structures but there are some cases with distant metastasis and local recurrence [1, 9, 10]. The pathological histology that predicts slow progression and dissociation of the clinical course leading to metastasis/recurrence is a feature of this disease.

Tubulocystic carcinoma of the bile duct is very unusual with regard to its histopathology, and no definite view has yet been obtained. We must carefully observe its clinical course as a nonclassifiable intrahepatic bile duct carcinoma. It may be recognized as a very rare tumor derived from the bile duct in the future.

5. Conclusion

We herein reported an extremely rare case of tubulocystic carcinoma that derived from the bile duct.

Acknowledgments

The authors are grateful to Professor Sohsuke Yamada for his comments on this case.

References

[1] M. B. Amin, G. T. MacLennan, R. Gupta et al., "Tubulocystic carcinoma of the kidney: clinicopathologic analysis of 31 cases of a distinctive rare subtype of renal cell carcinoma," *The American Journal of Surgical Pathology*, vol. 33, no. 3, pp. 384–392, 2009.

[2] T. Nakajima, Y. Kondo, M. Miyazaki, and K. Okui, "A histopathologic study of 102 cases of intrahepatic cholangiocarcinoma: histologic classification and modes of spreading," *Human Pathology*, vol. 19, no. 10, pp. 1228–1234, 1988.

[3] Y. Nakanuma, H. Minato, T. Kida, and T. Terada, "Pathology of cholangiocellular carcinoma," in *Primary Liver Cancer in Japan*, pp. 39–50, Springer, 1992.

[4] D. Snover, D. Ahnen, R. Burt, and R. Odze, *WHO classification of tumours of the digestive system*, IARC, Lyon, France, 2010.

[5] P. Masson, *Tumeurs Humaines 1955. Human Tumors, Histology, Diagnosis and Technique*, 1970.

[6] S. Azoulay, A. Vieillefond, F. Paraf et al., "Tubulocystic carcinoma of the kidney: A new entity among renal tumors," *Virchows Archiv*, vol. 451, no. 5, pp. 905–909, 2007.

[7] M. Zhou, X. J. Yang, J. I. Lopez et al., "Renal tubulocystic carcinoma is closely related to papillary renal cell carcinoma: implications for pathologic classification," *The American Journal of Surgical Pathology*, vol. 33, no. 12, pp. 1840–1849, 2009.

[8] A. O. Osunkoya, A. N. Young, W. Wang, G. J. Netto, and J. I. Epstein, "Comparison of gene expression profiles in tubulocystic carcinoma and collecting duct carcinoma of the kidney," *The American Journal of Surgical Pathology*, vol. 33, no. 7, pp. 1103–1106, 2009.

[9] X. J. Yang, M. Zhou, O. Hes et al., "Tubulocystic carcinoma of the kidney: Clinicopathologic and molecular characterization," *The American Journal of Surgical Pathology*, vol. 32, no. 2, pp. 177–187, 2008.

[10] A. Lopez-Beltran, J. C. Carrasco, L. Cheng, M. Scarpelli, Z. Kirkali, and R. Montironi, "2009 update on the classification of renal epithelial tumors in adults," *International Journal of Urology*, vol. 16, no. 5, pp. 432–443, 2009.

32

Young Man with Hepatomegaly: A Case of Glycogenic Hepatopathy

Walid Abboud ⓘ,[1] Saif Abdulla,[1] Mohammed Al Zaabi,[2] and Ramzi Moufarrej[3]

[1]*Department of Internal Medicine, Zayed Military Hospital, Abu Dhabi, UAE*
[2]*Department of Gastroenterology, Zayed Military Hospital, Abu Dhabi, UAE*
[3]*Department of Critical Care, Zayed Military Hospital, Abu Dhabi, UAE*

Correspondence should be addressed to Walid Abboud; wamd7@hotmail.com

Academic Editor: Manuela Merli

Glycogenic hepatopathy is a rare but potentially reversible condition characterized by hepatomegaly and elevated liver enzymes occurring in poorly controlled type 1 diabetes mellitus patients and often requires a liver biopsy to confirm the diagnosis. We present the case of a young man who was admitted with diabetic ketoacidosis in the setting of poorly controlled diabetes mellitus type 1 and was noted to have significantly elevated transaminases that continued to worsen despite appropriate treatment of the diabetic ketoacidosis. A liver biopsy confirmed the diagnosis of glycogenic hepatopathy and the patient improved with diabetes control. The aim of this report is to shed light on possible causes of significant elevation of liver enzymes in patients presenting with diabetic ketoacidosis. In addition, we would like to raise awareness about the diagnosis, management, and prognosis of glycogenic hepatopathy and how to differentiate it from other hepatic conditions that have a similar presentation.

1. Introduction

Glycogenic hepatopathy presents with abdominal pain, hepatomegaly, and transaminasemia as a result of increased glycogen formation and deposition in the setting of excess levels of insulin and glucose. This condition remains poorly recognized among clinicians, which may lead to expensive and unnecessary testing and delaying appropriate management. In this case report, we reviewed the presentation, evaluation, and management of a patient who developed elevated liver enzymes after initiation of treatment of diabetic ketoacidosis. In addition, we present the thought process involved in the differential diagnosis and workup done for our patient leading to the final diagnosis of glycogenic hepatopathy.

2. Case Presentation

A 15-year-old boy was brought to the emergency department by his family for evaluation of abdominal pain associated with nausea and vomiting. His discomfort started one day earlier and was localized to the right upper quadrant of the abdomen. He described a constant pressure unrelated to food intake. He reported no change in urine or stools and no melena, dysphagia, anorexia, increase in abdominal girth, or change in his weight. He was lethargic and fatigued but had no pruritus, jaundice, night sweats, fever, easy bruising, or bleeding.

The patient's medical history was notable for type 1 diabetes mellitus for 6 years, which has been poorly controlled and was complicated by several episodes of diabetic ketoacidosis. There was no family history of diabetes mellitus, autoimmune diseases, or liver disorders. His medications included insulin Lantus 22 units at night and insulin Humalog 20 units three times daily before each meal. He admitted that he had not been consistently compliant with his medications. There was no history of new medication usage. He also denied the use of any over-the-counter medication or alcohol use. There was no recent travel and no sick contact. On physical examination, the patient was noted to be thin and in no acute distress and afebrile with heart rate of 109 beats per minute and blood pressure of 109/60 mm Hg. His weight was 37 kg and his height was 153 cm with a

TABLE 1: Liver enzymes and lactic acid results.

Tests	Day 1 (admission)	2	3	4	7	8	9	10	Reference range
ALT	262	214	226	286	405	433	423	304	16–63 U/L
AST	205	345	419	558	678	743	501	310	0–37 U/L
Lactate	3.2	5.3	4.7	3.4	1.6				0.4–2 mmol/L

body mass index (BMI) of 15.8 kg/m^2. The jugular venous pressure was not elevated. Examination of the heart and lungs was unremarkable. Abdominal examination revealed mildly distended abdomen with mild tenderness on palpation in the right upper quadrant. There was no rebound or guarding and Murphy's sign was absent. The liver was palpable 6 cm below the costal margin, with a smooth edge. The spleen was not palpable, and there was no evidence of ascites. Skin examination showed no palmar erythema, leg edema, spider angiomata, or evidence of pigmentation. There was a scant presence of axillary and pubic hair. The neurologic examination, including mental status, was normal.

3. Investigations

On presentation, blood glucose was 480 mg per deciliter (mg/dl). The serum sodium level was 137 mmol per liter (mmol/L), potassium was 4.1 mmol/L, chloride was 97 mmol/L, and bicarbonate was 19 mmol/L. The anion gap was calculated at 21. The blood urea nitrogen (BUN) was 29 mg/dl and the creatinine was 0.6 mg/dl. The arterial blood gas showed a pH of 7.25, partial pressure of carbon dioxide (PCO_2) of 30 mmHg, and partial pressure of oxygen (PO_2) of 95 mmHg. The liver enzymes were abnormal with the alanine aminotransferase (ALT) of 262 units per liter (U/L) (normal range: 16 to 63 U/L) and aspartate aminotransferase (AST) of 205 U/L (normal range: 0 to 37 U/L). The alkaline phosphatase was 139 U/L (normal range: <322 U/L), gamma-glutamyl transferase (GGT) was 122 U/L (normal range: 15–85 U/L), and the total bilirubin was 0.5 mg/dl (normal range: 0 to 1 mg/dl). Serum albumin was 4.1 g per deciliter and the amylase and lipase levels were within normal ranges. The acetaminophen level was undetectable. His lactate level was 3.2 mmol/L (normal range: 0.4–2 mmol/L). The prothrombin time and partial-thromboplastin time were both normal. The white cell count was 4,700 per cubic millimeter, with a normal differential count. The hemoglobin was 13.8 grams per deciliter, with mean corpuscular volume of 88 fL, and the platelet count was 383,000 per cubic millimeter. The urinalysis showed evidence of ketones. A radiograph of the chest showed no abnormal findings.

4. Inpatient Course

The patient was admitted to the hospital with the impression of diabetic ketoacidosis, most probably due to noncompliance with medications. The patient was started on insulin infusion and intravenous fluid with potassium chloride.

There was no evidence of sepsis or other causes that precipitated this event. He also had elevated liver enzymes and lactic acid with hepatomegaly, with no obvious etiology.

The patient's ketoacidosis resolved with treatment and he was shifted to his regular dose of insulin with good glycemic control achieved by the second day. He continued to have mild abdominal pain in the right side of the abdomen and his liver enzymes continued to rise significantly. The lactate level also worsened on the second day before slowly trending to normal range on day 7 (Table 1).

Given this rise in liver enzymes associated with abdominal pain and hepatomegaly in the setting of type 1 diabetes mellitus, we initiated the workup to evaluate the etiology behind this presentation. We ordered an ultrasound of the liver to evaluate for evidence of nonalcoholic fatty liver disease. Also, we sent investigation for iron deposition disorder and for autoimmune workup. We also tested for viral hepatitis serology, despite the fact that he had no previous history or risk factors for viral hepatitis. Other conditions considered in our differential diagnosis included medication-induced hepatitis, Wilson's disease, alpha-1 antitrypsin deficiency, glycogen storage disorder, Gaucher's disease, and secondary amyloidosis.

The results of the additional investigations were as follows: the serum iron was 104 μg per deciliter (normal range: 65–176), total iron-binding capacity was 392 μg per deciliter (normal range: 240–450), and ferritin was 141 nanograms per milliliter (normal range: 5–244). His total cholesterol was 218 mg/dl, triglycerides level was 141 mg/dl, high-density lipoprotein (HDL) was 41 mg mg/dl, and low-density lipoprotein (LDL) was 149 mg/dl. The glycated hemoglobin (HbA_{1c}) was 12.4%. Hepatitis A, B, and C, Epstein-Barr virus (EBV), and cytomegalovirus (CMV) serology all came back negative. The antimitochondrial antibody and anti-smooth muscle antibody were negative. Results for the ceruloplasmin serum test were in the normal range. The thyroid function was normal. Alpha-1 antitrypsin level was normal. Ultrasonography of the abdomen showed the liver to be enlarged with a bipolar length of 24 cm, with normal echogenicity. The gall bladder had normal wall thickness, with no stones or biliary dilatation. The spleen and kidneys appeared normal.

In conclusion, there was no evidence based on our investigation for the common causes of rising liver enzymes. Revising his previous medical history, the patient had several admissions with diabetic ketoacidosis associated with elevated liver enzymes. Also noted, his liver enzymes continued to rise before ultimately trending down around the ninth hospital day. The decision was then made to perform a liver biopsy.

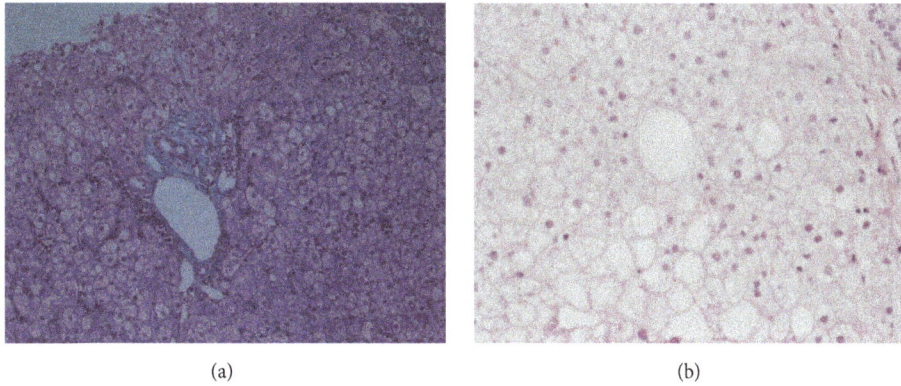

(a)   (b)

FIGURE 1: (a) Liver biopsy showing hepatocytic ballooning of moderate degree, with mild microvesicular and macrovesicular steatosis, and prominent glycogenated nuclei by PAS stain (magnification: ×40). (b) Hematoxylin and Eosin staining showing evidence of steatosis, nuclear glycogenosis, and lobular inflammation (magnification: ×100).

TABLE 2: Glycogenic hepatopathy versus hepatic steatosis.

Condition	Glycogenic hepatopathy	Hepatic steatosis
Association	Type 1 diabetes mellitus	Type 2 diabetes mellitus
Treatment	Insulin and better glycemic control	Weight loss
Complication	Unlikely cirrhosis	Complicated by cirrhosis

The liver biopsy results showed mild macrovesicular and microvesicular steatosis with mild portal and lobular inflammation. Periodic acid-Schiff staining revealed increased overall intracellular glycogen content with the presence of glycogenated nuclei. The biopsy findings were consistent with glycogenic hepatopathy (Figure 1).

5. Discussion

Glycogenic hepatopathy was first described in 1930 by Mauriac as "hepatic glycogenosis, characterized by hepatic glycogen deposition in patients with poorly controlled type 1 diabetes mellitus" [1]. Mauriac's original description of this syndrome was for children with features of hepatomegaly, abdominal pain, abnormal liver enzymes, elevated cholesterol, and growth retardation with delayed puberty. However, it was later recognized to occur in both adults [2] and children [3]. In addition, elevation of lactic acid has been increasingly recognized and reported to occur in glycogenic hepatopathy [4].

While the pathophysiology of glycogenic hepatopathy or Mauriac syndrome is not fully understood, the most accepted theory is that the presence of insulin and excess glucose activates glycogen synthase phosphatase into activated glycogen synthase, an enzyme required for the conversion of glucose-1-phosphate to glycogen. This activation promotes glycogen formation and storage in the liver and blocks glycogenolysis, increasing hepatic glycogen stores during hyperglycemia. Insulin is administered as the main treatment for hyperglycemia, driving glycogen synthesis further and inhibiting gluconeogenesis and glycogenolysis, resulting in increasing hepatocyte glycogen stores. Glycogen overload ultimately leads to hepatomegaly and elevated liver enzymes [5, 6]. Elevated levels of glucose and insulin in prepubertal diabetic patients results in a state of hypercortisolism, which explains the pubertal and growth delays [3, 7]. The exact mechanism for lactic acidosis reported in glycogenic hepatopathy is poorly understood [4, 8]. It is felt that the reduction in gluconeogenesis in the liver and the resultant reduction in conversion of pyruvate to glucose may drive the anaerobic reaction of pyruvate to lactate. Therapy with insulin would further reduce gluconeogenesis and increase lactic acid formation, explaining the increase of lactic acidosis observed with early therapy of glycogenic hepatopathy [9]. In a case series conducted by Torbenson et al. which studied 14 patients with biopsy-proven glycogenic hepatopathy, all the patients had type 1 diabetes and 13 patients had abnormal liver-function tests. Hepatomegaly was evident by imaging in 9 patients and 6 patients had elevated HbA$_{1c}$ levels. Steatosis was present in only 2 patients [7].

The diagnosis of glycogenic hepatopathy is usually supported by the following features: poorly controlled type 1 diabetes mellitus, abdominal pain, hepatomegaly, abnormal levels of liver enzymes, and the improvement of the liver enzymes with insulin therapy. The reversibility of the elevation in liver enzymes with rigorous glucose control usually occurs within 2 to 4 weeks [10]. Elevated lactic acid may exist with or without evidence of hypoperfusion [11]. The test to confirm the diagnosis is the liver biopsy. Treatment involves the use of adequate doses of insulin to achieve rigorous glucose control.

It is important to differentiate glycogenic hepatopathy from hepatic steatosis and from other inherited glycogen storage disorders (Tables 2 and 3). While hepatic steatosis is

TABLE 3: Glycogenic hepatopathy versus glycogen storage disorder.

Condition	Glycogenic hepatopathy	Glycogen storage disorder
Etiology	Acquired	Inherited
Course	Reversible	Irreversible

TABLE 4: Height, weight, HbA_{1c}, and BMI on follow-up visits.

	7/2015 (admission)	4/2016	2/2017	Units
Height cm/(percentile)	153/(8.7)	159/(8.5)	163/(18.7)	cm
Weight kg/(percentile)	37/(2.94)	45/(8.85)	54/(22.7)	kg
BMI/ (percentile)	15.8/(3.8)	17.8/(18.1)	21.5/(61.8)	kg/m^2
HbA_{1c}	12.4	9.8	10.2	%

more commonly associated with obesity and type 2 diabetes mellitus and could potentially lead to liver cirrhosis, glycogenic hepatopathy is classically seen in type 1 diabetes mellitus patients and it is highly unlikely to lead to liver cirrhosis [6, 12, 13].

On further follow-up visits, the patient was more compliant with his medical care and his diabetes was under better control with the surveillance of the endocrinology department. He did not show any further rise in his liver enzymes. With HbA_{1c} trending down with treatment, the growth indicators including height, weight, and BMI showed gradual improvement (Table 4).

6. Conclusion

Our patient fulfills several criteria for glycogenic hepatopathy, including history of poorly controlled type 1 diabetes mellitus and physical findings of hepatomegaly confirmed by abdominal ultrasonography. In addition, he had elevated liver enzymes and lactic acidosis in the absence of hypoperfusion, both of which responded to insulin therapy and glucose control. With other common etiologies of liver disease such as infectious, autoimmune, metabolic, or drug-induced etiologies ruled out, the characteristic histological findings noted on the liver biopsy showing the increased intracellular glycogen content and the glycogenated nuclei confirmed the diagnosis.

The reversibility of liver enzymes with intensive insulin therapy, in our case, is particularly important given that it is consistent with the diagnosis and prognosis of this condition. This case reinforces the importance of recognizing the features of glycogenic hepatopathy for proper management. Glycogen hepatopathy has an excellent prognosis with improved glycemic control.

Ethical Approval

Ethical approval was obtained from the ethics committee at Zayed Military Hospital.

Disclosure

The work was not supported or funded by any drug company. Dr. Abboud is the main author. The manuscript has not been published previously, in any language, in whole or in part, and is not currently under consideration elsewhere.

Acknowledgments

The authors thank Dr. Ali Al-Za'abi, Head of Department of Pathology at Zayed Military Hospital. The authors also thank Rashida Augustine Elliott and acknowledge the Medical Education Department at Zayed Military Hospital.

References

[1] P. Mauriac, "Gros ventre, hepatomegalie, troubles de la croissance chez les enfants diabetiques traites depuis plusieurs annes par l'insuline," *Gazette Hebdomadaire des Sciences Médicales de Bordeaux*, vol. 26, pp. 402–410, 1930.

[2] R. Chatila and A. B. West, "Hepatomegaly and abnormal liver tests due to glycogenosis in adults with diabetes," *Medicine*, vol. 75, no. 6, pp. 327–333, 1996.

[3] E. Fitzpatrick, C. Cotoi, A. Quaglia, S. Sakellariou, M. E. Ford-Adams, and N. Hadzic, "Hepatopathy of Mauriac syndrome: a retrospective review from a tertiary liver centre," *Archives of Disease in Childhood*, vol. 99, no. 4, pp. 354–357, 2014.

[4] M. C. G. J. Brouwers, J. C. Ham, E. Wisse et al., "Elevated lactate levels in patients with poorly regulated type 1 diabetes and glycogenic hepatopathy: a new feature of mauriac syndrome," *Diabetes Care*, vol. 38, no. 2, pp. e11–e12, 2015.

[5] N. Parmar, M. Atiq, L. Austin, R. A. Miller, T. Smyrk, and K. Ahmed, "Glycogenic hepatopathy: thinking outside the box," *Case Reports in Gastroenterology*, vol. 9, no. 2, pp. 221–226, 2015.

[6] C. F. J. Munns, R. B. McCrossin, M. J. Thomsett, and J. Batch, "Hepatic glycogenosis: Reversible hepatomegaly in type 1 diabetes," *Journal of Paediatrics and Child Health*, vol. 36, no. 5, pp. 449–452, 2000.

[7] M. Torbenson, Y.-Y. Chen, E. Brunt et al., "Glycogenic hepatopathy: an underrecognized hepatic complication of diabetes mellitus," *The American Journal of Surgical Pathology*, vol. 30, no. 4, pp. 508–513, 2006.

[8] M. Chen, T. Y. Kim, and A. M. Pessegueiro, "Elevated lactate levels in a non-critically ill patient," *The Journal of the American Medical Association*, vol. 313, no. 8, pp. 849-850, 2015.

[9] J. B. Jeppesen, C. Mortensen, F. Bendtsen, and S. Møller, "Lactate metabolism in chronic liver disease," *Scandinavian Journal of Clinical & Laboratory Investigation*, vol. 73, no. 4, pp. 293–299, 2013.

[10] B. Krishnan, S. Babu, J. Walker, A. B. Walker, and J. M. Pappachan, "Gastrointestinal complications of diabetes mellitus," *World Journal of Diabetes*, vol. 4, no. 3, pp. 51–63, 2013.

[11] K. S. Deemer and G. F. Alvarez, "A Rare Case of Persistent Lactic Acidosis in the ICU: Glycogenic Hepatopathy and Mauriac Syndrome," *Case Reports in Critical Care*, vol. 2016, pp. 1–4, 2016.

[12] A. Abaci, O. Bekem, T. Unuvar et al., "Hepatic glycogenosis: a rare cause of hepatomegaly in Type 1 diabetes mellitus," *Journal of Diabetes and its Complications*, vol. 22, no. 5, pp. 325–328, 2008.

[13] R. M. Hudacko, A. V. Manoukian, S. H. Schneider, and B. Fyfe, "Clinical resolution of glycogenic hepatopathy following improved glycemic control," *Journal of Diabetes and its Complications*, vol. 22, no. 5, pp. 329-330, 2008.

33

Hepatotoxicity Associated with Use of the Weight Loss Supplement *Garcinia cambogia*: A Case Report and Review of the Literature

Jiten P. Kothadia ⓘ,[1] **Monica Kaminski,**[2]
Hrishikesh Samant,[3] **and Marco Olivera-Martinez**[4]

[1]*Nazih Zuhdi Transplant Institute, INTEGRIS Baptist Medical Center, 3300 NW Expressway, Oklahoma City, OK 73112, USA*
[2]*Department of Internal Medicine, Coney Island Hospital, 2601 Coney Island Avenue, Brooklyn, NY 11235, USA*
[3]*Division of Gastroenterology and Hepatology, Louisiana State University Health Sciences Center, Shreveport, LA 71103, USA*
[4]*Department of Gastroenterology and Hepatology, University of Nebraska Medical Center, 982000 Nebraska Medical Center, Omaha, NE 68198, USA*

Correspondence should be addressed to Jiten P. Kothadia; kothadia.jiten@gmail.com

Academic Editor: Fumio Imazeki

The use of herbal and dietary supplements for weight loss is becoming increasingly common as obesity is becoming major health problem in the United States. Despite the popularity of these natural supplements, there are no guidelines for their therapeutic doses and their safety is always a concern. *Garcinia cambogia* extract with its active ingredient "hydroxycitric acid" is a component of many weight loss regimens. It suppresses fatty acid biosynthesis and decreases appetite. However, its prolonged use in weight maintenance is unknown. Here we describe a case of acute hepatitis after the use of *Garcinia cambogia* for weight loss.

1. Introduction

In the United States, dietary supplements (DS) are being used more commonly as a strategy for weight loss [1–3]. The National Health and Nutrition Examination Survey (NHANES) 2003–2006 showed the use of DS in as many as 50% of Americans and 70% of adults above the age of 70 years [3, 4]. Many consumers have a false sense of security that these products are "natural" and thus safe for use [2, 3, 5]. In reality, many of these DS do not have established guidelines for safe doses and their use is not as tightly regulated by the United States (US) Food and Drug Administration (FDA) as pharmaceuticals [1, 3, 5]. For pharmaceuticals to be approved for the market, there is a process of close scientific scrutiny including a demonstration of safety and efficacy; no such scrutiny is applied to dietary supplements as they are considered as food products [1, 4]. Some DS also have been associated with significant side effects and case reports of DS causing such health injuries are increasing [2, 5]. It is often challenging to determine the causative agent, as many

of these DS are made up of a variety of compounds that may change with time [3]. Although direct causality is difficult to confirm, the US Drug Induced Liver Injury Network (DILIN) has reported that herbal supplements attributed liver injury has increased in the past ten years and ranges from 2% to 16% of all reported hepatotoxicity [3, 4]. In particular, DS known to cause liver injury include Hydroxycut, *Camellia sinensis* (green tea extract), Herbalife products, usnic acid, LipoKinetix, 1,3-Dimethylamylamine, uncoupling protein-1, vitamin A, OxyELITE pro, and anabolic steroids [4].

Garcinia cambogia (GC) is a component of many dietary supplements for weight loss. *GC* is a tropical fruit that grows in South East Asia and Africa and has been found to contain hydroxycitric acid (HCA) in its rind [3, 6, 7]. This active ingredient is an inhibitor of adenosine triphosphate (ATP) citrate lyase, which is an enzyme involved in fatty acid biosynthesis and glycogen storage. It also causes suppression of appetite [2, 8]. Thus, *GC/HCA* is often added to weight loss products [3, 4, 7]. Its potential to cause health hazard remains controversial, but there has been evidence in animal studies to show that *GC* is linked to causing oxidative stress, inflammation, and hepatic fibrosis [3, 4, 7].

2. Case Discussion

A 36-year-old female with no significant medical history presented with a 3-day history of low-grade fever, nausea, vomiting, and abdominal pain. She reported that she had been following a 500 Kcal diet and was taking GC for four weeks to lose weight. She also complained of fatigue, anorexia, and jaundice. The patient denied any history of recent blood transfusion, illicit drug use, or family history of liver disease. She denied alcohol consumption and was in a monogamous heterosexual relationship.

On physical examination, she had scleral icterus, cutaneous jaundice, and tender hepatomegaly measuring 2 cm below the costal margin. Abnormal laboratory results included white blood cell count of 2.73×10^3 cells/μL (4–11) and platelet count of 78×10^3 cells/μL (150–400), aspartate aminotransferase (AST) of 5340 U/L (15–41), alanine aminotransferase (ALT) of 5615 U/L (7–52), alkaline phosphatase of 104 U/L (32–91), total bilirubin of 7.4 mg/dl (0.3–1.0), and direct bilirubin of 4.9 mg/dl (0.0–0.4). Serologies for hepatitis A, hepatitis B, hepatitis C, autoimmune markers (anti-nuclear antibody, anti-smooth muscle antibodies, anti-mitochondrial antibody, and anti-liver kidney microsomal 1 antibody), human immunodeficiency virus, rapid plasma reagin test, cytomegalovirus, Epstein-Barr virus, Herpes Simplex virus, and Parvovirus were negative. Serum ceruloplasmin, alpha-fetoprotein, and alpha-1 antitrypsin levels were normal. Abdominal Doppler ultrasound showed mild echotexture coarsening in the liver and small ascites.

Considering her recent exposure to herbal medications, we suspected drug induced liver injury and used updated RUCAM (Roussel Uclaf Causality Assessment Method) scale to calculate its probability. Patient's RUCAM score came out to be 8 points, which is consistent with probable drug induced liver injury [9]. GC was discontinued and conservative management was initiated. Significant clinical improvement and the downward trend of liver function tests obviated the need for liver biopsy. The patient was discharged on hospital day 6. At follow-up visit two weeks later, her liver function tests had returned to normal (Figure 1).

3. Discussion

The use of dietary supplements with a perception that such use is safe is becoming increasingly popular in USA [2, 16]. Also, with the epidemic of obesity in US, many people have considered DS as a treatment remedy for weight loss [20]. However, there are no guidelines for their use and the FDA does not tightly regulate these DS for their safety. Several DS have been associated with acute liver injury, including fulminant liver failure requiring liver transplantation [2, 16].

According to the US Congress, DS is defined as a product taken by mouth which contains dietary ingredients to supplement the regular diet. These dietary ingredients include vitamins, herbs, minerals, amino acids, enzymes, metabolites, extracts, or concentrates [16]. Under the Dietary

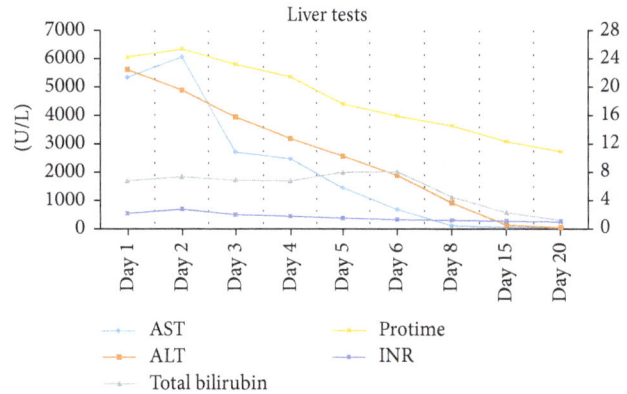

FIGURE 1: Changes in liver tests during hospitalization are plotted from admission at day 1 to day 20.

Supplement Health and Education Act (DSHEA), the FDA has the responsibility of demonstrating that a DS is harmful before it can take action to restrict or remove it from the market. In contrast, the pharmaceutical company must prove the safety of the medication it is manufacturing by clinical trials before the FDA will grant their approval [16].

In 2009, the FDA issued a notice against a popular supplement, *Hydroxycut*, due to the associated liver injury and one reported death [2, 3]. *GC* is one of the many ingredients contained in this compound, but it is not clear which ingredient of *Hydroxycut* compound was responsible for the liver damage [1, 21]. Furthermore, only 8 of the 14 marketed *Hydroxycut* products contained hydroxycitric acid (HCA) which is also the active component of *GC* [21]. Despite this information, many *Hydroxycut* products are still available online. In our patient, Omnitrition International, INC manufactured the GC supplement and contained GC extract 1000 mg (standardized to 50% HCA) and Potassium 150 mg per serving (2 capsules).

GC is a tropical fruit that grows in Southeastern Asia and Western Africa and contains active ingredient HCA [1, 2, 22]. Studies in both experimental mice and humans have shown fat loss and decrease in body weight [1]. Fat loss and weight reduction occur through many mechanisms including prevention of the conversion of carbohydrates to fatty acids by the inhibition of fatty acid biosynthesis through block of the ATP citrate lyase enzyme, which in turn leads to increased hepatic glycogen synthesis, and finally suppression appetite leading to decreased food intake [3, 21]. Appetite is suppressed further by the increased release of serotonin which is a neurotransmitter associated with eating behavior [21]. HCA has been on sale for almost two decades and there appear to be no reports of human liver toxicity other than those mentioned above regarding the product *Hydroxycut* of which HCA is a component [1, 6, 22].

Kim et al. studied the use of GC in a population of C57BL/6J mice fed a high-fat diet (45 kcal% fat) [1, 21, 22]. After a prolonged duration of observation over 16 weeks, it was determined that the use of *GC* promoted fatty acid oxidation and decreased fatty acid synthesis, leading to the amelioration of adipogenesis [1, 7]. They also showed

Table 1: Summary of patients with *Garcinia cambogia* related liver injury, characteristics, presentation, pattern of liver injury, and clinical outcome.

Author (year) [ref.]	Number Of cases	Age	Sex	Duration of GC containing supplement use	Presenting symptoms	Pattern of liver injury	Updated RUCAM score	Number of cases that underwent liver transplant	Mortality
Stevens et al. [10] (2005)	2	28.5*	M	5 weeks; 5 days	Fatigue, jaundice	Hepatocellular; cholestatic	8¥	0	0
Jones and Andrews [11] (2007)	1	19	M	120 days	Nausea, vomiting, and jaundice	Hepatocellular	7	0	0
Laczek and Duncan [12] (2008)	3	24.33*	M	60-90 days	Malaise, jaundice, and pruritus	2 hepatocellular; 1 cholestatic	8¥	0	0
Dara et al. [13] (2008)	2	36.5*	F	7 days; 14 days	Nausea, vomiting, fatigue, anorexia, and abdominal pain	Hepatocellular	8¥	0	0
Shim and Saab [14] (2009)	1	28	M	90 days	Fatigue, jaundice	Hepatocellular	8	0	0
Fong et al. [15] (2010)	8	30.9*	6M; 2 F	7 to 56 days	Nausea, vomiting, fatigue, and itching abdominal pain	Hepatocellular	7-8¥ NA for 3 patients needing transplant	3	0
Danan and Teschke [9] (2010)	1	19	M	7 days	Fever, fatigue, myalgia, arthralgia, and rash	Cholestatic	7	0	0
Sharma et al. [16] (2014)	1	27	M	Unknown	Nausea, vomiting, abdominal pain, and jaundice	Hepatocellular	7	0	0
Lee et al. [17] (2014)	1	39	F	2 days	Abdominal pain, anorexia, nausea, dyspepsia, fatigue, and jaundice	Hepatocellular	8	0	0
Melendez-Rosado et al. [7] (2015)	1	42	F	7 days	Nausea, abdominal pain	Hepatocellular	7	0	0
Corey et al. [2] (2016)	1	52	F	25 days	Jaundice, decreased appetite, fatigue, and confusion	Hepatocellular	NA	1	0
Smith et al. [18] (2016)	1	26	M	7 days	Jaundice, fatigue	Hepatocellular	NA	1	0
Lunsford et al. [19] (2016)	1	34	M	150 days	Nausea, vomiting, abdominal pain, and dark urine	Hepatocellular	NA	1	0
Kothadia et al. (present case)	1	26	F	28 days	Fever, nausea, vomiting, abdominal pain, malaise, fatigue, and jaundice	Hepatocellular	8	0	0

*Mean age; M: male; F: female; GC: *Garcinia cambogia*; ¥mean score; NA: not applicable.

that it induced oxidative stress, inflammation, and hepatic fibrosis as well as hepatic collagen accumulation and lipid peroxidation [1, 22]. Contrary to other published studies performed on animals and humans, this study by Clouatre and Preuss found HCA of GC to have a protective effect on the liver [22]. Thus, the form of HCA regarding strength, extraction process, residual compounds, and so forth may create a difference in study outcomes and requires definition [22].

Although there have been studies that show the weight loss benefit of GC, randomized, double-blind, placebo-controlled trial by Heymsfield et al. showed no significant change in fat mass and body weight observed over those using a placebo at 12 weeks [23]. A recent systematic review and meta-analysis by Onakpoya et al. showed that GC extract could cause short-term weight loss, but its overall effect on long-term weight is uncertain [24].

While it is difficult to prove causation in any drug-induced liver injury (DILI), in our case, hepatotoxicity was seen after taking GC and significant improvement in the liver function tests was seen after its discontinuation. Also, the absence of any other etiologies including infectious, autoimmune, and metabolic causes proven by comprehensive testing was suggestive of the fact that GC was the probable cause of the hepatotoxicity. Our patient was not tested for hepatitis E as hepatitis E is rare in the United States as a cause of acute liver failure. Also, clinical history was not classical for hepatitis E. We have summarized similar cases of hepatotoxicity secondary to GC reported till now in literature in Table 1 [2, 7, 10–20]. All of these cases presented with nonspecific symptoms such as nausea, vomiting, malaise, abdominal pain, and jaundice. The pattern of liver injury was hepatocellular in the majority of cases except for 3 cases that presented with cholestatic pattern. Six patients (24%) required orthotopic liver transplant. These cases indicate the need for better postmarketing surveillance and highlight the importance of reporting such cases to assist this process further.

DS induced liver injury often continues to remain a diagnosis of exclusion once viral hepatitis, autoimmune causes, and metabolic disturbances are excluded [2, 3]. Thus it is important to keep in mind that there may be further workup required to diagnose a DILI [2]. Despite this caveat, it is of benefit to obtain a thorough history of herbal or dietary supplements when the etiology of liver injury is unclear, both for the benefit of choosing appropriate therapy for the patient and for the future of drug development [2].

4. Conclusion

Although DS are often perceived to be natural and safe, they frequently have harmful side effects and can result in significant morbidity and mortality. This case depicts hepatotoxicity that was associated with the use of weight loss supplement GC. The physician should always ask about the use of DS as many patients may fail to disclose this information. Our case indicates the need for better postmarket surveillance and highlights the importance of reporting such cases to assist this process further.

Authors' Contributions

Jiten P. Kothadia, M.D., contributed to concept and design, acquisition of available literature, and drafting of the case report. Monica Kaminski, M.D., contributed to drafting of the case report and manuscript proofreading. Hrishikesh Samant, M.D., contributed to manuscript proofreading. Marco Olivera-Martinez, M.D., contributed to critical revision of the manuscript for important intellectual content.

References

[1] Y.-J. Kim, M.-S. Choi, Y. B. Park, S. R. Kim, M.-K. Lee, and U. J. Jung, "Garcinia cambogia attenuates diet-induced adiposity but exacerbates hepatic collagen accumulation and inflammation," *World Journal of Gastroenterology*, vol. 19, no. 29, pp. 4689–4701, 2013.

[2] R. Corey, K. T. Werner, A. Singer et al., "Acute liver failure associated with Garcinia cambogia use," *Annals of Hepatology*, vol. 15, no. 1, pp. 123–126, 2016.

[3] E. X. Zheng and V. J. Navarro, "Liver Injury from Herbal, Dietary, and Weight Loss Supplements: a Review," *Journal of Clinical and Translational Hepatology*, vol. 3, no. 2, pp. 93–98, 2015.

[4] M. García-Cortés, M. Robles-Díaz, A. Ortega-Alonso, I. Medina-Caliz, and R. J. Andrade, "Hepatotoxicity by Dietary Supplements: A tabular Listing and Clinical Characteristics," *International Journal of Molecular Sciences*, vol. 17, no. 4, article no. 537, 2016.

[5] V. J. Navarro, H. Barnhart, H. L. Bonkovsky et al., "Liver injury from herbals and dietary supplements in the U.S. Drug-Induced Liver Injury Network," *Hepatology*, vol. 60, no. 4, pp. 1399–1408, 2014.

[6] A. Lobb, "Hepatoxicity associated with weight-loss supplements: A case for better post-marketing surveillance," *World Journal of Gastroenterology*, vol. 15, no. 14, pp. 1786-1787, 2009.

[7] J. Melendez-Rosado, D. Snipelisky, G. Matcha, and F. Stancampiano, "Acute hepatitis induced by pure garcinia cambogia," *Journal of Clinical Gastroenterology*, vol. 49, no. 5, pp. 449-450, 2015.

[8] J. Heo, M. Seo, H. Park et al., "Gut microbiota Modulated by Probiotics and Garcinia cambogia Extract Correlate with Weight Gain and Adipocyte Sizes in High Fat-Fed Mice," *Scientific Reports*, vol. 6, Article ID 33566, 2016.

[9] G. Danan and R. Teschke, "RUCAM in drug and herb induced liver injury: the update," *International Journal of Molecular Sciences*, vol. 17, no. 1, p. 14, 2016.

[10] T. Stevens, A. Qadri, and N. N. Zein, "Two patients with acute liver injury associated with use of the herbal weight-loss supplement hydroxycut [7]," *Annals of Internal Medicine*, vol. 142, no. 6, pp. 477-478, 2005.

[11] F. J. Jones and A. H. Andrews, "Acute liver injury associated with the herbal supplement hydroxycut in a soldier deployed to Iraq," *American Journal of Gastroenterology*, vol. 102, no. 10, pp. 2357-2358, 2007.

[12] J. Laczek and M. Duncan, "Three cases of acute hepatitis in patients taking Hydroxycut (R) bodybuilding supplement," in *American Journal of Gastroenterology*, Nature Publishing Group, New York, NY, USA, 2008.

[13] L. Dara, J. Hewett, and J. K. Lim, "Hydroxycut hepatotoxicity: A case series and review of liver toxicity from herbal weight loss supplements," *World Journal of Gastroenterology*, vol. 14, no. 45, pp. 6999–7004, 2008.

[14] M. Shim and S. Saab, "Severe hepatotoxicity due to hydroxycut: A case report," *Digestive Diseases and Sciences*, vol. 54, no. 2, pp. 406–408, 2009.

[15] T.-L. Fong, K. C. Klontz, A. Canas-Coto et al., "Hepatotoxicity due to hydroxycut: A case series," *American Journal of Gastroenterology*, vol. 105, no. 7, pp. 1561–1566, 2010.

[16] T. Sharma, L. Wong, N. Tsai, and R. D. Wong, "Hydroxycut(®) (herbal weight loss supplement) induced hepatotoxicity: a case report and review of literature.," *Hawaii Medical Journal*, vol. 69, no. 8, pp. 188–190, 2010.

[17] J. L. Lee, H. P. Shin, J. W. Jeon, J. M. Cha, K. R. Joo, and J. I. Lee, "A Case of Toxic Hepatitis by Weight-Loss Herbal Supplement Containing Garcinia cambogia," *Soonchunhyang Medical Science*, vol. 20, no. 2, pp. 96–98, 2014.

[18] R. J. Smith, C. Bertilone, and A. G. Robertson, "Fulminant liver failure and transplantation after use of dietary supplements," *Medical Journal of Australia*, vol. 204, no. 1, pp. 30–32.e1, 2016.

[19] K. E. Lunsford, A. S. Bodzin, D. C. Reino, H. L. Wang, and R. W. Busuttil, "Dangerous dietary supplements: Garcinia cambogia-Associated hepatic failure requiring transplantation," *World Journal of Gastroenterology*, vol. 22, no. 45, pp. 10071–10076, 2016.

[20] D. Kaswala, S. Shah, N. Patel, S. Raisoni, and S. Swaminathan, "Hydroxycut-induced liver toxicity," *Annals of Medical and Health Sciences Research*, vol. 4, no. 1, pp. 143–145, 2014.

[21] L. O. Chuah, S. K. Yeap, W. Y. Ho, B. K. Beh, and N. B. Alitheen, "In vitro and in vivo toxicity of garcinia or hydroxycitric acid: A review," *Evidence-Based Complementary and Alternative Medicine*, vol. 2012, Article ID 197920, 12 pages, 2012.

[22] D. L. Clouatre and H. G. Preuss, "Hydroxycitric acid does not promote inflammation or liver toxicity," *World Journal of Gastroenterology*, vol. 19, no. 44, pp. 8160–8162, 2013.

[23] S. B. Heymsfield, D. B. Allison, J. R. Vasselli, A. Pietrobelli, D. Greenfield, and C. Nunez, "*Garcinia cambogia* (hydroxycitric acid) as a potential antiobesity agent: a randomized controlled trial," *The Journal of the American Medical Association*, vol. 280, no. 18, pp. 1596–1600, 1998.

[24] I. Onakpoya, S. K. Hung, R. Perry, B. Wider, and E. Ernst, "The use of *Garcinia* extract (hydroxycitric acid) as a weight loss supplement: a systematic review and meta-analysis of randomised clinical trials," *Journal of Obesity*, vol. 2011, Article ID 509038, 9 pages, 2011.

34

Tumor Regression in HCC Patient with Portal Vein Tumor Thrombosis after Intraportal Radiofrequency Thermal Ablation

Malkhaz Mizandari,[1] **Tamta Azrumelashvili,**[1] **Natela Paksashvili,**[1] **Nino Kikodze,**[2]
Ia Pantsulaia,[2] **Nona Janikashvili,**[2] **and Tinatin Chikovani**[2]

[1]*Department of Interventional Radiology, Tbilisi State Medical University, High Technology University Clinic, 0144 Tbilisi, Georgia*
[2]*Department of Immunology, Tbilisi State Medical University, 0177 Tbilisi, Georgia*

Correspondence should be addressed to Nona Janikashvili; njanikashvili@tsmu.edu

Academic Editor: Melanie Deutsch

Hepatocellular carcinoma (HCC) is the third leading cause of cancer-related death worldwide. Portal vein tumor thrombosis (PVTT) is a frequent entity in HCC, which strictly limits the gold standard treatment options such as surgical resection and transarterial chemoembolization. Therefore, the prognosis of patients with PVTT is extremely poor and an emergence of seeking an alternative option for intervention is inevitable. We present a case of a 60-year-old male patient with HCC induced PVTT who was subjected to the intraportal RFA and stenting-VesOpen procedure. No additional medical intervention was performed. The repeated CT performed 5 months after the VesOpen procedure revealed significant decrease of the tumor size, patent right, and main portal vein and a recanalization of the left portal vein, which was not processed. At this time point, liver functional tests, appetite, and general condition of the patient were improved evidently. This report designates the RFA as an instrumental option of therapeutic intervention for HCC patients with PVTT.

1. Introduction

Hepatocellular carcinoma (HCC) is the most common primary liver cancer, the sixth most common cancer overall, and the third most common cause of cancer-related death worldwide [1–3]. Classical treatments for HCC include surgical resection, liver transplantation, and local ablative therapy [4, 5]. Liver transplantation is theoretically the best therapeutic choice, however, limited by the shortage of donor organs, and hepatectomy is considered the standard treatment for patients with preserved liver function [6, 7].

Portal vein thrombosis (PVT) is a common complication of HCC. The management of HCC patients with PVT is more challenging than the ones without PVT [8]. The presence of PVTT limits standard treatment options: liver transplantation and curative resection [9, 10]. Transarterial chemoembolization (TACE) is associated with an increased risk of ischemic liver necrosis in such cases and is, therefore, subjective to a select group of patients with good hepatic

function and adequate collateral circulation around the occluded portal vein [11]. Thus, the prognosis of inoperable cases of HCC with PVTT is extremely poor; the average life span after diagnosis is reported to be 3 to 6 months [12, 13].

Radiofrequency thermal ablation (RFA) may be considered as an attainable method in such condition. Details of the percutaneous PVTT ablation procedure, including its safety and feasibility, are previously described by our team [14, 15].

2. Case Presentation

A 60-year-old man was admitted with three weeks of fatigue and abdominal discomfort. He was documented to suffer from a hepatitis C induced liver cirrhosis (Child-Pugh B) and was admitted to our hospital for US-guided biopsy of the liver mass. CT scan reported a left lobe vascular mass (8-9 cm), with prominent venous phase washout. Sharply circumscribed, hypodense component of 3 cm in size was shown within this mass. Left PV total tumor thrombosis and

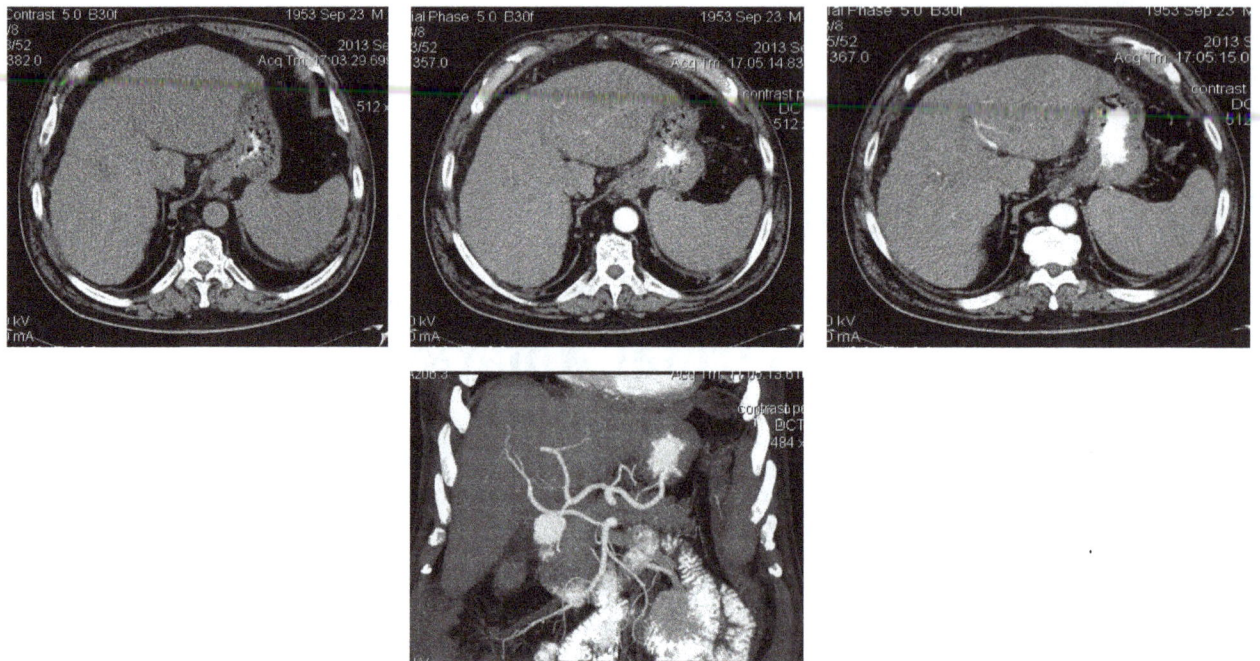

FIGURE 1: Preprocedure CT (native and arterial phase). Note: superior mesenteric artery type right hepatic artery; left lobe mass main feeder is left hepatic artery.

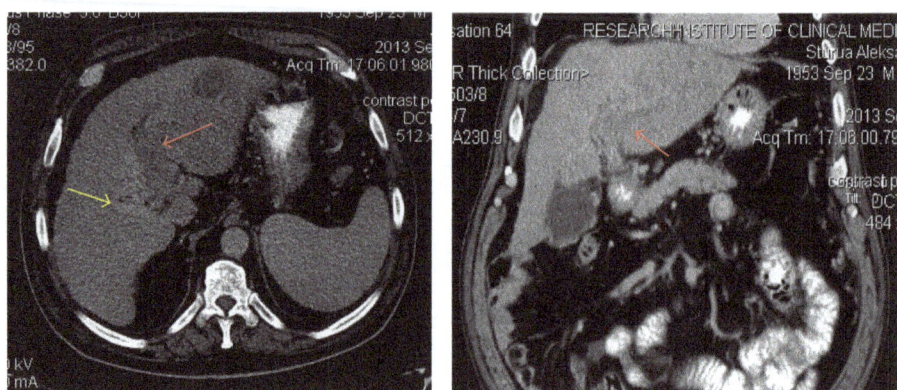

FIGURE 2: Preprocedure CT (portal phase): RPV patent branch (puncture "target" on VesOpen procedure), yellow arrow; completely obliterated LPV, red arrow.

PV cavernous transformation were also revealed. Thrombus was already protruding into the main PV, so that only right PV remained patent (Figures 1 and 2).

Blood tests revealed severe hypoalbuminemia and thrombocytopenia, moderate hypocoagulation, moderate changes of liver enzymes, and elevated α-fetoprotein (Table 1).

The patient first underwent a percutaneous ultrasound (US) guided biopsy of the left lobe mass (from small hypodense component). Morphological study of biopsy specimens revealed the diagnosis of HCC. Based on the existence of a PVTT, this patient was not subjected to the surgical resection and/or TACE procedure. The VesOpen procedure, aiming at normal blood flow restoration to the right PV, has been proven on MDT discussion.

The patient returned to the hospital a month later to undergo portal vein recanalization, via intraportal RFA and stenting-VesOpen procedure.

In VesOpen procedure, the right PV was accessed by 18 G puncture needle using real-time US guidance; contrast injection showed the portography "above" the thrombus, manifesting the PV thrombus "upper" border. 0.035-inch diameter wire was conducted through the thrombus into

Tumor Regression in HCC Patient with Portal Vein Tumor Thrombosis after Intraportal Radiofrequency...

169

TABLE 1: Blood test results.

Test	Result	Normal range
Chemistry		
Albumin (g/L)	25	35–52
AST (u/L)	99.8	<40
ALT (u/L)	76.0	<41
GGT (u/L)	158	10–70
Hematology		
Platelets (nL)	70	150–400
Coagulation		
PT (sec)	16.8	11–15
PT (%)	61.9	70–105
INR	1.48	1–1.3
Immunology		
AFP (m/L)	31577	≤5.8

SMV using 5 Fr guiding catheter and portography "below" the thrombus was performed, documenting the PV thrombus "lower" border. 8 Fr diameter introducer sheath was positioned and 8 Fr endoluminal device (RITA® Model 1500X RF Generator AngioDynamics, EMcision 8F VesOpen 2800) was introduced into the thrombus for 2-session processing. The 14 mm diameter self-expanding vascular stent (Zilver 635® Vascular Self-Expanding Stent | Cook Medical) was positioned into the thrombus and postdilated by balloon. Postprocedure portography showed the main PV patency complete restoration maintaining the normal blood flow into the right portal vein. The VesOpen procedure was completed with working track ablation by the same RF device.

The patient tolerated the procedure well; no intraprocedural complications were detected. On postprocedure follow-up (in 3 hours) fluid in small pelvis (blood) has been detected in 3 hours and as the amount was increasing slightly, small pelvis drainage has been performed and up to 800 cc blood was evacuated. The patient stayed in clinic for 36 hours and received the fresh frozen plasma and red blood cell mass infusion.

After being discharged from hospital, the patient was referred to the hematologist and hepatologist for further consultations and to prepare for a probable TACE.

Patient refused to undergo the TACE and visited the clinic only for the consultations 5 months later. His condition had been improved dramatically; albumin rose to 32 g/dL. Coagulation status and liver functional tests, appetite, and functional status had improved as well.

CT revealed that the LPV, which had initially been absolutely closed with thrombus and was not processed on VesOpen procedure, was now recanalized (without any anticoagulation or thrombolytic therapy). The left lobe bulging, which has previously been evaluated as a big HCC, was reduced. Only sharply circumscribed, hypodense small mass was seen (Figures 3 and 4). The patient refused to undergo the scheduled TACE.

18 months after the VesOpen procedure, the patient was referred to the hospital for heart problems and has proceeded blood tests which showed the normalized blood coagulation values: PT-14.0; PT%-85.6; INR-1.12. Unfortunately, patient was lost for the subsequent follow-up.

3. Discussion

RFA is a safe and effective modality for the treatment of focal malignant diseases in solid organs and has been used to achieve localized tumor necrosis in solid neoplasms for many years [16, 17]. It delivers a high amount of thermal energy to target tissue with curative or palliative intent, which can be monitored by a real-time ultrasonography or a computed tomography.

During RF, the energy passes between the electrodes and biological tissues to cause coagulation of a selected area. The high-frequency alternating electric current applied through the electrodes results in rapid movement of intracellular ions in opposite directions. Ionic motion creates frictional forces that generate heat around the electrodes and eventually around the tissue surrounding the catheter.

Supporting the release of a wide spectrum of tumor antigens by in situ tumor destruction, RFA is considered to be a strong adjuvant for initiating antitumor immune responses by virtue overcoming immune tolerance and leading to the presentation of otherwise cryptic neoplastic antigen [18–20]. A tumor-specific T-cell activation following RFA has been documented in the nonreactive neoplasm-bearing host [18]. In humans, post-RFA HCC regression has been associated with the increased dendritic cell infiltration and consequent tumor-specific T-cell responses [21]. RFA of HCC was found to trigger a functional transient activation of myeloid dendritic cells associated with increased serum levels of TNF-alpha and IL-1 beta with a sustained antitumor immune response [20]. In addition, animals treated with subtotal RFA showed significant elevation in tumor-specific class I and II responses to a male minor histocompatibility (HY) antigens and tumor regression [22]. Thus, by providing several "danger" signals to the immune cells, RFA includes an active immunotherapeutic effect in cancer which demands further exploration; moreover that therapeutic vaccination of HCC is still an awaited approach [23].

Liver synthetic function is one of the important factors determining the treatment option in patients with primary liver cancer, thereby directly influencing the long term prognosis of these patients. Improving liver synthetic function in these patients makes them suitable for better treatment options. Partial or complete recanalization of the PV following RFA of tumor thrombus improves liver function and makes these patients suitable for better treatment options like transarterial chemoembolization (TACE), local ablative therapies, or systemic therapy with sorafenib. This potentially improves survival in this group of patients who were initially not suitable for any tumor-specific treatment due to poor liver function.

In the presented case, RFA and stenting were done on RPV, expecting to have the clinical effect by RPV recanalization. Interestingly, however, the follow-up examination

Before

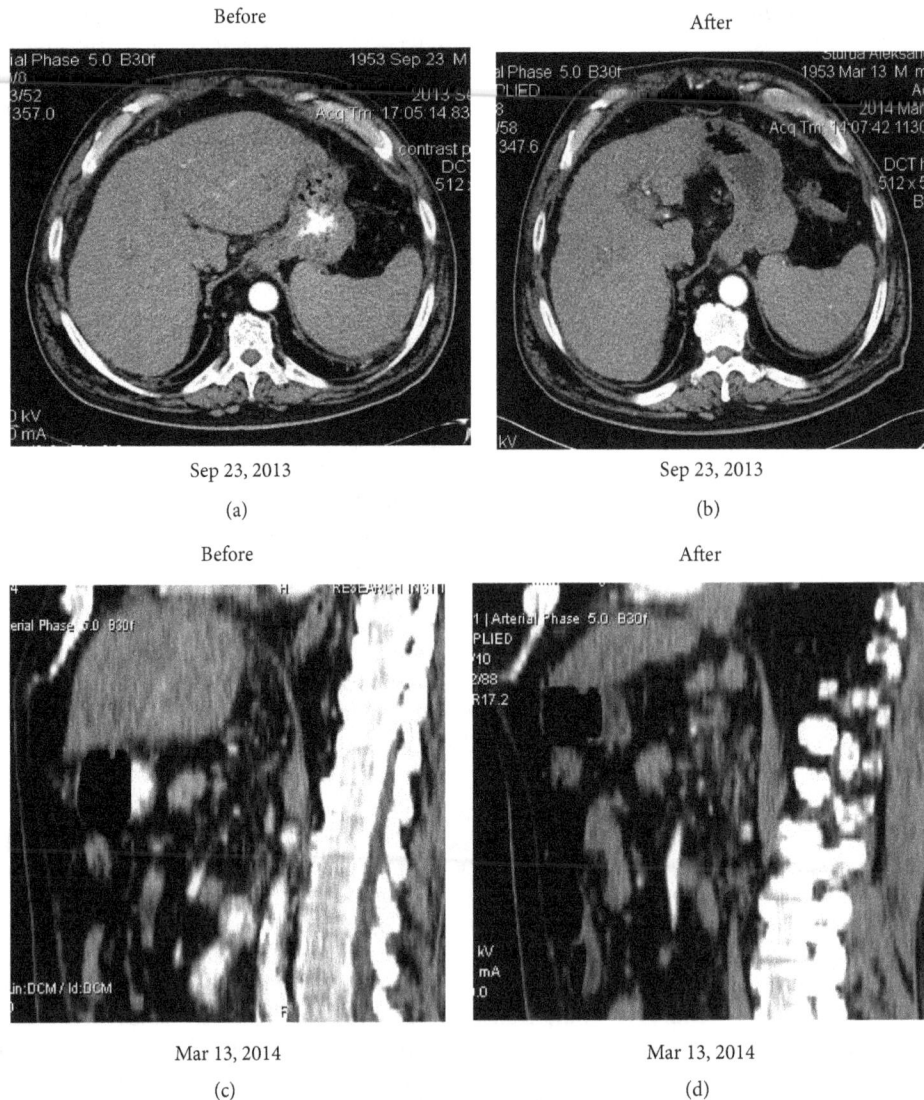

After

Sep 23, 2013

(a)

Sep 23, 2013

(b)

Before   After

Mar 13, 2014

(c)

Mar 13, 2014

(d)

FIGURE 3: Comparison: CT before and in 5 months after VesOpen procedure. Note the decreased size and normal shape of the left lobe.

showed that LPV was also recanalized and the left lobe tumor size decreased. As the LPV was not processed on VesOpen procedure, the only possible explanation of this effect is the antitumor immune response triggered by tumor thrombus RF processing.

4. Conclusion

In case of HCC with PVTT, RFA could be considered as an instrumental feasible procedure and the potential modulator of immune response against tumor.

Abbreviations

CT: Computed tomography
US: Ultrasound

PV: Portal vein
SMA: Superior mesenteric artery
RHA: Right hepatic artery
LHA: Left hepatic artery
RPV: Right portal vein
LPV: Left portal vein
PVT: Portal vein thrombosis
PVTT: Portal vein tumor thrombus
MDT: Multidisciplinary discussion
TACE: Transarterial chemoembolization
HCC: Hepatocellular carcinoma.

Before

After

(a)

(b)

After

(c)

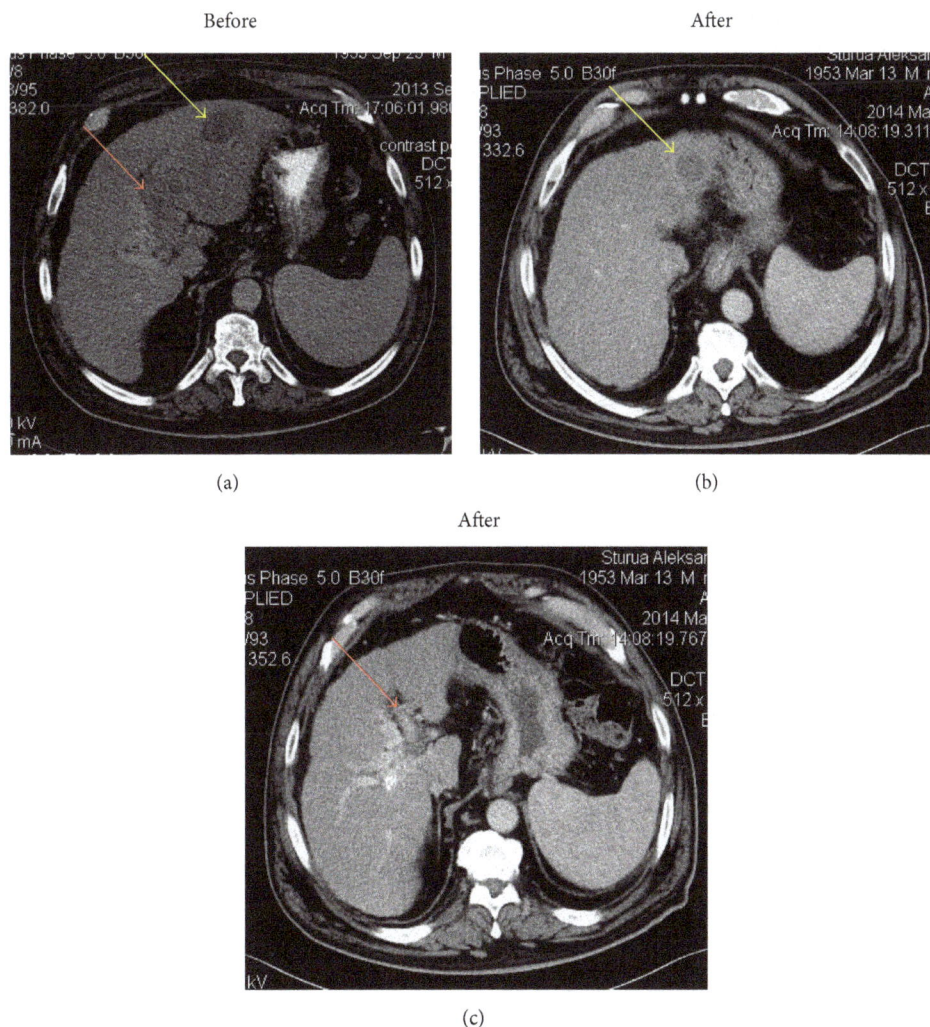

FIGURE 4: Comparison: CT before and in 5 months after VesOpen procedure. LPV (red arrow) is recanalized. The residual tumor is represented only by hypodense component, the size of which is decreased (yellow arrow).

References

[1] A. Forner, J. M. Llovet, and J. Bruix, "Hepatocellular carcinoma," *The Lancet*, vol. 379, no. 9822, pp. 1245–1255, 2012.

[2] J. Ferlay, H.-R. Shin, F. Bray, D. Forman, C. Mathers, and D. M. Parkin, "Estimates of worldwide burden of cancer in 2008: GLOBOCAN 2008," *International Journal of Cancer*, vol. 127, no. 12, pp. 2893–2917, 2010.

[3] J. D. Yang and L. R. Roberts, "Hepatocellular carcinoma: a global view," *Nature Reviews Gastroenterology & Hepatology*, vol. 7, no. 8, pp. 448–458, 2010.

[4] J. Bruix and M. Sherman, "Management of hepatocellular carcinoma: an update," *Hepatology*, vol. 53, no. 3, pp. 1020–1022, 2011.

[5] Z.-H. Gao, D.-S. Bai, G.-Q. Jiang, and S.-J. Jin, "Review of preoperative transarterial chemoembolization for resectable hepatocellular carcinoma," *World Journal of Hepatology*, vol. 7, no. 1, pp. 40–43, 2015.

[6] H. Y. Kim and J. W. Park, "Clinical trials of combined molecular targeted therapy and locoregional therapy in hepatocellular carcinoma: past, present, and future," *Liver Cancer*, vol. 3, pp. 9–17, 2014.

[7] Y.-B. Zheng, Q.-W. Meng, W. Zhao et al., "Prognostic value of serum vascular endothelial growth factor receptor 2 response in patients with hepatocellular carcinoma undergoing transarterial chemoembolization," *Medical Oncology*, vol. 31, no. 3, article 843, 2014.

[8] M. Quirk, Y. H. Kim, S. Saab, and E. W. Lee, "Management of hepatocellular carcinoma with portal vein thrombosis," *World Journal of Gastroenterology*, vol. 21, no. 12, pp. 3462–3471, 2015.

[9] M. Omata, L. A. Lesmana, R. Tateishi et al., "Asian Pacific Association for the study of the liver consensus recommendations on hepatocellular carcinoma," *Hepatology International*, vol. 4, no. 2, pp. 439–474, 2010.

[10] A. Forner, M. E. Reig, C. R. de Lope, and J. Bruix, "Current strategy for staging and treatment: the BCLC update and future prospects," *Seminars in Liver Disease*, vol. 30, no. 1, pp. 61–74, 2010.

[11] W.-Y. Lau, B. Sangro, P.-J. Chen et al., "Treatment for hepatocellular carcinoma with portal vein tumor thrombosis: the

emerging role for radioembolization using yttrium-90," *Oncology*, vol. 84, no. 5, pp. 311–318, 2013.

[12] J. M. Llovet, J. Bustamante, A. Castells et al., "Natural history of untreated nonsurgical hepatocellular carcinoma: rationale for the design and evaluation of therapeutic trials," *Hepatology*, vol. 29, no. 1, pp. 62–67, 1999.

[13] R. T.-P. Poon, S. T. Fan, I. O.-L. Ng, and J. Wong, "Prognosis after hepatic resection for stage IVA hepatocellular carcinoma: a need for reclassification," *Annals of Surgery*, vol. 237, no. 3, pp. 376–383, 2003.

[14] X. Feng, M. Pai, M. Mizandari et al., "Towards the optimization of management of hepatocellular carcinoma," *Frontiers of Medicine in China*, vol. 5, no. 3, pp. 271–276, 2011.

[15] M. Mizandari, G. Ao, Y. Zhang et al., "Novel percutaneous radiofrequency ablation of portal vein tumor thrombus: safety and feasibility," *CardioVascular and Interventional Radiology*, vol. 36, no. 1, pp. 245–248, 2013.

[16] M.-H. Chen, W. Yang, K. Yan et al., "Treatment efficacy of radiofrequency ablation of 338 patients with hepatic malignant tumor and the relevant complications," *World Journal of Gastroenterology*, vol. 11, no. 40, pp. 6395–6401, 2005.

[17] M. Toyoda, S. Kakizaki, K. Horiuchi et al., "Computed tomography-guided transpulmonary radiofrequency ablation for hepatocellular carcinoma located in hepatic dome," *World Journal of Gastroenterology*, vol. 12, no. 4, pp. 608–611, 2006.

[18] T. T. Wissniowski, J. Hünsler, D. Neureiter et al., "Activation of tumor-specific T lymphocytes by radio-frequency ablation of the VX2 hepatoma in rabbits," *Cancer Research*, vol. 63, no. 19, pp. 6496–6500, 2003.

[19] M. H. M. G. M. den Brok, R. P. M. Sutmuller, R. van der Voort et al., "*In situ* tumor ablation creates an antigen source for the generation of antitumor immunity," *Cancer Research*, vol. 64, no. 11, pp. 4024–4029, 2004.

[20] M. Y. Ali, C. F. Grimm, M. Ritter et al., "Activation of dendritic cells by local ablation of hepatocellular carcinoma," *Journal of Hepatology*, vol. 43, no. 5, pp. 817–822, 2005.

[21] S. A. Dromi, M. P. Walsh, S. Herby et al., "Radiofrequency ablation induces antigen-presenting cell infiltration and amplification of weak tumor-induced immunity," *Radiology*, vol. 251, no. 1, pp. 58–66, 2009.

[22] A. Zerbini, M. Pilli, A. Penna et al., "Radiofrequency thermal ablation of hepatocellular carcinoma liver nodules can activate and enhance tumor-specific T-cell responses," *Cancer Research*, vol. 66, no. 2, pp. 1139–1146, 2006.

[23] N. Kikodze, K. Mazmishvili, M. Iobadze et al., "Hepatocellular carcinoma: current and prospective immunotherapeutic strategies," *Georgian Medical News*, no. 246, pp. 78–84, 2015.

35

Severe Anemia with Hemoperitoneum as a First Presentation for Multinodular Hepatocellular Carcinoma: A Rare Event in Western Countries

Thein Swe,[1] **Akari Thein Naing,**[1] **Aama Baqui,**[2] **and Ratesh Khillan**[3]

[1]*Department of Internal Medicine, Interfaith Medical Center, Brooklyn, NY, USA*
[2]*Department of Pathology, Interfaith Medical Center, Brooklyn, NY, USA*
[3]*Division of Oncology, Interfaith Medical Center, Brooklyn, NY, USA*

Correspondence should be addressed to Thein Swe; mglay2004@gmail.com

Academic Editor: Tawesak Tanwandee

Hemoperitoneum due to spontaneous rupture of hepatocellular carcinoma is a life-threatening and rare condition in western countries with an incidence of less than 3% because of early detection of cirrhosis and neoplasm. Here, we describe a case of a 66-year-old male patient with altered mental status with hemorrhagic shock. Computed tomography scan of abdomen revealed hemoperitoneum and mass in liver. Patient underwent resection of liver tumor and biopsy revealed multinodular hepatocellular carcinoma. A high degree of suspicion is required where severe anemia and hemoperitoneum can be a first presentation for hepatocellular carcinoma especially in patients with chronic hepatitis C infection. Early diagnosis is crucial since mortality rates remain high for untreated cases.

1. Introduction

Hepatocellular carcinoma (HCC) is a hypervascular tumor with a high tendency for vascular invasion and can produce growth factors that induce neoangiogenisis. It is one of the most common types of cancer in the world accounting for about 500,000 of new cases diagnosed yearly [1, 2].

Spontaneous rupture of HCC was previously considered as problems of large tumor; however, small tumors with aggressive behavior are also at high risk. Symptoms may vary depending on location of tumor. Although rupture of deep tumors can present with asymptomatic or pain, a peripheral tumor can lead to hemoperitoneum with hemorrhagic shock in severe cases [3]. In the western countries, ruptured HCC is a rare condition with an incidence of less than 3% of HCC patients because of the earlier detection of HCC [2].

2. Case Presentation

A 66-year-old male with past medical history of chronic alcoholic and chronic hepatitis C (not sure if it was treated or not) was brought in by Emergency Medical Service (EMS) because of drowsiness and fatigue for 1 day. He denied any history of trauma.

Vital signs were pulse rate of 123 beats/minute, respiratory rate of 23 breaths/minute, and blood pressure of 82/55 mmHg. Physical examination revealed drowsy and pale patient that responded only to painful stimuli. Abdomen examination showed distended, tense abdomen with hypoactive bowel sounds. No organomegaly was found on palpation. Cardiovascular and chest examinations were within normal limits. No external bleeding source was identified.

laboratory tests showed white blood cells of 17.4×10^9/L, hemoglobin of 5 g/dL, hematocrit of 15%, platelet counts of 120,000/μL, mean corpuscular volume of 90.2 fL, absolute reticulocyte count of 63 K./μL (normal = 24–84 K./μL), haptoglobin of 68 mg/dL, bilirubin of 1.5 mg/dL, aspartate transaminase (AST) of 50 IU/L, alanine transaminase (ALT) of 103 IU/L and alkaline phosphatase of 90 IU/L, ammonia of 34 μmol/L, and tumor marker alpha fetoprotein level of 2556 ng/mL (normal = 0–8.3). Serum electrolytes, coagulation profile, amylase, and lipase were within normal limits.

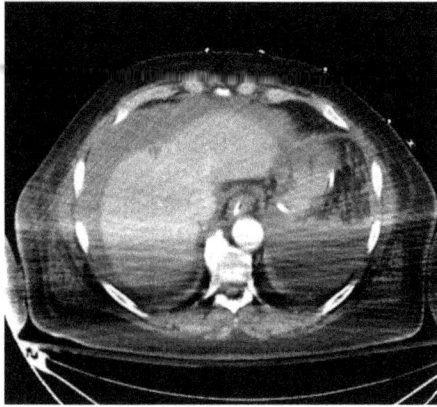

FIGURE 1: CT scan of abdomen and pelvic revealing hemoperitoneum and mass-like lesion in segment 4 of liver.

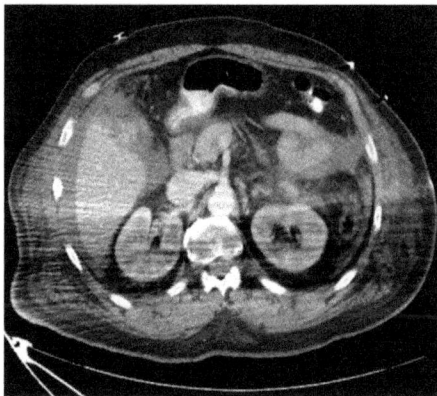

FIGURE 2: CT scan of abdomen and pelvic showing hemoperitoneum and mass-like density abutting gallbladder.

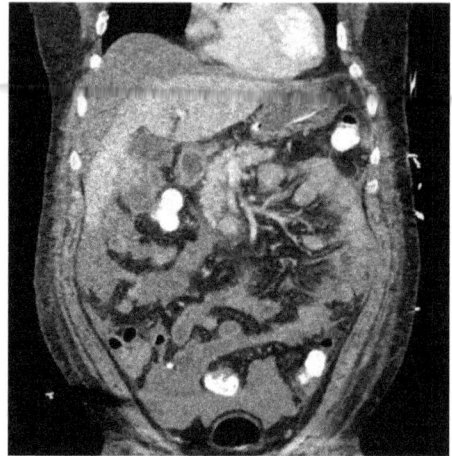

FIGURE 3: CT scan of abdomen and pelvic showing a mass at segment 5 of liver.

Baseline hemoglobin was 14.7 g/dL and hematocrit was 44% in 2011. Occult blood was negative.

Chest X-ray was unremarkable. Abdominal ultrasound revealed free peritoneal fluid and computed tomography (CT) scan of head showed no acute hemorrhage or infarct. CT scan of abdomen and pelvic revealed hemoperitoneum in the abdomen and pelvis and heterogeneous mass-like density abutting the gallbladder and lower right hepatic lobe (Figures 1, 2, and 3).

3. Treatment, Outcome, and Follow-Up

Patient was admitted to the intensive care unit (ICU) and treated with 4-litre bolus of normal saline intravenously and transfused a total of 4 units of pack red blood cells (PRBC). Patient underwent bland transcatheter arterial embolization (TAE). Microcatheter was used along with polyvinyl alcohol (PVA) particles injected into the hepatic artery. A sliding CT scanner system with interventional radiology features (IVR-CT) was used to take CT images during arterial infusion of contrast agents (CT during angiography). A mass was found to be exophytic from the edge of segment 5 of liver adjacent to the gallbladder bed. A small lesion in segment 4A of the liver

was also identified. Laparoscopic resections of segments 5 and 4A along with mass and cholecystectomy were performed.

Pathology report revealed that a tumor is segment 5 poorly differentiated 5.3 cm multinodular hepatocellular carcinoma with extensive microvascular invasions. It had approximately 85% necrosis and fibrosis. The tumor in segment 4A was 1.6 cm moderately differentiated multinodular hepatocellular carcinoma with extensive microvascular invasion. Background liver had portal and periportal fibrosis and focal fibrous septum formation. Hematoxylin and eosin (H & E) stained slides revealed evidence of background hepatitis C and grade 2 and stage 2 and multinodular poorly differentiated hepatocellular carcinoma, which was ruptured as evidenced by surrounding blood (Figures 4(a), 4(b), and 4(c)). Some of the hepatocellular carcinoma nodules showed area of steatosis (fatty change). No lymph node was submitted for examination. According to American Joint Committee on Cancer (AJCC), TNM Classification of Malignant Tumours (TNM) stage was T4NxMx, with direct invasion of adjacent organs other than the gallbladder or perforation of visceral peritoneum.

Patient condition improved along with stable vital signs. He tolerated diet gradually and was discharged from the hospital. Patient was called one week later after discharge and he denied any symptoms of postembolization syndrome such as nausea, pain, or fever. He was recommended follow-up with hematology and oncology clinic but was lost to follow-up.

4. Discussion

Spontaneous rupture of HCC is more prevalent in male with average age of around 45–75 years [3]. It is a life-threatening condition with a mortality rate at around 25%–75% [3, 4]. The mortality is even higher than that due to bleeding secondary to rupture of oesophageal varices [4]. About half of the cases of HCC occur in cirrhosis due to alcohol abuse while the remaining can be due to chronic hepatitis C and hepatitis B

(a)

(b)

(c)

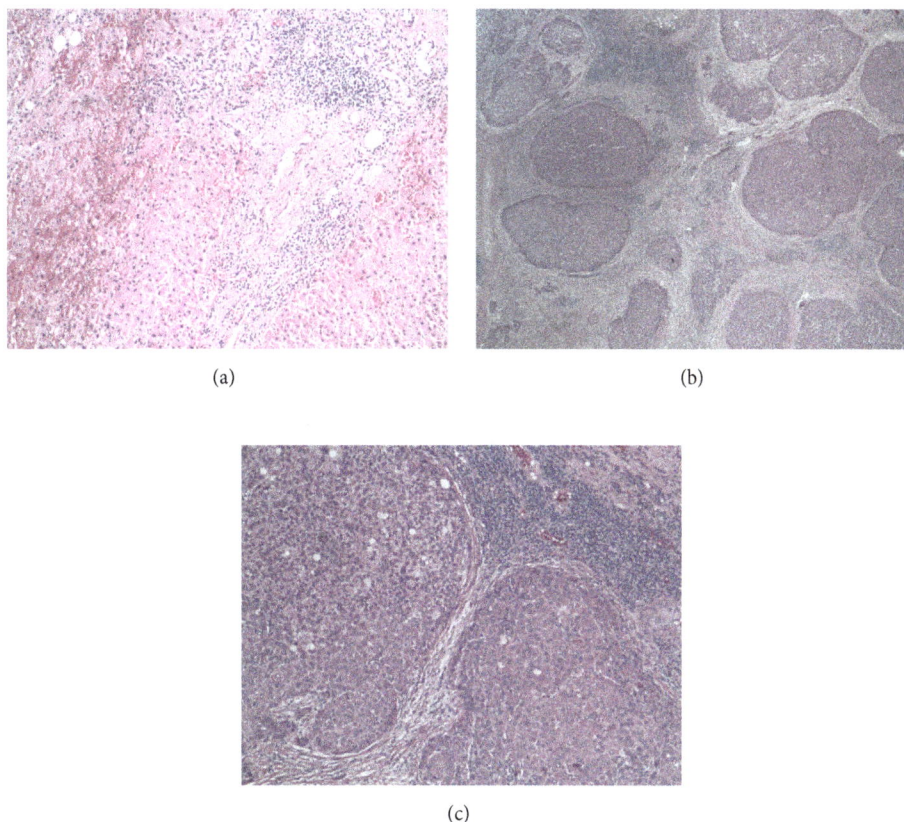

FIGURE 4: (a) H & E section (40x) shows the background normal liver cells showing mild to moderate portal triaditis and interface hepatitis (grade II) with most portal area infiltrated by many lymphocytes and few plasma cells as typical for hepatitis C. There is mild to moderate septal fibrosis that appears to be periportal and portal-portal (stage II). (b) H & E section (10x) shows multinodular hepatocellular carcinoma with fibrosis around the individual nodules. (c) H & E section (40x) shows poorly differentiated nature of the hepatocellular carcinoma with surrounding significant lymphocytic reaction.

infection since the incidence varies with geographic area and country's socioeconomic status [3].

The symptoms can range from severe abdominal pain to anemia, hemorrhagic shock, and eventually death if left untreated. Kanematsu et al. published a study that states that increased tumor size and extent of extrahepatic protrusion are correlated with an increased risk of rupture of HCC [5]. However, a study by Bassi et al. reported that size of the tumor did not correlate with severity of the hemoperitoneum [3]. It is assumed that a tear in the tumor surface or rupture of a feeding artery is the main reason for rupture of HCC and its complications such as hemoperitoneum [5]. The hepatic artery supplied small tumors and it was drained by the portal vein. Thus, a tamponade effect was created if there is obstruction of the main branches of the portal vein and portal hypertension which eventually lead to tumor rupture [6]. When tumors have an encompassing fibrous capsule which grow expansively, intratumoral pressure can be elevated leading to rupture. CT findings in ruptured HCC through hepatic capsule include discontinuity or disruption of hepatic surface abutting a HCC [5–7].

Management is dependent on hemodynamic status and resuscitation remains the first step in patients with shock.

TAE is the first choice of treatment in unstable patient with active intra-abdominal hemorrhage with a success rate of 90% [6]. It improves hemostasis and outcomes. One of the indications for elective surgical treatment is rupture of HCC at an early phase in the development of liver fibrosis because patients with rupture in the terminal phase of liver cirrhosis can be treated conservatively [4]. Conservative management can also be applied to stable patients at initial presentation. However, staged liver resection after securing hemostasis remains a definitive treatment [8]. Although transcatheter arterial chemoembolization (TACE) is recommended as the first line therapy for unresectable hepatic carcinoma, one of rare and serious complications of TACE is rupture of HCC. The predisposing factors are location of the tumor adjacent to the liver capsule, large tumor size, and total occlusion of the feeding artery [9].

Complications include repeated spontaneous rupture and intraabdominal HCC dissemination; however, it is not a contraindication for resection of primary tumor [6]. Prognostic factors to predict survival in the acute phase are serum bilirubin level, hemodynamic status on hospital admission, and preruptured disease state [8]. Tumor rupture itself is an impact on long term survival; however, individuals without portal venous thrombosis and decompensated liver cirrhosis and who underwent curative management had favorable outcome in a long term [10].

The incidence of ruptured HCC is a rare phenomenon accounting for <3% of HCC patients in western countries while incidence is higher in Asian countries in 2.3–26% of all HCC cases [11–15]. The reduced incidence in western countries is thought to be due to early detection of HCC with screening tests and low incidence of viral hepatitis B and hepatitis C. However, about 20–33% of the diagnosis of ruptured tumor is made only during an emergency exploratory laparotomy [16].

It is important to distinguish blood from simple fluid depending on amount of Hounsfield unit (HU) in CT scan images. The attenuation of fluids that have similar density as water such as bile, urine, and intestinal contents ranges from 0 to 15 HU [17]. However, blood usually has higher attenuation than other body fluids and unclotted extravascular blood usually has a measured attenuation of 30–45 HU whereas clotted blood is 45–70 HU [17].

In conclusion, spontaneous rupture of HCC is a rare condition in western countries because of early detection of cirrhosis and neoplasm. However, a high degree of suspicion is required where severe anemia and hemoperitoneum without history of trauma can be a first presenting sign for HCC. Early diagnosis is crucial since mortality rates remain high for untreated cases.

References

[1] J. M. Llovet, A. Burroughs, and J. Bruix, "Hepatocellular carcinoma," *The Lancet*, vol. 362, no. 9399, pp. 1907–1917, 2003.

[2] H. Yoshida, Y. Mamada, N. Taniai, and E. Uchida, "Spontaneous ruptured hepatocellular carcinoma," *Hepatology Research*, vol. 46, no. 1, pp. 13–21, 2016.

[3] N. Bassi, E. Caratozzolo, L. Bonariol et al., "Management of ruptured hepatocellular carcinoma: implications for therapy," *World Journal of Gastroenterology*, vol. 16, no. 10, pp. 1221–1225, 2010.

[4] A. Tanaka, R. Takeda, S. Mukaihara et al., "Treatment of ruptured hepatocellular carcinoma," *International Journal of Clinical Oncology*, vol. 6, no. 6, pp. 291–295, 2001.

[5] M. Kanematsu, T. Imaeda, Y. Yamawaki et al., "Rupture of hepatocellular carcinoma: predictive value of CT findings," *American Journal of Roentgenology*, vol. 158, no. 6, pp. 1247–1250, 1992.

[6] L. Veltchev, "Spontaneous rupture of hepatocellular carcinoma and hemoperitoneum management and long term survival," *Journal of IMAB*, vol. 1, pp. 53–57, 2009.

[7] B. G. Choi, S. H. Park, J. Y. Byun, S. E. Jung, K. H. Choi, and J.-Y. Han, "The findings of ruptured hepatocellular carcinoma on helical CT," *British Journal of Radiology*, vol. 74, no. 878, pp. 142–146, 2001.

[8] E. C. H. Lai and W. Y. Lau, "Spontaneous rupture of hepatocellular carcinoma: a systematic review," *Archives of Surgery*, vol. 141, no. 2, pp. 191–198, 2006.

[9] Z. Jia, F. Tian, and G. Jiang, "Ruptured hepatic carcinoma after transcatheter arterial chemoembolization," *Current Therapeutic Research, Clinical and Experimental*, vol. 74, pp. 41–43, 2013.

[10] W. H. Chan, C. F. Hung, K. T. Pan et al., "Impact of spontaneous tumor rupture on prognosis of patients with T4 hepatocellular carcinoma," *Journal of Surgical Oncology*, vol. 113, no. 7, pp. 789–795, 2016.

[11] N. Battula, M. Madanur, O. Priest et al., "Spontaneous rupture of hepatocellular carcinoma: a Western experience," *The American Journal of Surgery*, vol. 197, no. 2, pp. 164–167, 2009.

[12] C. Y. Chen, X. Z. Lin, J. S. Shin, C. Y. Lin, T. C. Leow, and T. T. Chang, "Spontaneous rupture of hepatocellular carcinoma. A review of 141 Taiwanese cases and comparison with nonrupture cases," *Journal of Clinical Gastroenterology*, vol. 21, no. 3, pp. 238–242, 1995.

[13] M. Miyamoto, T. Sudo, and T. Kuyama, "Spontaneous rupture of hepatocellular carcinoma: a review of 172 Japanese cases," *American Journal of Gastroenterology*, vol. 86, no. 1, pp. 67–71, 1991.

[14] C.-L. Liu, S.-T. Fan, C.-M. Lo et al., "Management of spontaneous rupture of hepatocellular carcinoma: single-center experience," *Journal of Clinical Oncology*, vol. 19, no. 17, pp. 3725–3732, 2001.

[15] F. Zhong, X. Cheng, K. He, S. Sun, J. Zhou, and H. Chen, "Treatment outcomes of spontaneous rupture of hepatocellular carcinoma with hemorrhagic shock: a multicenter study," *SpringerPlus*, vol. 5, no. 1, p. 1101, 2016.

[16] M. Islam, P. Deka, R. Kapur, and M. A. Ansari, "Non-bleeding spontaneous rupture of hepatocellular carcinoma," *Nigerian Journal of Surgery*, vol. 19, no. 2, pp. 82–84, 2013.

[17] M. Lubner, C. Menias, C. Rucker et al., "Blood in the belly: CT findings of hemoperitoneum," *Radiographics*, vol. 27, no. 1, pp. 109–125, 2007.

36

Clopidogrel-Induced Severe Hepatitis: A Case Report and Literature Review

Hesam Keshmiri, Anuj Behal, Shawn Shroff, and Charles Berkelhammer

Department of Medicine, Advocate Christ Medical Center, University of Illinois, Oak Lawn, IL 60453, USA

Correspondence should be addressed to Charles Berkelhammer; charlesberkel@aol.com

Academic Editor: Fumio Imazeki

Clopidogrel is a commonly prescribed antiplatelet agent that carries a rare risk of hepatotoxicity. We describe a case of severe clopidogrel-induced hepatitis with liver biopsy assessment. Prompt recognition and withdrawal of the offending agent are imperative to prevent progression and potentially fatal liver injury.

1. Introduction

Clopidogrel is a commonly used antiplatelet agent, yet only several cases of hepatotoxicity have been described [1–16]. Liver biopsies were not performed in many of these cases. We report a rare case of severe clopidogrel-induced hepatitis with histological assessment.

2. Case Description

A 34-year-old male with a history of coronary artery disease and remote coronary artery stent was placed on aspirin plus clopidogrel. His baseline liver biochemistries were normal. He had been on clopidogrel for 2 months 12 years ago without adverse effects but discontinued the medication on his own at that time due to nonadherence. Four and a half months after restarting clopidogrel, he presented with jaundice and fatigue. He denied fever, rash, arthralgias, or abdominal pain. His only other medications were aspirin and metoprolol, which he had been on for many years with normal liver biochemistries.

The patient was not on a statin. He denied recent alcohol or herbal medications. Physical examination was significant only for icterus. There was no hepatosplenomegaly, clubbing, rash, asterixis, or other stigmata of chronic liver disease.

Initial bilirubin was 5.7 mg/dL (normal 0.2–1.2 mg/dL), ALT 1,393 U/L (normal 7–48 U/L), AST 1,418 U/L (normal 7–48 U/L), alkaline phosphatase 130 U/L (normal 35–115 U/L),

INR 1.5, and partial prothrombin time 37 seconds (normal 15–37 seconds). Extensive serologies were negative to hepatitis A, hepatitis B, hepatitis C (including hepatitis C RNA), hepatitis E, IgM to cytomegalovirus and Epstein-Barr virus, anti-nuclear antibody, anti-smooth muscle antibody, anti-mitochondrial antibody, anti-liver kidney microsomal antibody, and ceruloplasmin.

Imaging studies were negative, and bile ducts were not dilated, including by ultrasound, computed tomography, and endoscopic retrograde cholangiopancreatography. No gallstones were present on any imaging modality. Liver biopsy revealed severe acute hepatitis with mixed inflammatory portal tract infiltrates including plasma cells, neutrophils and eosinophils, bile ductular reaction, patchy hepatocyte ballooning degeneration, and extensive periportal hepatocyte dropout, without fibrosis (Figure 1).

The patient was diagnosed with clopidogrel-induced severe hepatitis. Despite discontinuing clopidogrel, AST increased to 2,107 U/L, ALT to 1,567 U/L, and bilirubin to 37 mg/dL (predominately direct bilirubin). INR had increased to 2.1 despite empiric administration of vitamin K. A brief course of prednisone and ursodiol was initiated, with subsequent normalization of liver biochemistries.

3. Discussion

We describe a rare case of severe clopidogrel-induced hepatitis, with histological assessment. Our patient's drug-induced

TABLE 1: Clopidogrel-induced hepatitis: reported cases.

Cases	Latency/onset	Peak ALT (U/L)	Peak bilirubin (mg/dL)	Peak alkaline phosphatase (U/L)	Symptoms	Histology	Outcome
Keshmiri et al. 2016 (current)	135 days (4.5 months)	1567	37	130	Jaundice, fatigue	Hepatocellular	Recovery
Kapila et al. 2015 [9]	5 days	716	1.6	160	Nausea, vomiting, fever	No liver biopsy	Recovery
Pisapia et al. 2015 [2]	3 days	1603	24.5	408	Jaundice, arthralgia, papular rash	Mixed hepatocellular and cholestatic	Recovery
Monteiro et al. 2011 [13]	30 days	540	3.5	139	Nausea, vomiting	No liver biopsy	Recovery
Leighton et al. 2011 [11]	1 day	3626	3.3	364	Anorexia, jaundice, epigastric pain	Lymphoplasmacytic portal, interface and lobular hepatitis with no fibrosis	Recovery
Kastalli et al. 2010 [10]	19 days	336	4.7	186	Jaundice, abdominal pain	No liver biopsy	Death
Goyal et al. 2009 [3]	23 days	1011	7.3	1011	Abdominal pain, anorexia, jaundice	No liver biopsy	Recovery
Wiper et al. 2008 [4]	60 days	450	Normal	680	General malaise	No liver biopsy	Recovery
López-Vicente et al. 2007 [12]	30 days	204	1.0	682	Abdominal pain, fever	No liver biopsy	Recovery
Ng et al. 2006 [5]	3 days	536	1.5	247	Fever, chills Weight loss,	No liver biopsy	Recovery
Höllmüller et al. 2006 [1]	43 days	1003	20.8	221	anorexia, jaundice, nausea, abdominal pain	Mixed hepatocellular and cholestatic	Recovery
Chau et al. 2005 [7]	37 days	253	6.9	172	Jaundice	No liver biopsy	Recovery
Beltran-Robles et al. 2004 [6]	4 days	318	0.51	100	No symptoms mentioned	No liver biopsy	Recovery
Wolf et al. 2003 [16]	12 days	173	1.3	132	Fever, leukopenia, weakness	No liver biopsy	Recovery
Ramos Ramos et al. 2003 [14]	60 days	710	24.9	118	Jaundice	No liver biopsy	Recovery
Duran-Quintana et al. 2002 [8]	180 days	786	13	474	Icterus, hepatomegaly	No liver biopsy	Recovery
Willens 2000 [15]	21 days	507	3.0	636	Malaise, anorexia, myalgia, icterus	No liver biopsy	Recovery

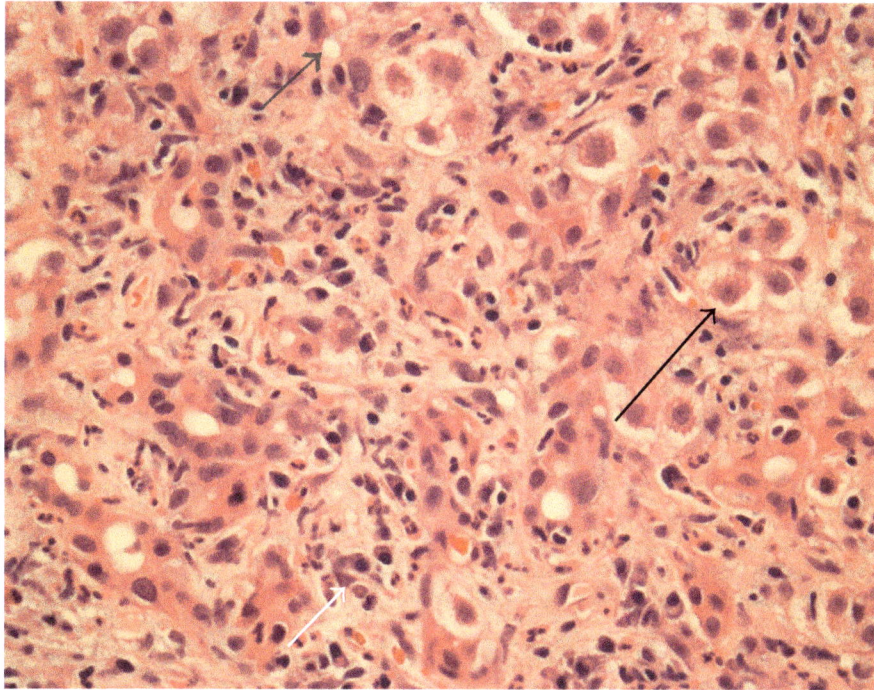

FIGURE 1: Liver biopsy showing severe acute hepatitis with mixed inflammatory portal tract infiltrate (white arrow), patchy hepatocyte ballooning degeneration (black arrow), and extensive periportal hepatocyte dropout (grey arrow).

hepatitis was particularly severe with jaundice (peak bilirubin 37 mg/dL), marked elevation of transaminases (peak ALT of 1,567 U/L), and coagulopathy (INR 2.1). This degree of hepatic injury portends an increased mortality and underscores the importance of early recognition and discontinuation of the offending agent.

Clopidogrel-induced hepatitis has been described [1–16]. Table 1 lists reported cases in reverse chronological order. The degree of liver injury has ranged from reversible liver injury and recovery [1–9, 11–16] to acute hepatic failure and death [10]. Onset of liver injury in these cases ranges between 3 and 180 days [1–16]. Rechallenge confirmed clopidogrel-induced hepatitis in some of these cases [2–5]. Our patient's Naranjo scale and RUCAM (Roussel Uclaf Causality Assessment Method) scores were both 8, indicating probable drug-induced hepatitis [17, 18].

Our patients liver biopsy revealed severe hepatocellular injury. This adds to the histological findings in clopidogrel-induced hepatitis, as liver biopsy was only performed in 3 of the previously reported cases [1, 2, 11]. Clopidogrel-induced liver injury can be cholestatic, hepatocellular [11], or mixed hepatocellular plus cholestatic [1, 2].

The exact mechanism of clopidogrel-induced hepatitis is unclear. The delayed onset of 4.5 months in our case suggests a toxic-metabolic etiology, whereas the inflammatory infiltrate and response to corticosteroids raise the possibility of a superimposed immune mediated mechanism of injury. Clopidogrel is a prodrug which is metabolized to inactive clopidogrel carboxylate (90%) and an active metabolite containing a mercapto group (10%) by cytochrome P450 3A4 and 2C19. In vitro studies suggest that the active metabolite is responsible for the hepatotoxicity and that high cytochrome 3A4 activities coupled with cellular glutathione depletion are potential risk factors [19]. Interestingly, an earlier antiplatelet agent, ticlopidine, has also been reported to cause drug-induced cholestatic hepatitis [20, 21].

Clopidogrel-induced hepatitis is a rare but potentially serious adverse effect. A high degree of clinical suspicion is required in patients presenting with abnormal liver biochemistries within a few months after starting clopidogrel. Prompt recognition and discontinuation of the offending agent are necessary, as progressive liver injury and even death can occur.

References

[1] I. Höllmüller, S. Stadlmann, I. Graziadei, and W. Vogel, "Clinico-histopathological characteristics of clopidogrel-induced hepatic injury: case report and review of literature," *European Journal of Gastroenterology and Hepatology*, vol. 18, no. 8, pp. 931–934, 2006.

[2] R. Pisapia, A. Abdeddaim, A. Mariano et al., "Acute hepatitis associated with clopidogrel: a case report and review of the literature," *American Journal of Therapeutics*, vol. 22, no. 1, pp. e8–e13, 2015.

[3] R. K. Goyal, D. Srivastava, and K.-D. Lessnau, "Clopidogrel-induced hepatocellular injury and cholestatic jaundice in an elderly patient: case report and review of the literature," *Pharmacotherapy*, vol. 29, no. 5, pp. 608–612, 2009.

[4] A. Wiper, M. Schmitt, and D. Roberts, "Clopidogrel-induced hepatotoxicity," *Journal of Postgraduate Medicine*, vol. 54, no. 2, p. 152, 2008.

[5] J. A. Ng, N. Goldberg, and M. J. Tafreshi, "Clopidogrel-induced hepatotoxicity and fever," *Pharmacotherapy*, vol. 26, no. 7, pp. 1023–1026, 2006.

[6] M. Beltran-Robles, E. Marquez Saavedra, D. Sanchez-Muñoz, and M. Romero-Gomez, "Hepatotoxicity induced by clopidogrel," *Journal of Hepatology*, vol. 40, no. 3, pp. 560–562, 2004.

[7] T. N. Chau, K. F. Yim, N. S. Mok et al., "Clopidogrel-induced hepatotoxicity after percutaneous coronary stenting," *Hong Kong Medical Journal*, vol. 11, no. 5, pp. 414–416, 2005.

[8] J. A. Duran-Quintana, M. Jimenez-Saenz, A. R. Montero et al., "Clopidogrel probably induced hepatic toxicity," *Medicina Clínica*, vol. 119, article 37, 2002 (Spanish).

[9] A. Kapila, L. Chhabra, A. D. Locke et al., "An indiosyncratic reaction to clopidogrel," *The Permanente Journal*, vol. 19, no. 1, pp. 74–76, 2015.

[10] S. Kastalli, S. El Aïdli, A. Zaïem, H. Ben Abdallah, and R. Daghfous, "Fatal liver injury associated with clopidogrel," *Fundamental & Clinical Pharmacology*, vol. 24, no. 4, pp. 433–435, 2010.

[11] S. P. Leighton, C. Gordon, and A. Shand, "Clopidogrel, Turkey and a red herring?" *BMJ Case Reports*, 2011.

[12] J. López-Vicente, C. Garfia, F. López-Medrano, and C. Yela, "Hepatic toxicity and clopidogrel-induced systemic inflammatory response syndrome," *Revista Espanola de Cardiologia*, vol. 60, no. 3, pp. 323–324, 2007.

[13] P. H. Monteiro, L. Dos Santos Pinheiro, L. Alvoeiro, M. Lucas, and R. M. Victorino, "Clopidogrel-induced liver failure," *JRSM Short Reports*, vol. 2, no. 5, p. 40, 2011.

[14] J. C. Ramos Ramos, J. Sanz Moreno, L. Calvo Carrasco, and J. de Dios García Díaz, "Clopidogrel-induced hepatotoxicity," *Medicina Clinica*, vol. 120, no. 4, pp. 156–157, 2003 (Spanish).

[15] H. J. Willens, "Clopidogrel-induced mixed hepatocellular and cholestatic liver injury," *American Journal of Therapeutics*, vol. 7, no. 5, pp. 317–318, 2000.

[16] I. Wolf, M. Mouallem, S. Rath, and Z. Farfel, "Clopidogrel-induced systemic inflammatory response syndrome," *Mayo Clinic Proceedings*, vol. 78, no. 5, pp. 618–620, 2003.

[17] C. A. Naranjo, U. Busto, E. M. Sellers et al., "A method for estimating the probability of adverse drug reactions," *Clinical Pharmacology & Therapeutics*, vol. 30, no. 2, pp. 239–245, 1981.

[18] G. Danan and C. Benichou, "Causality assessment of adverse reactions to drugs-I. A novel method based on the conclusions of international consensus meetings: application to drug-induced liver injuries," *Journal of Clinical Epidemiology*, vol. 46, no. 11, pp. 1323–1330, 1993.

[19] A. Zahno, J. Bouitbir, S. Maseneni, P. W. Lindinger, K. Brecht, and S. Krähenbühl, "Hepatocellular toxicity of clopidogrel: mechanisms and risk factors," *Free Radical Biology and Medicine*, vol. 65, pp. 208–216, 2013.

[20] Y. D. Skurnik, A. Tcherniak, K. Edlan, Z. Sthoeger, M. D. Martínez, and M. Larouche, "Ticlopidine-induced cholestatic hepatitis," *Annals of Pharmacotherapy*, vol. 37, no. 3, pp. 371–375, 2003.

[21] E. Mambelli, E. Mancini, S. Casanova, A. Di Felice, and A. Santoro, "Severe ticlopidine-induced cholestatic syndrome," *Blood Purification*, vol. 25, no. 5-6, pp. 441–445, 2008.

37

The Spiraling Case of a Yellow Chef: Isolated Hyperbilirubinemia

Karen Jiang,[1] Ahmad Najdat Bazarbashi,[2] Sami Dahdal,[3]
Adina Voiculescu,[4] and Natalia Khalaf[2]

[1]Division of Hospital Medicine, Department of Medicine, Brigham and Women's Hospital, Boston, MA, USA
[2]Division of Gastroenterology, Hepatology and Endoscopy, Brigham and Women's Hospital, Boston, MA, USA
[3]Department of Internal Medicine, St. John's Riverside Hospital, Yonkers, NY, USA
[4]Division of Renal Medicine, Department of Medicine, Brigham and Women's Hospital, Boston, MA, USA

Correspondence should be addressed to Natalia Khalaf; nataliakhalaf@gmail.com

Academic Editor: Ivan Gentile

Leptospirosis is a common bacterial disease in tropical regions of the world due to greater exposure to rodents and domestic animals; however, this condition can also occur in US urban areas, though it often goes unrecognized. Gastrointestinal symptoms are very commonly seen, and icteric leptospirosis is often confused for other conditions resulting in delayed diagnosis and worse outcomes. As mortality increases with more extensive hepatic involvement, gastroenterologists should be aware of the constellation of gastrointestinal symptoms related to leptospirosis, as it can occur in the absence of classic exposure history.

1. Introduction

Leptospirosis is a prevalent zoonotic disease caused by the spirochete bacteria *Leptospira*. A number of mammals serve as natural hosts, with human infection occurring after exposure to animal or environmental contact. The disease is most common in tropical regions of the world, with an incidence in tropical climates being an estimated 10 times higher than in more temperate climates. However, cases of human infection in urban settings within developed countries such as the US have also been reported [1, 2]. Experts believe the disease to be underreported, with an estimated 873,000 cases of human infections occurring worldwide each year, accounting for an estimated 48,600 deaths [3].

Making a timely diagnosis of leptospirosis is challenging as its presentation can be diverse and nonspecific. The majority of affected individuals (75-100%) will suffer from fever, rigors, myalgias, and headache after an average incubation period of 10 days. Gastrointestinal symptoms such as nausea, vomiting, and diarrhea occur in up to 50% of cases, with less common symptoms including cough, sore throat, arthralgias, conjunctival suffusion, skin rash, abdominal pain, and aseptic meningitis [4–7].

It is important for gastroenterologists to recognize key features of leptospirosis, which commonly presents with gastrointestinal (GI) symptoms. Presented here is a case of icteric leptospirosis characterized by intrahepatic cholestasis and renal failure, highlighting the often key role gastroenterologists play in the care of these patients.

2. Case Presentation

A 56-year-old healthy man presented to the emergency department in the summer season with three days of fatigue and bilateral thigh pain. He was born in Puerto Rico but resided in the Northeast Region of the US, where he worked as a chef in a major metropolitan city. He had no sick contacts, recent travel, or alcohol or drug use.

Laboratory data on presentation demonstrated a creatinine (Cr) of 1.73 mg/dL, creatinine kinase (CK) of 3494 U/L and platelet count of $68 \times 10^3/\mu L$ with initially normal liver function tests (LFTs). The patient was admitted for treatment of acute kidney injury from presumed rhabdomyolysis of unclear cause but subsequently developed low-grade fevers, leukocytosis, and worsening thrombocytopenia over the

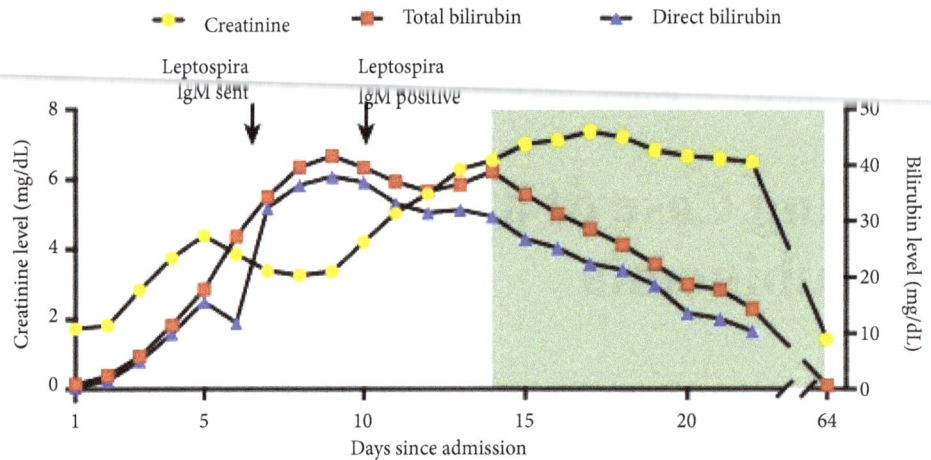

(a)

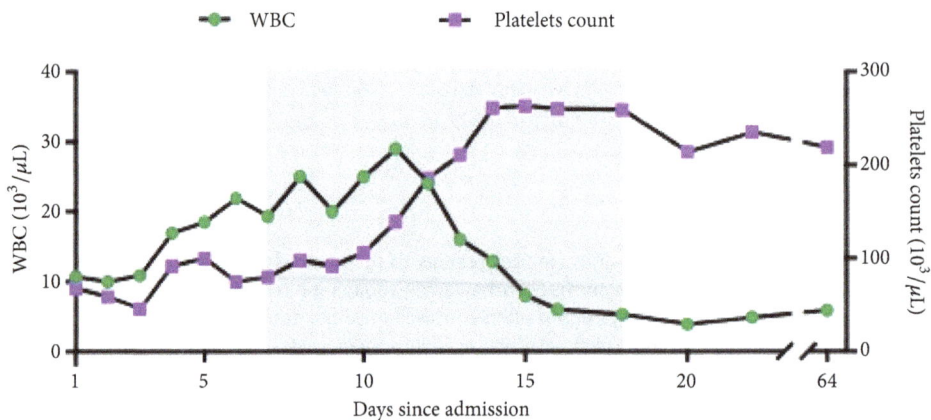

(b)

FIGURE 1: Multiorgan failure and response to treatments in patient with leptospirosis. (a) Creatinine, total bilirubin, and direct bilirubin levels during and after hospitalization. Shaded green area represents duration of cholestyramine and ursodiol treatment for bile cast nephropathy. (b) White-blood cell count (WBC) and platelet count during and after hospitalization. Shaded grey area represents duration of doxycycline treatment.

following days. His Cr worsened despite hydration and conservative management for which the patient underwent a renal biopsy on hospital day 4, with findings of acute tubular necrosis, interstitial hemorrhage, and capillaritis.

In addition to worsening renal function, he had an impressively rapid rise in his total and direct bilirubin with development of clinical jaundice over the subsequent days with laboratory values on hospital day 8 as follows: Cr of 4, total bilirubin of 41 mg/dL, and direct bilirubin of 38 mg/dL (Figure 1(a)). The GI consult service became involved in his care and on physical examination noted no evidence of chronic liver disease other than jaundice. The patient had no abdominal tenderness, hepatosplenomegaly, or asterixis. The bilirubin values were out of proportion to his other liver tests such as INR and albumin, which remained within normal values and AST/ALT and alkaline phosphatase values

wavered between mildly elevated (<2 times the upper limit of normal) and normal values. Based on the kidney biopsy results and significant hyperbilirubinemia, testing was done for bacteremia, influenza, tuberculosis, HIV, tick-borne diseases, Hantavirus infection, acute viral hepatitis (A, B, C, E, CMV, EBV, and VZV) and vasculitis, which were all negative or normal.

An abdominal ultrasound and MRI liver protocol/MCRP showed a normal hepatobiliary system. Given his impressive rise in bilirubin out of proportion to other LFTs in combination with renal failure and rhabdomyolysis, the GI service recommended antibody testing for leptospirosis, for which serum IgM antibodies were checked on hospital day 5. The following day, he was started on empiric doxycycline in liaison with infectious disease consultation at 100 mg intravenously twice daily. In the interim, a liver biopsy was done showing liver parenchyma with marked canalicular and intracellular cholestasis, accentuated in perivenular zone, and rare foci of bile duct injury and ductular proliferation. There was no evidence of significant steatosis, fibrosis or intracellular iron deposition with trichrome, reticulin, PAS-D, and iron stains being unrevealing.

On hospital day 10, the Leptospira IgM returned positive, consistent with the diagnosis of icteric leptospirosis. He was continued on doxycycline 100 mg twice daily with subsequent normalization of leukocyte and platelet counts (Figure 1(b)). In view of the positive Leptospira IgM antibody results, the liver tissue obtained from biopsy was reevaluated for spirochete organisms with special staining; however no organisms were found.

The patient completed a 10-day course of doxycycline but unfortunately suffered from bile cast nephropathy from severe hyperbilirubinemia with continued rise in Cr (Figure 1(a)), for which he was treated with cholestyramine and ursodiol. His liver function tests and kidney laboratory results began to improve thereafter, and he was discharged on hospital day 26. At six-week follow-up, his renal function improved (Cr of 1.4 mg/dL) and his LFTs had normalized. It was later discovered that the restaurant where the patient had been working had a rodent infestation, which were the most likely source of his infection.

3. Discussion

Leptospirosis is the one of the most prevalent zoonotic diseases globally but is rare and often under recognized in developed countries. It is important for clinicians to be aware that sporadic cases of leptospirosis can be seen in urban areas where the disease is spread through the urine of rodents and domestic animals [8]. While some patients will only experience self-limited symptoms such as mild fever, myalgias, and fatigue, others suffer more severe disease states such as Weil's disease, as highlighted in the case. Weil's disease is characterized by multiorgan failure including liver failure, renal failure, and pulmonary hemorrhage. Other clinical manifestations include central nervous system and cardiac and ocular involvement [9]. Severe manifestations of leptospirosis are treated with antibiotics such as penicillin or doxycycline [10].

Recognizing the clinical manifestations of leptospirosis is critical for initiating treatment in a timely fashion. While the overall median mortality rate of leptospirosis is 2.2%, it is significantly more fatal once renal failure or jaundice develops, with mortality rates rising to 12% and 19%, respectively [10]. Gastroenterologists are often involved in the care of affected patients given the variety of GI symptoms people can develop, ranging from abdominal pain, vomiting, and diarrhea to more severe complications such as pancreatitis, acalculous cholecystitis, enteritis, peritonitis, and liver failure [11]. Diagnostic options for leptospirosis include serological testing such as agglutination testing and enzyme linked immunosorbent assays (ELISA); microscopic examination (dark field microscopy, silver staining, and Warthin-starry stain); molecular testing with PCR; and culture of organisms [12].

Our patient's presentation highlights the fact that leptospirosis can cause isolated direct hyperbilirubinemia or direct hyperbilirubinemia out of proportion to other LFT values. Jaundice in leptospirosis is a unique feature that remains incompletely understood; however intrahepatic cholestasis, duodenitis resulting in ampulla of Vater obstruction, and indirect hyperbilirubinemia from hemorrhage have all been described as causes of jaundice with this condition [13]. In mouse models, Leptospira bacteria have been seen to invade the intercellular junctions of host hepatocytes resulting in disruption of cellular junctions within bile canaliculi [14]. While awareness of the disease and a high clinical suspicion is required to identify this condition in a timely fashion, liver biopsy can be helpful, as this may reveal congested sinusoids, leptospiral attachment to and invasion of the perijunctional region between hepatocytes, and a lack of normal adhesion between hepatocytes with hepatocyte apoptosis. Damage to hepatocytes and disruption of their intercellular junction is thought to lead to bile leak from the canaliculi and into the sinusoidal blood vessels, thus causing direct hyperbilirubinemia [15]. The patient's liver biopsy revealed marked parenchymal and canalicular cholestasis, which can be seen with leptospirosis as well as a variety of other conditions. We hypothesize that the patient's liver biopsy did not reveal evidence of spirochetes on special staining because the patient was receiving treatment with empiric doxycycline prior to liver biopsy.

Treatment of leptospirosis depends on its clinical severity. Mild cases can be treated as an outpatient with penicillin, doxycycline, or azithromycin, with intravenous doxycycline, ceftriaxone, or cefotaxime recommended for more severe cases in hospitalized patients. Although not found to impact mortality, antimicrobial therapy may be associated with faster clinical resolution of symptoms [16]. Our patient was treated with doxycycline in discussion with our infectious disease colleagues given the broad differential diagnosis the patient had on admission including concern for tick-borne illnesses, for which doxycycline would be a preferred agent.

Our case is unique in that Weil's disease developed in a patient residing in an urban city in the US without obvious exposure history. Icteric leptospirosis can be confused for other hepatic conditions such as viral hepatitis, malaria, and sepsis [11] and should be considered in the differential diagnosis of patients presenting with both severe renal and liver injury, even in the absence of classic exposure history.

Disclosure

Karen Jiang and Ahmad Najdat Bazarbashi shared co-first authorship. Natalia Khalaf is article guarantor.

Authors' Contributions

Karen Jiang, Ahmad Najdat Bazarbashi, Sami Dahdal, Adina Voiculescu, and Natalia Khalaf contributed to literature review and drafting and critically revising the manuscript. All authors gave final approval of the version to be published.

References

[1] World Health Organization, *Report of the First Meeting of the Leptospirosis Burden Epidemiology Reference Group, Geneva*, World Health Organization, Geneva, Switzerlands, 2010.

[2] R. A. Hartskeerl, M. Collares-Pereira, and W. A. Ellis, "Emergence, control and re-emerging leptospirosis: dynamics of infection in the changing world," *Clinical Microbiology and Infection*, vol. 17, no. 4, pp. 494–501, 2011.

[3] World Health Organization, "Global burden of human leptospirosis and cross-sectoral interventions for its prevention and control," http://www.pmaconference.mahidol.ac.th/dmdo-cuments/2013-PMAC-Poster-P9-Bernadette%20Abela-Ridder.pdf,

[4] N. B. Vanasco, M. F. Schmeling, J. Lottersberger, F. Costa, A. I. Ko, and H. D. Tarabla, "Clinical characteristics and risk factors of human leptospirosis in Argentina (1999-2005)," *Acta Tropica*, vol. 107, no. 3, pp. 255–258, 2008.

[5] J. P. Sanford, "Leptospirosis—time for a booster," *The New England Journal of Medicine*, vol. 310, no. 8, pp. 524-525, 1984.

[6] S. J. Berman, C. C. Tsai, K. Holmes, J. W. Fresh, and R. H. Watten, "Sporadic anicteric leptospirosis in South Vietnam: a study in 150 patients," *Annals of Internal Medicine*, vol. 79, no. 2, pp. 167–173, 1973.

[7] A. R. Katz, V. E. Ansdell, P. V. Effler, C. R. Middleton, and D. M. Sasaki, "Assessment of the clinical presentation and treatment of 353 cases of laboratory-confirmed leptospirosis in hawaii 1974-1998," *Clinical Infectious Diseases*, vol. 33, no. 11, pp. 1834–1841, 2001.

[8] J. M. Vinetz, G. E. Glass, C. E. Flexner, P. Mueller, and D. C. Kaslow, "Sporadic urban leptospirosis," *Annals of Internal Medicine*, vol. 125, no. 10, pp. 794–798, 1996.

[9] P. Vijayachari, A. P. Sugunan, and A. N. Shriram, "Leptospirosis: an emerging global public health problem," *Journal of Biosciences*, vol. 33, no. 4, pp. 557–569, 2008.

[10] A. J. Taylor, D. H. Paris, P. N. Newton, and J. M. Vinetz, "A systematic review of the mortality from untreated leptospirosis," *PLOS Neglected Tropical Diseases*, vol. 9, no. 6, 2015.

[11] C. Vaishnavi, *Infections of the Gastrointestinal System*, chapter 42: Gastrointestinal Manifestations of Leptospirosis by Raja Veerapandian, 2013.

[12] P. N. Levett, "Leptospirosis," *Clinical Microbiology Reviews*, vol. 14, no. 2, pp. 296–326, 2001.

[13] R. Higgins and G. Cousineau, "The pathogenisis of leptospirosis II. Jaundice in experimental leptospirosis in guinea pigs," *The Canadian Journal of Comparative Medicine*, vol. 41, no. 2, pp. 182–187, 1977.

[14] S. Miyahara, M. Saito, T. Kanemaru, S. Y. A. M. Villanueva, N. G. Gloriani, and S.-I. Yoshida, "Destruction of the hepatocyte junction by intercellular invasion of Leptospira causes jaundice in a hamster model of Weil's disease," *International Journal of Clinical and Experimental Pathology*, vol. 95, no. 4, pp. 271–281, 2014.

[15] D. A. Haake and P. N. Levett, "Leptospirosis in humans," *Current Topics in Microbiology and Immunology*, vol. 387, pp. 65–97, 2015.

[16] D. M. Brett-Major and R. Coldren, "Antibiotics for leptospirosis," *Cochrane Database of Systematic Reviews*, vol. 2, 2012.

38

A Case of Primary Hepatic Lymphoma and Related Literature Review

Yonghua Liu, Jinhong Jiang, Qinli Wu, Qiaolei Zhang, Yehui Xu, Zhigang Qu, Guangli Ma, Xiaoqiu Wang, Xiaoli Wang, Weimei Jin, and Bingmu Fang

Department of Hematology, Sixth Affiliated Hospital of Wenzhou Medical University, Lishui City, Zhejiang 323000, China

Correspondence should be addressed to Bingmu Fang; fbm636@163.com

Academic Editor: Mario Pirisi

Objective. Primary hepatic lymphoma is a rare disease. And the clinical manifestations of this disease are nonspecific. The objective of this paper is to improve clinicians' understanding of this disease. *Methods.* We analyzed the clinical characteristics of a case of primary hepatic lymphoma in association with hepatitis B virus infection and reviewed the literature. *Conclusion.* The clinical manifestations of primary hepatic lymphoma are nonspecific. And it is easily misdiagnosed. Postoperative radiotherapy of patients with early stage was previously speculated to achieve favorable improvement. The application of targeted therapeutic drugs, chemotherapy, or combined local radiotherapy has become the first-line treatment strategy.

1. Background

Primary hepatic lymphoma (PHL) refers to tumor confined in the liver at the early stage of lymphoma without infiltration of other locations. PHL is a rare disease, with an incidence of only 0.1% for malignant liver tumors. This disease also accounts for 0.4% of all primary extranodal lymphoma and 0.016% of all non-Hodgkin's lymphoma [1]. PHL of diffuse large B-cell lymphoma (PHL-DLBCL) is more infrequent. The clinical manifestations of PHL-DLBCL are nonspecific. Hence, the condition is difficult to distinguish from primary liver cancer, liver metastases, granulomatous pseudotumor, and other diseases and is thus easily misdiagnosed. To improve clinicians' understanding of this disease, the diagnosis and treatment course of a case of PHL in our hospital were discussed in detail.

2. Case Introduction

A 61-year-old male was admitted because of "fatigue and abdominal distension for over 50 days." The patient presented with a 6 kg weight loss (12%) and experienced fatigue and abdominal distension from an unknown cause since 50 days prior to admission. The patient showed no signs of skin pruritus or yellow discoloration of the skin or eyes. Despite his symptoms, the patient did not initially seek medical consultation. He was then admitted in a local hospital from June 6 to June 12, 2014 because of fever. The patient suffered from chills and sweating, and his body temperature fluctuated at 37.4–38.9°C. He was diagnosed with "cholecystitis, fatty liver, hepatomegaly, and fever (unknown)." He was then treated with cefoperazone/sulbactam sodium for the inflammation, pantoprazole to relieve hyperacidity, and polyene phosphatidylcholine to protect the liver, all of which afforded the patient with no improvement of condition. The patient sought consultation in one of the top three local hospitals on June 19. His signs and symptoms of fatigue, abdominal distension, and yellow urine aggravated, along with the decrease in urine amount. At the time, the patient presented with a urine output of less than 500 mL/24 h, with concurrent skin pruritus, icteric skin and sclerae, occasional cough, and severe bilateral lower extremities edema. He also experienced slight chest tightness and hence was admitted to the hospital.

Upon admission, routine blood examination obtained the following results: white blood cell count, 9.3×10^9/L; neutrophil absolute value, 4.9×10^9/L; hemoglobin, 128 g/L; and platelet count, 171×10^9/L. Meanwhile, analysis of serum biochemistry revealed the following levels: albumin, 28 g/L; ALT, 128 U/L; AST, 109 U/L; total bilirubin, 12.5 μmol/L; direct

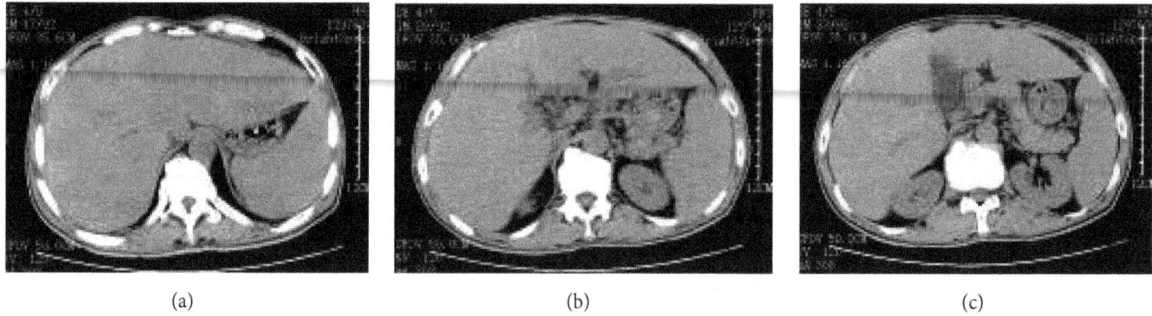

FIGURE 1: Epigastrium CT before treatment. Note: the liver outline was significantly more prominent. The liver edge was less smooth. Liver parenchymal density was uneven. Patchy low-density shadows were observed, especially in the left live. Multiple quasicircular low-density foci appeared in the right lobe of the liver. The spleen was enlarged to about seven rib units. The density was uniform.

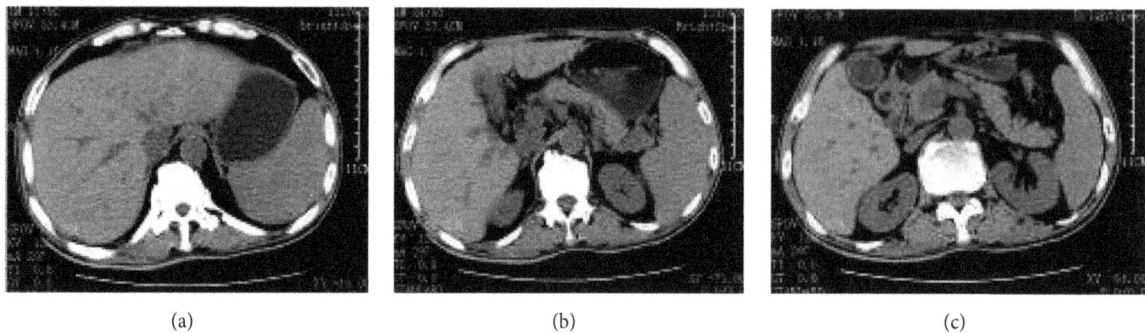

FIGURE 2: Epigastrium CT after treatment. Note: the liver outline was significantly more prominent. The liver edge was less smooth. Liver parenchymal density was uniform. Multiple quasicircular low-density foci were found in the right lobe of the liver, but no intensified low-density focus was noted. The largest diameter was about 5.5 mm. The spleen was enlarged to approximately seven rib units. The density was uniform. Compared with the CT findings on July 11, the liver density increased and the density was more uniform.

bilirubin, 2.7 μmol/L; indirect bilirubin, 125 μmol/L; hydroxybutyrate dehydrogenase, 1093 U/L; lactate dehydrogenase, 1387 U/L; and Total Bile Acids (TBA), 2.461 μmol/L. The liver fibrosis index is as follows: hyaluronic acid, 1162.2 μg/L; type IV collagen, 279.4 μg/L; type III collagen, 659.8 μg/L; and laminin, 149 μg/L. The blood ammonia level was 365 μmol/L, whereas that of C-reactive protein was 136.4 mg/L. Coomb's test was negative. Hepatitis B screening tested positive for three components: HBV-DNA, $3.1E + 02$ copy/mL. Chest computed tomography (CT) scan revealed the following findings: (1) small fibrotic foci at the middle lobe of the right lung and lingular segment of the superior lobe of the left lung and (2) emphysema in the superior lobe of the right lung and calcified foci at the superior lobe of the left lung. No swollen lymph nodes were found by ultrasound on the bilateral neck, supraclavicular, subaxillary, and inguinal regions. Abdominal CT (July 11, 2014) displayed (1) hepatosplenomegaly, ascites, patchy low-density shadows in the liver (especially in the left liver), and multiple low-density lesions in the right lobe of liver; (2) gallbladder wall thickening; and (3) prostate calcification (Figure 1). The patient was treated with entecavir dispersible tablet 0.5 mg qd, oral administration of antiviral drugs, and drugs for liver protection and diuresis. The liver progressively enlarged, with a significant increase in bilirubin. The patient underwent liver biopsy. Pathological

examination showed the following results: heteromorphic lymphocytes were observed in the hepatic sinusoid and portal area. The nuclei were round or oval. The cells displayed single or multiple nucleoli. The nuclear mitotic figure was common. For immunohistochemistry, LCA, CD20, and BCL-6 were diffusely strongly positive; CD79a and Mum-1 were locally weakly positive; the Ki-67 labeling index was about 60%; and CK, CD68, CD34, Hepaar-1, CD3, CD43, CD10, and ALK were negative; HBs-Ag and HBc-Ag were negative (Figure 3). Bone marrow morphology and biopsy showed no signs of lymphoma infiltration. On the basis of clinical, laboratory, and pathological examinations, the patient was diagnosed with primary hepatic non-Hodgkin's lymphoma staged IVA (DLBCL, non-GCB), chronic viral hepatitis (B), and decompensated cirrhosis. CHOP (cyclophosphamide, doxorubicin, vincristine, and prednisone) scheme chemotherapy was then initiated on July 17 with the following agents: IFO, 2 g (Days 1 and 8); THP, 60 mg (Day 1); DXM, 10 mg (Days 1 to 5); and VDS, 4 mg (Days 1, 8, and 15). The chemotherapeutic course was uneventful. The liver significantly shrunk in three days after chemotherapy was completed. The CT review after the first chemotherapy (August 11) showed that the liver significantly decreased in size, and liver density became uniform (Figure 2). These findings suggest that the treatment was satisfactory and achieved partial remission. The R-CHOP

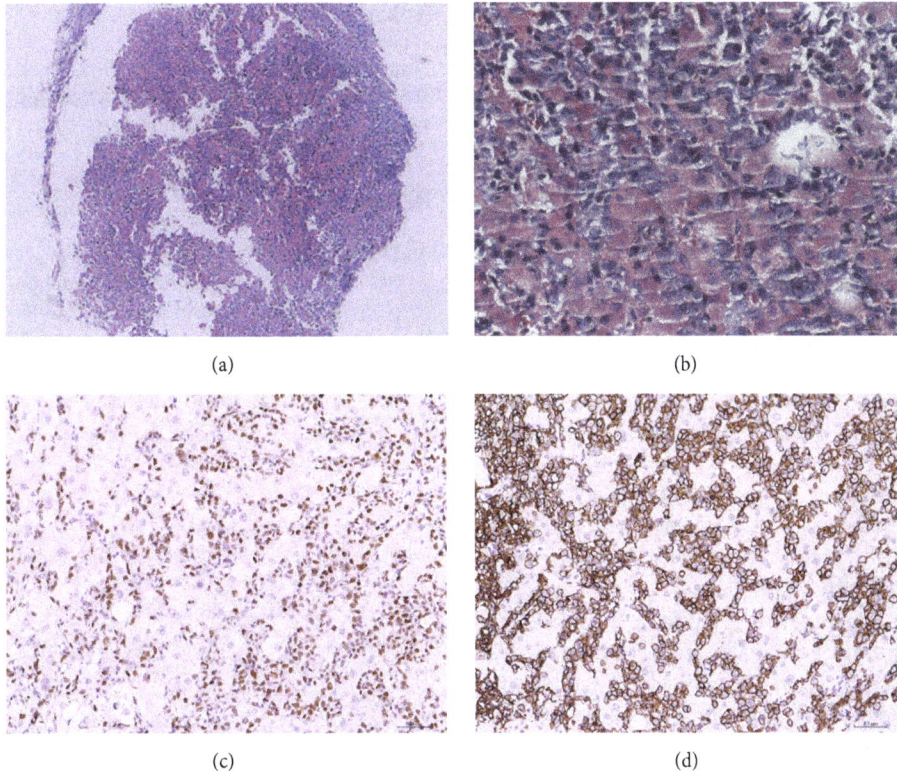

FIGURE 3: Liver biopsy pathology and histochemistry (hematoxylin-eosin staining,). (a) and (b) Heteromorphic lymphocytes were observed in the hepatic sinusoid and portal area. The nuclei were round or oval. The cells presented with one or multiple nucleoli. The nuclear mitotic figure was common, low, and high magnifications ($\times 4$, $\times 40$, resp.). (c) BCL-6 was diffusely strongly positive. (d) CD20 was diffusely strongly positive.

scheme was adopted for six cycles (CHOP with rituximab injection, 500 mg [Day 0]); the other drugs included were the same as those mentioned above). No new lesion was noted, and the patient has lived for nearly 2 years till now of disease-free-survival.

3. Literature Review

Primary hepatic lymphoma (PHL) refers to the lesion only confined to the liver at the early stage of lymphoma. Infiltrations of lymph nodes, spleen, bone marrow, and other organs must be excluded at the onset. The patient's clinical characteristics include abdominal distension, fatigue, abnormal liver function, and progressive hepatomegaly. This patient was diagnosed with non-Hodgkin's lymphoma by liver biopsy. The pathological type was DLBCL. The involvement of other locations was excluded by superficial lymph node examination, bone marrow morphology and biopsy, and radiologic examinations. The diagnosis of PHL-DLBCL was confirmed.

3.1. Epidemiological Analysis of PHL. PHL may occur at any age but more commonly in males of about 50 years old. The male-to-female ratio for the disease incidence is about 3 : 1 [2]. Liver involvement accounts for about 15%–17% of non-Hodgkin's lymphoma. However, primary liver non-Hodgkin's lymphoma is extremely rare, accounting for 0.4%

of all primary extranodal lymphoma and 0.016% of all cases of non-Hodgkin's lymphoma. The etiology of PHL is uncertain and may include virus infection (HIV, AIDS, HBV, HCV, and EBV), autoimmune diseases, and immune inhibitor application [3]. Its mechanism potentially involves T lymphocyte loss of inherent immune surveillance and function after viral infection or application of immunosuppressive agents. This occurrence may result in unrestrained lymphopoiesis, thereby forming lymphoma.

3.2. Clinical Manifestations of PHL. The clinical manifestations of PHL are nonspecific. Most patients seek consultation because of fatigue, loss of appetite, night sweats, low-grade fever, and weight reduction. Some patients show hepatomegaly, abdominal pain, or liver function abnormalities. Disease progression is rapid. Several patients suffer from hepatic encephalopathy early, resulting in coma and even death [2, 4]. In our case, the onset of disease was acute. The patient experienced abdominal distension and fatigue and sustained low fever, hepatomegaly, and progressive increase of bilirubin, which were rapidly relieved by treatment. The patient's clinical characteristics were consistent with that of primary hepatic non-Hodgkin's lymphoma. For laboratory indices, most PHL patients show elevated ALT and AST levels by two to three times of the normal value, which is also significantly increased with the increase in bilirubin and

HDL. However, AFP and CEA levels are usually normal, in contrast to those in primary liver cancer and liver metastasis.

A common radiologic finding in the disease is liver space-occupying lesions. Most patients show single lesions, as well as multiple space-occupying lesions. Some patients sustain diffuse liver lesions, displayed in radiologic examination as hepatomegaly without liver space-occupying lesion. PHL radiologic manifestations often involve a nonuniform liver texture. The central mass mainly shows low-density shadows in CT and sometimes multilobar or patchy low-density shadows, which are peripherally intensified after enhancement. These low-density radiologic findings differ from those of other solid hepatic tumors. This result may be explained by the lesser vascularization of the lymphoma compared with other tumors, resulting in tissue necrosis during the disease process. MRI revealed high-density T1 and high-signal T2. The radiologic performance of the patient showed that the liver was obviously enlarged and the liver texture was not uniform, combined with patchy low-density shadows, which was consistent with literature reports [5, 6].

Most hepatic lymphomas are derived from B-lymphocyte cells, whereas the minority originates from T lymphocytes. The diagnosis should depend on liver tissue biopsy, including immunohistochemistry. PHL patients with liver function abnormality, hepatomegaly, or space-occupying lesions but with normal AFP and CEA must be suspected of liver lymphoma. Laparoscopic examination or percutaneous liver biopsy is highly necessary. However, tissue necrosis is often associated with liver lymphoma; hence, fine needle aspiration biopsy may provide false negative results. PHL was often misdiagnosed as other conditions, such as embryonic sarcoma, inflammatory pseudotumor, or granulomatous hepatitis. Occasionally, immunohistochemistry still cannot sufficiently obtain a satisfactory diagnosis. Cellular immunology, gene rearrangement, cell genetics, and molecular biology related to PHL should be explored to assist diagnosis and determine prognosis.

3.3. PHL Treatment. Postoperative radiotherapy of patients with early PHL was previously speculated to achieve favorable improvement [7]. However, with the continuous development of chemotherapeutic regimens, especially the application of targeted therapeutic drugs, chemotherapy or combined local radiotherapy has become the first-line treatment of PHL. The chemotherapy regimen often applied is mainly based on CHOP [8]. Our patient was diagnosed with PHL-DLBCL. The single-course treatment with CHOP combined with rituximab was significant. The liver was significantly reduced in size, and the low-density lesions were significantly decreased. In a previous study, the follow-up visits of 24 PHL cases after 20 years by the Anderson Cancer Center in the United States revealed a complete remission rate of 85% through chemotherapy and an event-free five-year survival of 70% [9].

PHL is an extremely rare condition in clinical practice. Moreover, PHL-DLBCL is rarely reported worldwide. A considerable number of prospective, randomized controlled clinical trials are lacking and must be further conducted.

Acknowledgments

This paper is funded by Science and Technology Department of Zhejiang Province (no. 2012C33110) and Lishui Science and Technology Bureau (no. 2012JYZB79).

References

[1] X.-W. Yang, W.-F. Tan, W.-L. Yu et al., "Diagnosis and surgical treatment of primary hepatic lymphoma," *World Journal of Gastroenterology*, vol. 16, no. 47, pp. 6016–6019, 2010.

[2] N. K. Gatselis and G. N. Dalekos, "Hepatobiliary and pancreatic: primary hepatic lymphoma," *Journal of Gastroenterology and Hepatology*, vol. 26, no. 1, p. 210, 2011.

[3] K. Kikuma, J. Watanabe, Y. Oshiro et al., "Etiological factors in primary hepatic B-cell lymphoma," *Virchows Archiv*, vol. 460, no. 4, pp. 379–387, 2012.

[4] Y.-J. Ma, E.-Q. Chen, J. Wang, and H. Tang, "Progress in research of primary hepatic lymphoma," *World Chinese Journal of Digestology*, vol. 18, no. 26, pp. 2790–2793, 2010.

[5] J. Gao, J. Liu, L. Hou et al., "Report of one case of primary hepatic T cell lymphoma," *Chinese Medical Imaging Technology*, vol. 28, no. 11, p. 1952, 2012.

[6] Z. Li, J. He, Y. Zhu, and X. Wu, "CT manifestation of primary liver lymphoma," *Medical Imaging Technology*, vol. 24, no. 10, pp. 1762–1764, 2014.

[7] K. Miyashita, N. Tomita, H. Oshiro et al., "Primary hepatic peripheral T-cell lymphoma treated with corticosteroid," *Internal Medicine*, vol. 50, no. 6, pp. 617–620, 2011.

[8] Y.-J. Ma, E.-Q. Chen, X.-B. Chen, J. Wang, and H. Tang, "Primary hepatic diffuse large b cell lymphoma: a case report," *Hepatitis Monthly*, vol. 11, no. 3, pp. 203–205, 2011.

[9] E. J. Steller, M. S. van Leeuwen, R. van Hillegersberg et al., "Primary lymphoma of the liver—a complex diagnosis," *World Journal of Radiology*, vol. 4, no. 2, pp. 53–57, 2012.

39

Hepatic Sclerosing Hemangioma with Predominance of the Sclerosed Area Mimicking a Biliary Cystadenocarcinoma

Hiroyuki Sugo ⓘ,[1] Yuki Sekine,[1] Shozo Miyano,[1] Ikuo Watanobe ⓘ,[1] Michio Machida,[1] Kuniaki Kojima ⓘ,[1] Hironao Okubo,[2] Ayako Ura,[3] Kanako Ogura,[3] and Toshiharu Matsumoto[3]

[1]Department of General Surgery, Juntendo University Nerima Hospital, Japan
[2]Department of Gastroenterology, Juntendo University Nerima Hospital, Japan
[3]Department of Diagnostic Pathology, Juntendo University Nerima Hospital, Japan

Correspondence should be addressed to Hiroyuki Sugo; sugo@juntendo.ac.jp

Academic Editor: Fumio Imazeki

We report here an extremely rare case of hepatic sclerosing hemangioma mimicking a biliary cystadenocarcinoma. A previously healthy 39-year-old woman was referred to our hospital because of a large tumor in the liver. Abdominal computed tomography revealed early peripheral ring enhancement in the arterial phase and slight internal heterogeneous enhancement in the delayed phase. Magnetic resonance imaging revealed a tumor with low intensity in the T1-weighted image and very high intensity in the fat-saturated T2-weighted image. The patient underwent hepatectomy for a possible malignant liver tumor. Grossly, the tumor appeared as a white, solid, and cystic mass (weighted 1.1 kg and measured 170×100×80 mm) that was elastic, soft, and homogeneous with a yellowish area. Histological examination showed that the tumor mostly consisted of fibrotic areas with hyalinization. The typical histology of cavernous hemangioma was confirmed in part, and the tumor was diagnosed as a sclerosing hemangioma with predominancy of the sclerosed area. A review of 20 cases reported previously revealed that only 2 (10%) patients were diagnosed as having sclerosing hemangioma preoperatively.

1. Introduction

Hemangioma is the most common type of benign hepatic tumor [1]. Hemangioma degeneration can occur through an increase in the degree of fibrosis and thrombosis of its vascular channels, a condition known as sclerosing and/or hyalinizing hemangioma [2]. This can then lead to the end stage, known as the involution stage, in which the hemangioma becomes completely sclerosed and/or hyalinized [3, 4]. Sclerosing hemangioma is an extremely rare type of benign hepatic tumor, which mimics hepatic malignancies such as metastatic liver tumor or cholangiocarcinoma [5, 6]. We present herein a case of sclerosing hemangioma in a 39-year-old woman and review the relevant literature, with special reference to pathological features.

2. Case Presentation

A previously healthy 39-year-old woman was referred to our hospital because of a cystic lesion in the liver demonstrated by abdominal ultrasonography (US). Laboratory studies, including liver function tests, and tumor markers were also within the normal limits. Serological markers for hepatitis B or C viral infection were undetectable. Abdominal US revealed a well demarcated, heterogeneously low-echoic mass 170 mm in diameter in right lobe of the liver. Abdominal computed tomography (CT) during hepatic arteriography (CTHA) revealed early ring enhancement in the peripheral area in the arterial phase and slight internal heterogeneous enhancement in the delayed phase (Figures 1(a) and 1(b)). Magnetic resonance imaging (MRI) showed that the tumor had low signal intensity on T1-weighted images and some foci of high signal intensity on T2-weighted images. Gadolinium

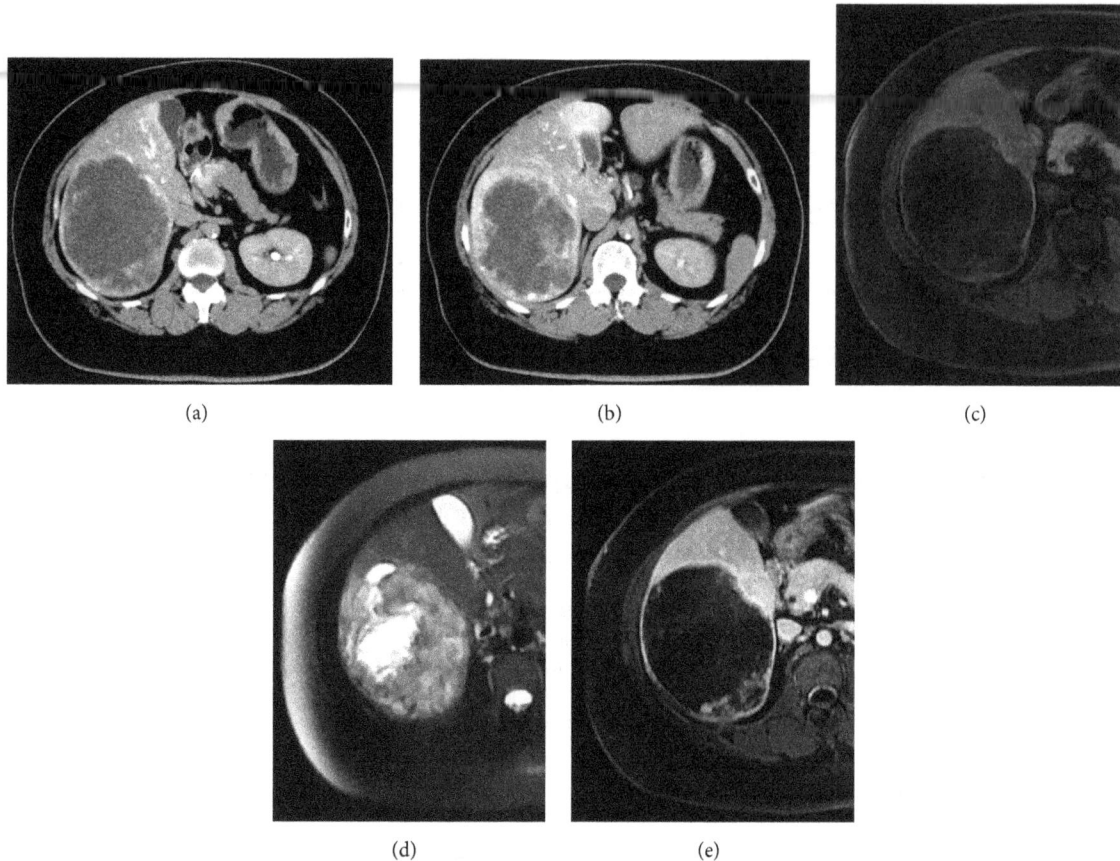

(a)   (b)   (c)

(d)   (e)

FIGURE 1: **Abdominal computed tomography during hepatic angiography and magnetic resonance imaging.** Arterial phase CT scan shows a geographic lesion in the right lobe of the liver with a rim and nodular enhancement (a), and the delayed phase of CT reveals heterogeneous enhancement in the peripheral area of the mass with a gradual centripetal enhancement pattern (b). The tumor shows low signal intensity on T1-weighted images (c) and some high-signal intensity nodules on T2-weighted images (d). EOB-MRI shows no uptake in the corresponding area (e).

ethoxybenzyl (Gd-EOB) MRI revealed no uptake in the corresponding area (Figures 1(c), 1(d), and 1(e)). Abdominal angiography demonstrated a large avascular region in the liver corresponding to the tumor, although no typical features of cavernous hemangioma were evident (Figure 2). 18-Fluorodeoxyglucose positron emission tomography (FDG-PET) revealed no abnormal FDG uptake. With these radiological findings, malignant liver tumor could not be excluded, such as biliary cystadenocarcinoma, cholangiocarcinoma, mesenchymal tumors, and hepatocellular carcinoma associated with cystic formation.

The patient underwent posterior sectionectomy. Intraoperative examination revealed a relatively soft dark red tumor (Figure 3(a)); the resected specimen weighed 1.1 kg and measured as 170×100×80 mm. The cut surface of the tumor revealed a white, solid, and cystic mass that was elastic, soft, and homogeneous with a yellowish area considered to be myxoid degeneration (Figure 3(b)). Histological examination showed that the tumor mostly consisted of sclerotic area and cavernous hemangioma area is partly observed (Figure 4(a)). Sclerotic area presents diffuse fibrosis (Figure 4(b)) and the typical histology of cavernous hemangioma was confirmed in some parts. In addition,

marked increase and dilation of medium sized veins with cavernous form were frequently noted in the surrounding areas of tumor (Figure 4(c)). The increased and dilated veins show positivity of CD31 immunostaining being a marker of endothelium (Figure 4(d)). The pathologic features were consistent with sclerosing hemangioma. The postoperative course was uneventful, and the patient was discharged on postoperative day 10.

3. Discussion

Hepatic sclerosing and sclerosed hemangiomas are very rare benign tumor, but the mechanism responsible for the degenerative changes in hepatic cavernous hemangioma has not been well clarified. Makhlouf and Ishak have reported that there are distinct clinical and histological differences between sclerosing and sclerosed hemangiomas; they suggested that recent hemorrhages and hemosiderin deposits, rich in mast cells are present in sclerosing hemangioma [2]. In the present case, histological examination revealed that the tumor was a sclerosing hemangioma composed mainly of a sclerosed area resulting from changes secondary to ischemic necrosis, venous occlusion by thrombi, and hemorrhage.

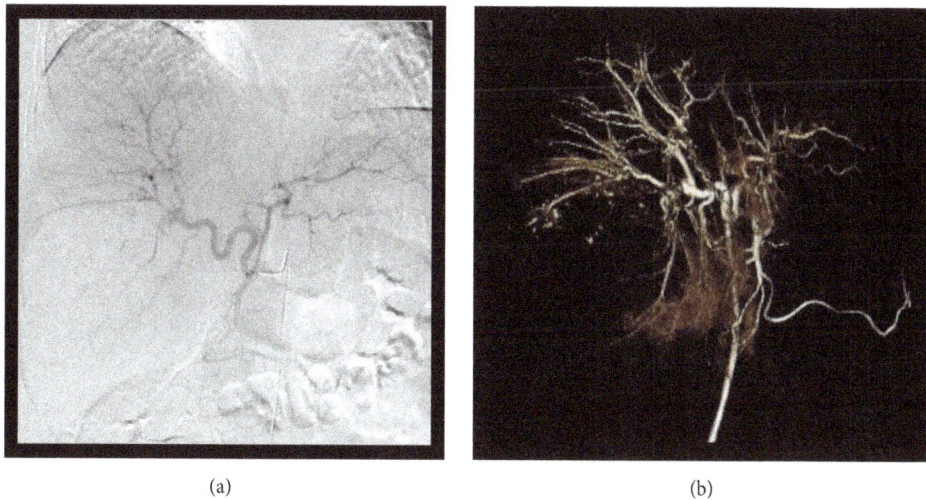

FIGURE 2: **Abdominal angiography.** (a) Common hepatic angiography image. (b) Three-dimensional image obtained by common hepatic angiography. Hepatic angiography shows a large avascular region in the liver corresponding to the tumor.

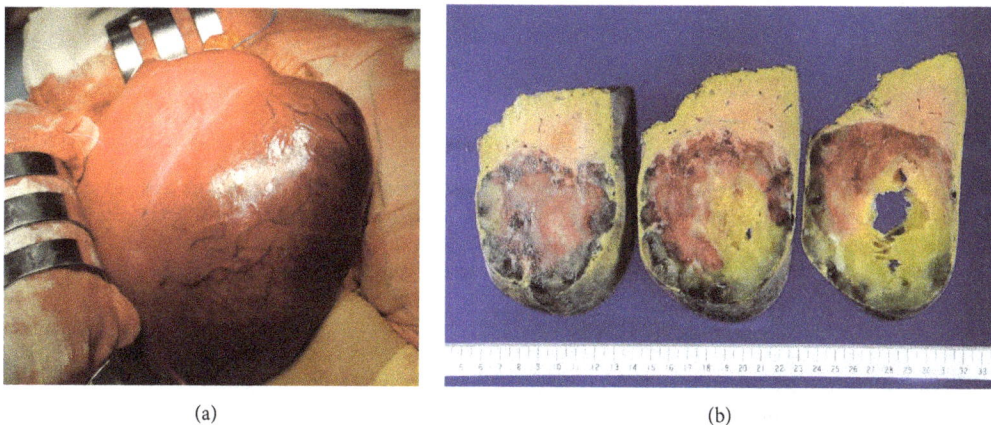

FIGURE 3: **Intraoperative findings and macroscopic findings of the resected tumor.** Exploration of the abdominal cavity showed a relatively soft, dark red tumor (a). The cut surface demonstrated a white solid and cystic mass (170×100×80 mm in size) that was elastic, soft, and homogeneous with multiple hemorrhagic foci (b).

These features support the contention that sclerosed and sclerosing hemangiomas are fundamentally similar lesions and may represent different stages in the development of the same lesion. From a clinical viewpoint, they also reported that patients with sclerosing hemangioma were younger, and had larger tumors that tended to present as a mass, occurring much more frequently in the right lobe [2]. The clinical features of the present case were well consistent with that report, and we finally diagnosed the lesion as a sclerosing hemangioma on the basis of the histological findings.

Hepatic sclerosing hemangiomas are caused by degenerative changes such as thrombus formation, necrosis, and scar formation within liver cavernous hemangioma, and such varieties of pathological characteristics make precisely radiological diagnosis very difficult [6]. On the other hand, the radiological findings of sclerosing and sclerosed hemangiomas have rarely been reported. In our case, CT showed only marginal enhancement in the peripheral area in the

arterial phase and slight internal heterogeneous enhancement in the delayed phase, mimicking adenocarcinoma. MRI showed low intensity on T1-weighted images and some high-signal intensity nodules on T2-weighted images, categorized as non-specific, and not excluding biliary cystadenocarcinoma, mesenchymal tumors with necrosis. Regarding imaging examinations, Yamashita et al. reported that sclerosing hemangiomas exhibit only marginal enhancement on CTHA, whereas the majority of the tumor presents as a perfusion defect [7]. Based on a review of sclerosing and sclerosed hemangiomas, Miyamoto et al. described that MRI revealed a low-intensity signal on T1-weighted images and a high-intensity signal on T2-weighted images [8]. Cheng et al. reported that hyalinized hemangiomas had a signal intensity lower than cerebrospinal fluid on T2-weighted images, lack of early enhancement, and slight peripheral enhancement in the late phase [3]. The collagen-rich and relatively acellular mature fibrous tissue generally has lower signal intensity

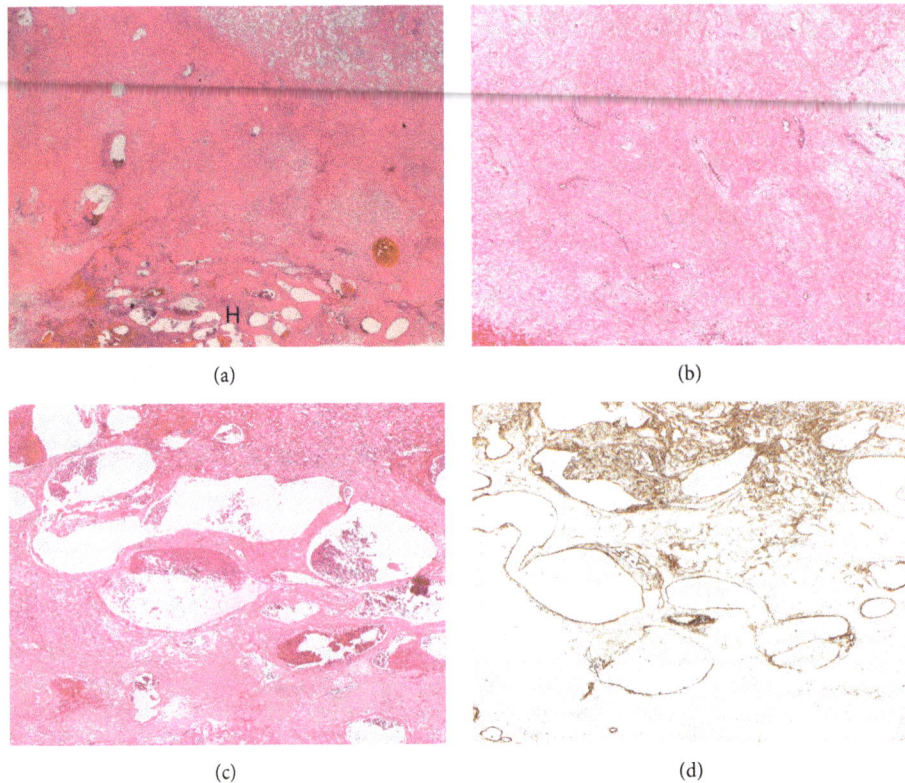

FIGURE 4: **Histological appearances of sclerosing hemangioma.** (a) Sclerotic area is manly present and cavernous hemangioma area (indicated by H) is partly observed. (Loupe image, HE stain). (b) Sclerotic area presents diffuse fibrosis. (HE stain, x40). (c) Histology of cavernous hemangioma. Note increase and dilation of medium sized veins with cavernous form in b (HE stain, x40). (d) The increased and dilated veins show positivity of CD31 immunostaining being a marker of endothelium in (c) (x40).

than muscle on T2-weighted images because of a decreased free water content and a low mobile proton density. Such radiological findings might lead to a preoperative diagnosis of hypovascular adenocarcinoma, including biliary cystade-nocarcinoma, cholangiocarcinoma, metastatic liver cancer, mesenchymal tumors, and hepatocellular carcinoma. Preoperatively, abdominal angiography was also performed in this case. To our knowledge, there have been no previous reports that present hepatic angiography image findings of sclerosing hemangioma. This showed a large avascular region in the liver corresponding to the tumor and no typical features of cavernous hemangioma. Ultimately, diagnosis is difficult based on these findings of angiography.

The use of surgical resection for hepatic sclerosing hemangioma is controversial. Most of the tumors reported previously were resected due to preoperative misdiagnosis as hepatic malignancies. Behbahani et al. have shown that knowledge of the appearance of atypical hemangioma and its inclusion in the differential diagnosis of hepatic lesions can alter patient management, being an important aspect to consider before invasive therapies are planned [9]. On the other hand, in fine-needle aspirates, the smears tend to be hemorrhagic, and sometimes only blood is aspirated. Miyamoto et al. have suggested that hepatic resection should be chosen for the management of hepatic sclerosing hemangioma at present [8]. They consider that percutaneous

needle biopsy is not acceptable because of the possibility of dissemination of cancer cells if the tumor proves to be malignant.

Including the present case, only 20 cases of hepatic sclerosing hemangioma have been reported in the English literature with detailed information on the patients (Table 1) [3, 4, 7, 10–23] A review of these 20 cases revealed that the average size of the tumor was 86.4 mm, ranging from 8 to 170 mm, and that the mean age of the patients was 63 years, ranging from 39 to 84 years. Our present patient was a very young woman aged 39 years, and the tumor was 170 mm in diameter and weighed 1.1 kg, making this patient the youngest and the tumor the largest to have been reported so far. Of these 20 patients, only 2 (10%) were diagnosed as having sclerosing hemangioma preoperatively.

Sclerosing hemangioma is extremely difficult to differentiate from other hepatic tumors. Further studies in more patients with this tumor are needed to provide an appropriate differential diagnosis of patients of having atypical hemangioma. Therefore, it is critical to be familiar with sclerosing hemangiomas, which leads to preoperative biopsy or intraoperative frozen section to avoid unnecessary extended hepatic resection of this rare benign tumor. However, if tumor malignancy cannot be ruled out in spite of biopsy, hepatic resection should remain the choice for diagnostic surgery at present.

TABLE 1: Cases of hepatic sclerosing hemangioma in the English literature.

Age/sex	Author.	Age/sex	Number of tumor	Size (mm)	CT	MRI (T1/T2)	Preoperaitve diagnosis	Treatment
1986	Takayasu et al.	62F	Solitary	50	Ring E	NA	NA	Surgery
1992	Haratake et al.	65F	Solitary	26	Ring E	NA	Meta/HCC	Surgery
1995	Cheng et al.	NA	Solitary	30	Ring E	Low/Slightly high	Malignant tumor	Surgery
1995	Shim et al.	41F	Solitary	130	Partly filled in	NA	Angiosarcoma	Surgery
2000	Yamashita et al.	67F	Solitary	50	Ring E	High/high	Meta	Surgery
2001	Aibe et al.	67F	Solitary	40	Delayed E	High/high	Meta	Surgery
2005	Lee et al.	65F	Solitary	55	Ring E	Low/moderate	HCC, IHCC, atypical hemangioma	Surgery
2008	Mori et al.	77F	Solitary	95	Ring E	Low/high	IHCC, FLC	Surgery
2008	Choi et al.	63M	Solitary	45	Multifocal patchy E	Low/intermediate	HCC, IHCC, atypical hemangioma	Surgery
2009	Lauder et al.	72M	Solitary	NA	Mild contrast E	NA	Meta	Surgery
2009	Lauder et al.	84M	Solitary	NA	Hypodense	NA	Meta	Surgery
2010	Jin et al.	52M	Solitary	21	Ring E	Low/Slightly high	HCC, Hemangioma	Surgery
2011	Papafragkakis et al.	52F	Solitary	75	Intralesional E	NA	NA	Surgery
2011	Shin YM	50M	Solitary	100	Patch E	Low/high		Obsevation
2012	Yamada et al.	75M	Solitary	8	Ring E	Low/Slightly high	Meta	Surgery
2013	Song et al.	63F	Solitary	91	Ring E	NA	Atypical hemangioma, Meta, HCC	Surgery
2013	Shimada et al.	63M	Solitary	10	Ring E	Low/Slightly high		Surgery
2015	Wakasugi et al.	67F	Multiple	11,28	Ring E	Low/hetero	Meta, HCC	Surgery
2017	Behbahani et al.	70M	Multiple	NA	Ring E	NA		Obsevation
2018	Sugo et al.	39F	Solitary	170	Ring E	Low/Slightly high	Biliary Cystadenocarcinoma	Surgery

E: enhancement, Meta: metastasis, HCC: hepatocellular carcinoma, IHCC: intrahepatic cholangiocarcinoma, FLC: fibromellar HCC.

References

[1] P. J. Karhunen, "Benign hepatic tumours and tumour like conditions in men," *Journal of Clinical Pathology*, vol. 39, no. 2, pp. 183–188, 1986.

[2] H. R. Makhlouf and K. G. Ishak, "Sclerosed hemangioma and sclerosing cavernous hemangioma of the liver: A comparative clinicopathologic and immunohistochemical study with emphasis on the role of mast cells in their histogenesis," *Journal of Liver*, vol. 22, no. 1, pp. 70–78, 2002.

[3] H. C. Cheng, S. H. Tsai, J. H. Chiang, and C. Y. Chang, "Hyalinized liver hemangioma mimicking malignant tumor at MR imaging.," *American Journal of Roentgenology*, vol. 165, no. 4, pp. 1016-1017, 1995.

[4] J. S. Song, Y. N. Kim, and W. S. Moon, "A sclerosing hemangioma of the liver.," *Clinical and Molecular Hepatology*, vol. 19, no. 4, pp. 426–430, 2013.

[5] T. Ishi, O. Takahara, and I. Sano, "Sclerosing hemangioma of the liver," *Nagasaki Medical Journal*, vol. 70, pp. 23–26, 1995.

[6] D. J. Doyle, K. Khalili, M. Guindi, and M. Atri, "Imaging features of sclerosed hemangioma," *American Journal of Roentgenology*, vol. 189, no. 1, pp. 67–72, 2007.

[7] Y.-I. Yamashita, M. Shimada, K.-I. Taguchi et al., "Hepatic sclerosing hemangioma mimicking a metastatic liver tumor: Report of a case," *Surgery Today*, vol. 30, no. 9, pp. 849–852, 2000.

[8] S. Miyamoto, A. Oshita, Y. Daimaru, M. Sasaki, H. Ohdan, and A. Nakamitsu, "Hepatic Sclerosed Hemangioma: A case report and review of the literature," *BMC Surgery*, vol. 17, pp. 15–45, 2015.

[9] S. Behbahani, J. C. Hoffmann, R. Stonebridge, and S. Mahboob, "Clinical case report: Sclerosing hemangioma of the liver, a rare but great mimicker," *Radiology Case Reports*, vol. 11, no. 2, pp. 58–61, 2016.

[10] K. Takayasu, N. Moriyama, Y. Shima et al., "Atypical radiographic findings in hepatic cavernous hemangioma: Correlation with histologic features," *American Journal of Roentgenology*, vol. 146, no. 6, pp. 1149–1153, 1986.

[11] J. Haratake, A. Horie, and Y. Nagafuchi, "Hyalinized Hemangioma of the Liver," *American Journal of Gastroenterology*, vol. 87, no. 2, pp. 234–236, 1992.

[12] K. S. Shim, J. M. Suh, Y. S. Yang et al., "Sclerosis of hepatic cavernous hemangioma: CT findings and pathologic correlation," *Journal of Korean Medical Science*, vol. 10, no. 4, pp. 294–297, 1995.

[13] H. Aibe, H. Honda, T. Kuroiwa et al., "Sclerosed hemangioma of the liver," *Abdominal Imaging*, vol. 26, no. 5, pp. 496–499, 2001.

[14] V. T. W. Lee, M. Magnaye, H. W. Tan, C. H. Thng, and L. L. P. J. Ooi, "Sclerosing haemangioma mimicking hepatocellular carcinoma," *Singapore Medical Journal*, vol. 46, no. 3, pp. 140–143, 2005.

[15] H. Mori, T. Ikegami, S. Imura et al., "Sclerosed hemangioma of the liver: Report of a case and review of the literature," *Hepatology Research*, vol. 38, no. 5, pp. 529–533, 2008.

[16] Y. J. Choi, K. W. Kim, E.-Y. Cha, J.-S. Song, E. Yu, and M.-G. Lee, "Sclerosing liver haemangioma with pericapillary smooth muscle proliferation: Atypical CT and MR findings with pathological correlation," *British Journal of Radiology*, vol. 81, no. 966, pp. e162–e165, 2008.

[17] S.-Y. Jin, "Sclerosed hemangioma of the liver," *Korean Journal of Hepatology*, vol. 16, no. 4, pp. 410–413, 2010.

[18] C. Lauder, G. Garcea, H. Kanhere, and G. J. Maddern, "Sclerosing haemangiomas of the liver: two cases of mistaken identity," *HPB Surgery*, vol. 2009, Article ID 473591, 3 pages, 2009.

[19] H. Papafragkakis, M. Moehlen, M. T. Garcia-Buitrago, B. Madrazo, E. Island, and P. Martin, "A case of a ruptured sclerosing liver hemangioma," *International Journal of Hepatology*, vol. 2011, Article ID 942360, 5 pages, 2011.

[20] Y. M. Shin, "Sclerosing hemangioma in the liver," *Korean Journal of Hepatology*, vol. 17, no. 3, p. 242, 2011.

[21] S. Yamada, M. Shimada, T. Utsunomiya et al., "Hepatic screlosed hemangioma which was misdiagnosed as metastasis of gastric cancer: Report of a case," *Journal of Medical Investigation*, vol. 59, no. 3-4, pp. 270–274, 2012.

[22] Y. Shimada, Y. Takahashi, H. Iguchi et al., "A hepatic sclerosed hemangioma with significant morphological change over a period of 10 years: A case report," *Journal of Medical Case Reports*, vol. 7, no. 5, 139 pages, 2013.

[23] M. Wakasugi, S. Ueshima, M. Tei et al., "Multiple hepatic sclerosing hemangioma mimicking metastatic liver tumor successfully treated by laparoscopic surgery: Report of a case," *International Journal of Surgery Case Reports*, vol. 8, pp. 137–140, 2015.

40

Laparoscopic Resection of Cholecystocolic Fistula and Subtotal Cholecystectomy by Tri-Staple in a Type V Mirizzi Syndrome

Fahri Yetişir,[1] **Akgün Ebru Şarer,**[2] **Hasan Zafer Acar,**[3] **Omer Parlak,**[1] **Basar Basaran,**[1] **and Omer Yazıcıoğlu**[1]

[1]*Atatürk Research and Training Hospital, General Surgery Department, Ankara, Turkey*
[2]*Atatürk Research and Training Hospital, Anesthesiology and Reanimation Department, Ankara, Turkey*
[3]*Natomed Private Hospital, General Surgery Department, Ankara, Turkey*

Correspondence should be addressed to Fahri Yetişir; drfahriyetisir@hotmail.com

Academic Editor: Pier Cristoforo Giulianotti

The Mirizzi syndrome (MS) is an impacted stone in the cystic duct or Hartmann's pouch that mechanically obstructs the common bile duct (CBD). We would like to report laparoscopic subtotal cholecystectomy (SC) and resection of cholecystocolic fistula by the help of Tri-Staple™ in a case with type V MS and cholecystocolic fistula, for first time in the literature. A 24-year-old man was admitted to emergency department with the complaint of abdominal pain, intermittent fever, jaundice, and diarrhea. Two months ago with the same complaint, ERCP was performed. Laparoscopic resection of cholecystocolic fistula and subtotal cholecystectomy were performed by the help of Tri-Staple. At the eight-month follow-up, he was symptom-free with normal liver function tests. In a patient with type V MS and cholecystocolic fistula, laparoscopic resection of cholecystocolic fistula and SC can be performed by using Tri-Staple safely.

1. Introduction

Mirizzi syndrome (MS) is a rare cause of intermittent or constant obstructive jaundice, where an impacted stone in the cystic duct or Hartmann's pouch mechanically obstructs the common bile duct (CBD). MS was first described in 1948, as a repeated inflammation of the gallbladder due to an impacted gallstone. This leads to the formation of adhesions between the gallbladder and the CBD resulting in anatomic distortion of these structures [1]. It generally occurs in females with advanced age. Incidence of MS is 0.3–5.7%. Few articles have described the coexistence of MS and cholecystoenteric fistula [2]. Csendes' MS classification system has been renewed. Depending on the degree of involvement of the biliary tract, the patients may be grouped into five distinct groups and coexistence of cholecystoenteric fistula and MS was classified as type V [2]. MS and cholecystoenteric fistulas are rare and late complications of gallstone disease [3, 4]. The most common type of biliary enteric fistula is cholecystoduodenal (75%); cholecystocolic fistula is the next common (10–20%),

with a variety of other types being less common (15%) [5]. Symptoms are similar to that of acute and chronic cholecystitis, with or without jaundice and diarrhea [1].

It is important to identify MS and fistula formation before surgery or at least during surgery because of serious morbidity and mortality related to the condition [3]. Correct surgical approach and management are very important for MS as chronic biliary tree inflammation and bile duct anatomic alteration necessitate a rigorous technique [5].

Laparoscopic subtotal cholecystectomy (SC) is considered to be a safe option in severe cholecystitis with frozen anatomy within Calot's triangle where there is a potential risk of causing injury to the common bile duct (CBD) [6]. Laparoscopic stapling devices are an effective method for performing LSC or dividing a dilated cystic duct or neck of gallbladder due to its ease and speed of application [7].

According to our knowledge there is no reported data about laparoscopic treatment of type V MS. We would like to report laparoscopic SC and resection of cholecystocolic fistula by the help of endoscopic stapler (Covidien Endo GIA

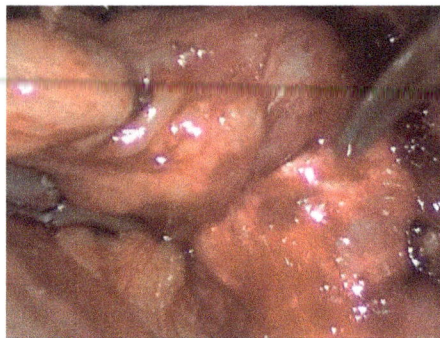

FIGURE 1: Cholecystocolic fistula between fundus of gallbladder and hepatic flexure of colon is seen.

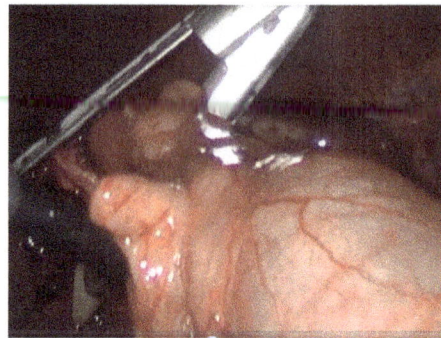

FIGURE 2: Resection of the cholecystocolic fistula by the help of the vascular Tri-Staple is seen (Covidien Endo GIA Reinforced Reload with Tri-Staple Technology).

Reinforced Reload with Tri-Staple Technology) in a case with type V MS with cholecystocolic fistula.

2. Presentation of Case

A 24-year-old man was admitted to emergency department with the complaint of abdominal pain, intermittent fever, jaundice, and diarrhea for the last five days. Pain especially was present at right upper quadrant and epigastric region. In his past history, there was no operation and chronic disease. He had been admitted 2 months ago with the same complaint and hospitalized for cholelithiasis and choledocolithiasis. Endoscopic retrograde cholangiopancreatography (ERCP) was performed. Endoscopic papillotomy was applied and sludge was removed by ERCP. Five days later, total bilirubin level decreased from 3.1 to 1.2 mg/dL (normal 0.2–1 mg/dL), and the patient was discharged from gastroenterology department. His vital parameters were as follows: blood pressure (BP): 110/50 mmHg, heart rate (HR): 88, and fever: 37.7°C. On abdominal examination, there was evidence of icterus and sensitiveness and rebound was positive at right hypochondrium. In biochemical analysis, total bilirubin was 2.6 mg/dL, conjugated bilirubin 1.8 (normal < 0.2 mg/dL), serum glutamic oxaloacetic transaminase (SGOT) 60 U/L (5–40 U/L), serum glutamic-pyruvic transaminase (SGPT) 71 U/L (normal 5–40 U/L), alkaline phosphatase 287 U/L (<106 U/L), and glutamyl transferase 130 U/L (<45 U/L). LDH was 277 U/L, lipase 155 U/L, amylase 134 U/L, and CRP 7 mg/dL; in total blood count, WBC was 12.000 K/Ul. Abdominal ultrasound showed that so many calculi were present in gallbladder and a large calculus was located in cystic duct. He underwent emergent laparoscopic operation. The final diagnosis was made intraoperatively.

2.1. Surgical Technique. He underwent operation under general anesthesia. Classical 4 trocars entries were used. There were dense adhesions between colon, duodenum, gallbladder, and omentum in the right subhepatic space. After gentle dissection, first cholecystocolic fistula between fundus of gallbladder and hepatic flexure of colon was observed (Figure 1). After visualization of boundaries of cholecystocolic fistula, its resection was performed by the help of the vascular Tri-Staple (Covidien Endo GIA™ Reinforced Reload with

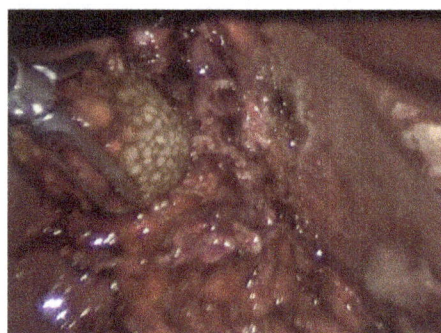

FIGURE 3: Extraction of large impacted stone from cholecystocholedochal fistula trough opening of fundus is seen.

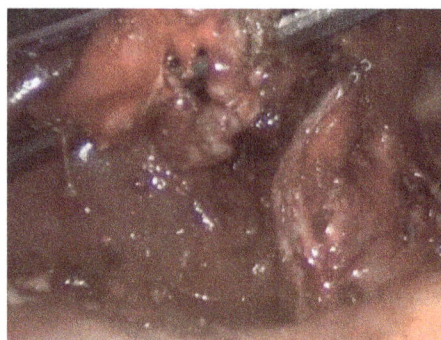

FIGURE 4: Applied Tri-Staple line is seen on stump.

Tri-Staple Technology) (Figure 2). It was seen that there was no narrowing at resection side of colon. Later there were significant difficulties in dissecting the gallbladder neck and Calot's triangle and further dissection would expose the patient to a higher risk of common bile duct injury or hemorrhage; the cystic duct and artery could not be isolated. The operative method was changed and dissection was started from fundus and anterior wall of fundus was resected. All gallstones were extracted one by one through an incision in the fundus of gallbladder. At the end large impacted stone was also extracted (Figure 3). After extracting this large impacted stone, excessive amount of bile drainage came from this fistula. Irrigation of common bile duct with

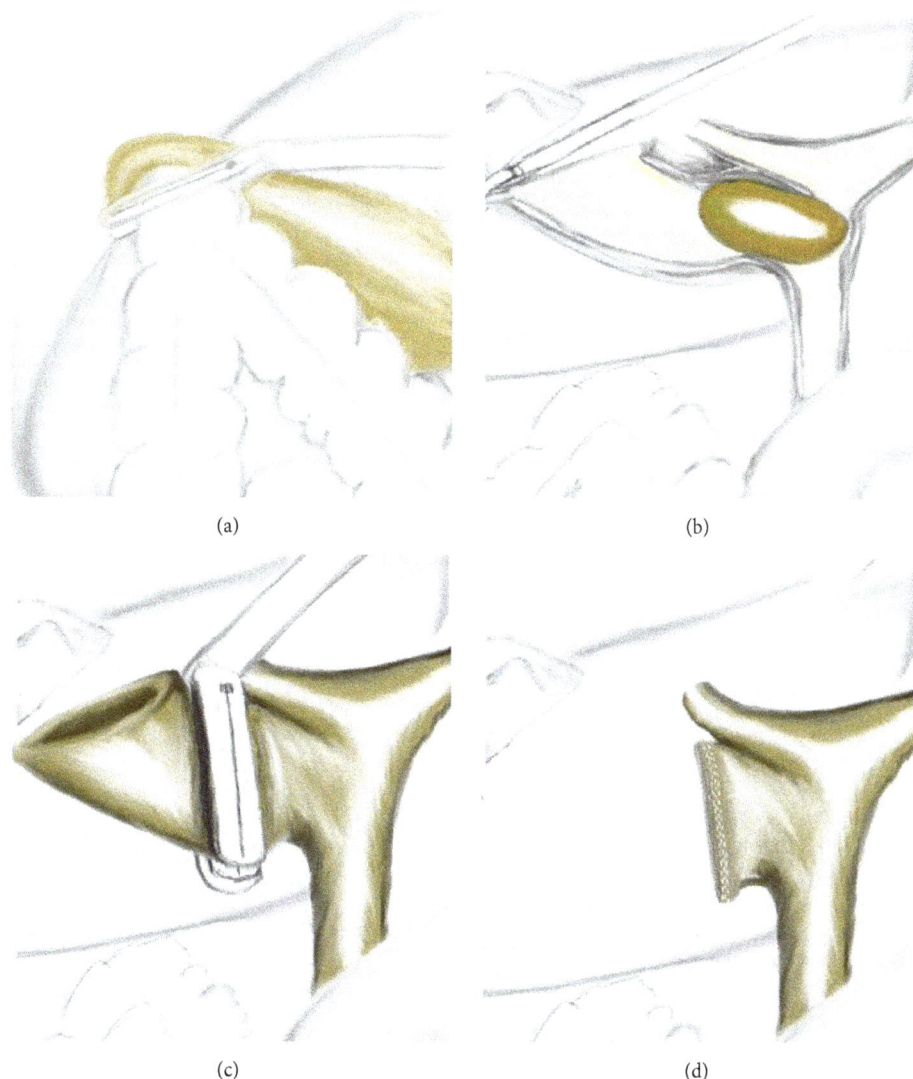

(a) (b) (c) (d)

FIGURE 5: Schematic illustration of the case: (a) illustration is seen during the resection of cholecystocolic fistula by Tri-Staple. (b) Impacted stone is seen in the cholecystocholedochal fistula like type IV Mirizzi syndrome, illustration is drown as anterior surface of gallbladder and biliary was opened. (c) Subtotal cholecystectomy line by Tri-Staple is seen. (d) After completion of the subtotal cholecystectomy, stump of gallbladder and staple line on stump is seen.

saline was performed via fistula opening. There were no other stones. A subtotal cholecystectomy was done by stapling over infundibulum of gallbladder with medium thick Tri-Staple (Figure 4). All the resection steps were summarized in illustration (Figure 5). Resection of the remnant posterior part of fundus could be completed by harmonic scalpel. After irrigation with saline, one drainage was placed near to the gallbladder stump. Postoperative course was uneventful and patient was discharged 5 days after the operation. At the eighth-month follow-up, there was no problem. He was symptom-free with normal liver function tests.

3. Discussion

During laparoscopic treatment of this case, two important problems were facilitated by using laparoscopic stapler; one

of them is resection of cholecystocolic fistula and second one is subtotal cholecystectomy. By the help of stapler resection of cholecystocolic fistula was performed laparoscopically without injuring or narrowing the colon. After extracting impacted stone and irrigating CBD with saline subtotal cholecystectomy was undertaken by applying a staple across gallbladder infundibulum safely. Before subtotal cholecystectomy to understand anatomical structure of external bile duct using cholangiogram or choledochoscopy could be better but we could not perform both of them due to technical insufficiencies. Suturing the gallbladder stump would be an acceptable alternative if stapler could not be applied.

Open surgery for MS is accepted. The reported conversion rate to open cholecystectomy was remarkably high, with a range of 37–78% [8]. As the type of MS increases, conversion rate increases with concordance. There is no reported data in literature about laparoscopic treatment of a case with type V MS and cholecystocolic fistula.

There are so many treatment modalities for MS. It can be changed according to patient, type of MS, and experience of surgeon and gastroenterologist to apply ERCP. If the patient has high risk for surgery, endoscopic treatment can also be tried [9]. Laparoscopic or open SC can be used safely by dividing across Hartmann's pouch, infundibulum, or dilated cystic duct. Another safe option is the drainage of the remnant pouch after performing a partial cholecystectomy. The proper surgical treatment mentioned in literature is partial cholecystectomy and a biliary drainage procedure (Roux-en-Y anastomosis), with open surgical procedure especially in types III and IV MS [10].

There are two most important issues for SC; one of them is the formation of residual gallstones in the remnant gallbladder. Symptomatic gallstone disease recurrence was reported to be 2.2–5%. These complications can be treated successfully by endoscopic papillotomy or completion with cholecystectomy. Another one is gallbladder cancer which is found in 0.2–0.8% of patients undergoing laparoscopic cholecystectomy [10, 11].

Chaudery et al. reported two laparoscopic subtotal cholecystectomies by using stapler and both of them had acute pancreatitis approximately 6 weeks after this operation. The episodes of pancreatitis described in their cases were thought to be associated with contained residual stones in the remnant pouch. At the end they advised that laparoscopic SC with stapler should be done after extracting all stones and irrigating CBD via the opening of the fundus [7]. In our case no complication occurred, because first all the stone was removed and irrigation of CBD was done; after that reticulating endoscopic stapler was applied to close infundibulum of gallbladder in a good exposure by using 30°C scope. Another factor may be the application of the endoscopic papillotomy by ERCP before surgery for preventing from this kind of complication.

4. Conclusion

Laparoscopic resection of cholecystocolic fistula and subtotal cholecystectomy can be performed by using Tri-Staple safely in a patient with type V MS and cholecystocolic fistula.

References

[1] D. C. Desai and R. D. Smink Jr., "Mirizzi syndrome type II: is laparoscopic cholecystectomy justified?" *Journal of the Society of Laparoendoscopic Surgeons*, vol. 1, no. 3, pp. 237–239, 1997.

[2] M. A. Beltran, A. Csendes, and K. S. Cruces, "The relationship of Mirizzi syndrome and cholecystoenteric fistula: validation of a modified classification," *World Journal of Surgery*, vol. 32, no. 10, pp. 2237–2243, 2008.

[3] A. Abou-Saif and F. H. Al-Kawas, "Complications of gallstone disease: mirizzi syndrome, cholecystocholedochal fistula, and gallstone ileus," *The American Journal of Gastroenterology*, vol. 97, no. 2, pp. 249–254, 2002.

[4] M. A. Beltran and A. Csendes, "Mirizzi syndrome and gallstone ileus: an unusual presentation of gallstone disease," *Journal of Gastrointestinal Surgery*, vol. 9, no. 5, pp. 686–689, 2005.

[5] M. S. Faridi and A. Pandey, "Mirizzi syndrome type II with cholecystoduodenal fistula: an infrequent combination," *Malaysian Journal of Medical Sciences*, vol. 21, no. 1, pp. 69–71, 2014.

[6] I. Sinha, M. Lawson Smith, P. Safranek, T. Dehn, and M. Booth, "Laparoscopic subtotal cholecystectomy without cystic duct ligation," *British Journal of Surgery*, vol. 94, no. 12, pp. 1527–1529, 2007.

[7] M. Chaudery, T. Hunjan, A. Beggs, and D. Nehra, "Pitfalls in the use of laparoscopic staplers to perform subtotal cholecystectomy," *BMJ Case Reports*, 2013.

[8] R. Mithani, W. H. Schwesinger, J. Bingener, K. R. Sirinek, and G. W. W. Gross, "The Mirizzi syndrome: multidisciplinary management promotes optimal outcomes," *Journal of Gastrointestinal Surgery*, vol. 12, no. 6, pp. 1022–1028, 2008.

[9] R. E. England and D. F. Martin, "Endoscopic management of Mirizzi's syndrome," *Gut*, vol. 40, no. 2, pp. 272–276, 1997.

[10] D. Henneman, D. W. da Costa, B. C. Vrouenraets, B. A. Van Wagensveld, and S. M. Lagarde, "Laparoscopic partial cholecystectomy for the difficult gallbladder: a systematic review," *Surgical Endoscopy*, vol. 27, no. 2, pp. 351–358, 2013.

[11] J. A. E. Philips, D. A. Lawes, A. J. Cook et al., "The use of laparoscopic subtotal cholecystectomy for complicated cholelithiasis," *Surgical Endoscopy and Other Interventional Techniques*, vol. 22, no. 7, pp. 1697–1700, 2008.

41

Intrahepatic Cholangiocarcinoma Masquerading as Acute Fatty Liver of Pregnancy: A Case Report and Review of the Literature

Ayman Qasrawi (ID),[1] **Omar Abughanimeh,**[1] **Mouhanna Abu Ghanimeh** (ID),[2] **Simran Arora-Elder,**[3] **Osama Yousef,**[4] and **Tarek Tamimi**[4]

[1]*Internal Medicine Department, University of Missouri-Kansas City School of Medicine, Kansas City, MO, USA*
[2]*Internal Medicine Department, Division of Gastroenterology, Henry Ford Hospital, Detroit, MI, USA*
[3]*Division of Hematology/Oncology, University of Maryland Medical Center, Baltimore, MD, USA*
[4]*Division of Gastroenterology, University of Missouri-Kansas City School of Medicine, Kansas City, MO, USA*

Correspondence should be addressed to Ayman Qasrawi; ahqasrawi@gmail.com

Academic Editor: Pier Cristoforo Giulianotti

Cholangiocarcinoma (CCA) is an uncommon cancer and accounts only for 3% of all gastrointestinal malignancies. In this report, we present a case of an intrahepatic cholangiocarcinoma masquerading as acute fatty liver of pregnancy (AFLP). A 38-year-old female who is 36-week pregnant presented with a 1-week history of headache, nausea, vomiting, and right upper abdominal pain, along with hepatomegaly. Laboratory investigations were remarkable for mild leukocytosis, hyperbilirubinemia, proteinuria, and elevated transaminases and prothrombin time. Ultrasound of the liver revealed hepatomegaly, fatty infiltration, and a right hepatic lobe mass. Based on the overall picture, AFLP was suspected, and the patient underwent delivery by Cesarean section. However, bilirubin and liver enzyme levels gradually increased after delivery. MRI revealed a large dominant hepatic mass along with multiple satellite lesions in both lobes. Biopsy revealed the presence of intrahepatic CCA. CCA presenting during pregnancy is extremely rare with only 9 other cases reported in the literature. Therefore, the signs and symptoms can be easily confused with other more common disorders that occur during pregnancy.

1. Introduction

Cholangiocarcinoma (CCA) is an uncommon malignancy that arises from the epithelial cells of the biliary tree. CCA accounts for approximately 3% of all gastrointestinal malignancies [1, 2] and has a high mortality rate, given its late diagnosis and refractoriness to therapy [3]. On average, CCAs have a 5-year survival rate of 5–10% [4]. CCA presents extremely rarely during pregnancy and can mimic other disorders, such as obstructive cholestasis or HELLP syndrome [5, 6], which can lead to delayed diagnosis. We present a case of intrahepatic CCA that mimicked acute fatty liver of pregnancy (AFLP) and was subsequently diagnosed after delivery.

2. Case Presentation

A 38-year-old female with morbid obesity and chronic hypertension presented in her fourth pregnancy at 36 weeks of gestation with a 1-week history of mild headache, nausea, epigastric and right upper quadrant pain, and dark urine. The pain started gradually but was constant and sharp in nature. Upon physical examination, she was jaundiced. The abdominal exam was remarkable for hepatomegaly and a gravid uterus. The neurological exam was normal. The patient denied use of any hepatotoxic medications. Her labs were completely normal about three weeks earlier. Initial laboratory workup showed a leucocyte count of 12.0 × 10^9/L (70% neutrophils), platelet count of 450 × 10^9/L, hemoglobin of 11.5 g/dL, total bilirubin of 6.4 mg/dl (direct fraction 5.0 mg/dL), aspartate aminotransferase (AST) of 83 U/L, alanine aminotransferase (ALT) of 87 U/L, alkaline phosphatase (ALP) of 319 U/l, glucose of 66 mg/dL, LDH of 679 U/L, uric acid of 4.2 mg/dL, and total serum bile acids of 71 μmol/L (ref. 0–19 μmol). Prothrombin time was 17 seconds with an international normalized ratio (INR) of 1.4. Viral hepatitis serology, autoimmune marker, and

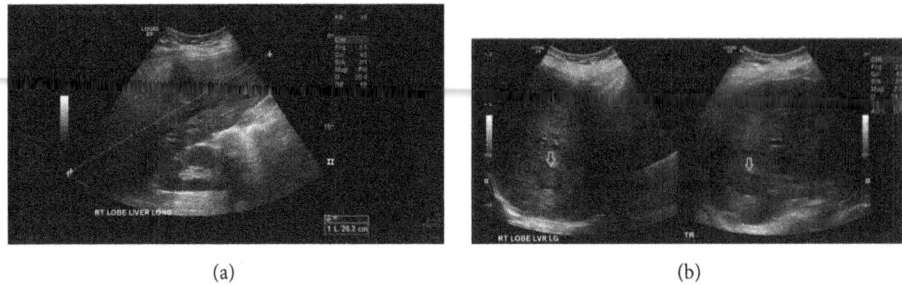

FIGURE 1: Liver ultrasound. (a) demonstrates the size of the liver measured to be about 26.2 cm. (b) demonstrates the hypoechoic mass in the right hepatic lobe (green arrows). The mass measured 2.8 cm.

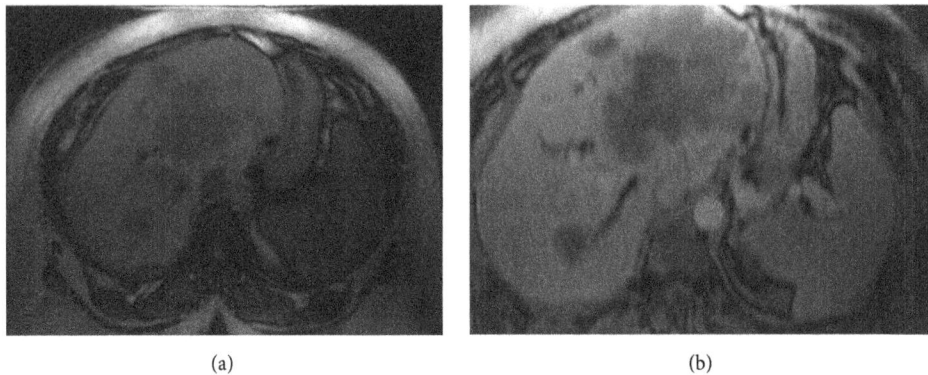

FIGURE 2: MRI of the liver and abdomen showing the large hepatic mass. (a) T1-weighted image. (b) T2-weighted image. The mass is involving the majority of the left hepatic lobe, measuring approximately $11.2 \times 9.2 \times 5.8$ cm. There are multiple additional satellite lesions within the left hepatic lobe. There is an additional similar-appearing smaller T2 hyperintense lesion within the right hepatic lobe, measuring approximately 2.8×2.1 cm.

ceruloplasmin test results were unremarkable. The urine protein-to-creatinine ratio was elevated with 24 hours of collection for urine protein, 1300 mg/day; her 24-hour urine protein was 180 mg/day prior to pregnancy. Ultrasonography showed marked hepatomegaly (~27 cm), fatty infiltration of the liver, and a right hepatic hypoechoic 2.8 cm mass (Figure 1). Moreover, the liver exhibited heterogenous echotexture along with areas of nodular contour. Given the patients' clinical presentation, biochemical profile, and imaging findings, the obstetricians suspected AFLP. The patient underwent delivery by Cesarean section; however, bilirubin and liver enzyme levels gradually increased after delivery. Magnetic resonance imaging (MRI) of the liver was obtained three days after delivery for further evaluation of the mass and worsening liver function (Figure 2). MRI showed a heterogeneous T2 hyperintense mass involving the majority of the left hepatic lobe, measuring approximately $11.2 \times 9.2 \times 5.8$ cm. There was an additional similar, smaller lesion within the right hepatic lobe, measuring approximately 2.8×2.1 cm. There were additional satellite lesions within the left hepatic lobe. There was mild, diffuse intrahepatic biliary dilation. Serum tumor markers were obtained and showed elevated cancer antigen 19-9 (CA19-9) of >10,000 U/ml, CEA of 160.5 ng/mL (normal up to 5.20), and α-fetoprotein (AFP) of 1,135 ng/mL. US guided biopsy tissue obtained from the smaller right hepatic mass showed adenocarcinoma with an

immunohistochemical profile consistent with cholangiocarcinoma. A CT scan of the chest showed multiple bilateral pulmonary nodules suspicious for metastasis. Total bilirubin started to increase gradually, up to 14.0 mg/dL. The patient underwent placement of percutaneous biliary drains with subsequent improvement of her total bilirubin to 4.0 mg/dL. She was then started on palliative chemotherapy with gemcitabine; however, this was complicated by recurrent episodes of cholangitis with multidrug-resistant organisms. She also developed progressive disease and peritoneal carcinomatosis and was subsequently transitioned into hospice care. She died around six months after her original presentation.

3. Discussion

CCAs can be classified based on their anatomical location, as intrahepatic, perihilar, or distal extrahepatic [3]. The majority of CCAs are either perihilar or distal, with intrahepatic disease responsible for <10% of the cases [2, 7]. CCA risk factors include, but are not limited to, primary sclerosing cholangitis, choledocholithiasis, long-standing ulcerative colitis, infestation with *Clonorchis sinensis*, Caroli's disease, and congenital hepatic fibrosis [2, 3, 8]. In most patients, there is no identifiable cause of CCA [2]. The clinical features of CCAs differ according to their clinical location [2, 4]. In general, they are asymptomatic in the early stages and symptomatic cases usually indicate advanced disease [2, 3]. Extrahepatic tumors usually present with painless jaundice from biliary obstruction [2, 4]; on the other hand, intrahepatic CCAs are less likely to cause jaundice. Common CCA symptoms include abdominal pain, fatigue, cachexia and/or fever, and night sweats [2–4]. Intrahepatic CCAs can be an incidental finding, when imaging is obtained, as part of the workup of abnormal liver blood tests [9].

Liver diseases complicate the courses of ~3% of all pregnancies and some of them can have severe consequences [9–11]. They often have very similar presentations. The most important pregnancy-specific presentations are preeclampsia, eclampsia, hyperemesis gravidarum, AFLP, intrahepatic cholestasis of pregnancy, and HELLP syndrome [11, 12]. Additionally, the differential diagnosis includes other disorders that are unrelated to pregnancy, such as drugs, toxins, and viral hepatitis. AFLP is a rare but life-threatening disease that occurs mostly in the third trimester [11]. The usual symptoms of AFLP are nausea, vomiting, and epigastric pain [11, 12] and the notable laboratory features include leukocytosis, moderate elevation in liver enzymes, hyperbilirubinemia, coagulopathy, hyperuricemia, hypoglycemia, and proteinuria [11–13]. Ultrasound features include increased echogenicity, indicating fatty infiltration and sometimes ascites [11, 14]. Swansea criteria can also be used to aid the diagnosis [11].

The majority of liver masses identified during pregnancy are more commonly benign [15], for example, hemangiomas, adenomas, hamartomas, and focal nodular hyperplasia [15, 16]. Only a few cases of hepatocellular carcinoma were reported in the literature [15]; given the rarity of malignant liver lesions in pregnancy and that the presenting symptoms of malignancy may be confused with the common symptoms of pregnancy, the diagnosis is often delayed [5, 15]. In addition, diagnostic and interventional modalities are limited in pregnancy, which might be another limiting factor in early diagnosis [16].

CCA is extremely rare during pregnancy. We searched the PubMed database and found 9 cases in 8 reports of CCA in pregnancy from 1975 to 2015 [5, 6, 17–22]. We analyzed the 9 cases and the present case. The age of the women ranged from 25 to 38. Five of the cases were diagnosed in the second trimester and one in the third. In our case and in the case reported by Zelissen et al., the symptoms started in the pregnancy but the correct diagnosis was established postpartum [18]. In one of the cases reported by Purtilo et al., the patient died from meningitis during pregnancy and was found to have incidental CCA during autopsy [17]. In the other case reported by Purtilo et al., a postpartum woman had a positive pregnancy test and a metastatic malignancy. The diagnosis was confused with choriocarcinoma due to ectopic secretion of human chorionic gonadotropin; the correct diagnosis was established during autopsy [17]. Common presenting symptoms and signs were nausea, vomiting, abdominal pain, pruritus, jaundice, hepatomegaly, and/or a palpable mass; interestingly, one of the cases presented as spinal cord compression [21]. In the cases with reported laboratory values, the liver enzymes (AST/ALT) were normal or slightly elevated. Total bilirubin was elevated in five cases (range:

3.6–15.9 mg/dL). Other abnormal lab results were malignant hypercalcemia in one case and elevated bile acids in another [5, 18]. The diagnosis mimicked obstetric cholestasis in one case [5], HELLP in another [6], and acute fatty liver of pregnancy in our case. The prognosis was generally poor: six of the women died shortly, up to 6 months, after diagnosis. Pregnancy may adversely affect the prognosis of hepatocellular carcinoma, as gestational immune suppression may be an enabling factor in tumor progression [23]. This might be also true for CCA but cannot be proven due to the paucity of reported cases.

In conclusion, CCA presenting during pregnancy is extremely rare; however, the signs and symptoms can be easily confused with other more common disorders that occur in pregnant women. In addition, pregnancy might limit the diagnostic modalities, which can lead to delayed diagnosis and potentially worse outcomes.

Disclosure

This manuscript is a detailed description of a previous abstract which was presented at the annual meeting of the American College of Gastroenterology (ACG) 2016 in Las Vegas and it was published as an abstract in a special supplement of the American Journal of Gastroenterology.

Authors' Contributions

Dr. Ayman Qasrawi wrote and edited the manuscript. Dr. Omar Abughanimeh, Dr. Mouhanna Abu Ghanimeh, and Dr. Simran Arora-Elder wrote the case presentation, reviewed the literature, and created the images. Dr. Osama Yousef and Dr. Tarek Tamimi revised and edited the final manuscript.

References

[1] J.-N. Vauthey and L. H. Blumgart, "Recent advances in the management of cholangiocarcinomas," *Seminars in Liver Disease*, vol. 14, no. 2, pp. 109–114, 1994.

[2] B. R. A. Blechacz and G. J. Gores, "Cholangiocarcinoma," *Clinics in Liver Disease*, vol. 12, no. 1, pp. 131–150, 2008.

[3] J. M. Banales, V. Cardinale, G. Carpino et al., "Expert consensus document: Cholangiocarcinoma: current knowledge and future perspectives consensus statement from the European Network for the Study of Cholangiocarcinoma (ENS-CCA)," *Nature Reviews Gastroenterology & Hepatology*, vol. 13, no. 5, pp. 261–280, 2016.

[4] C. D. Anderson, C. W. Pinson, J. Berlin, and R. S. Chari, "Diagnosis and treatment of cholangiocarcinoma," *The Oncologist*, vol. 9, no. 1, pp. 43–57, 2004.

[5] S. Sadoon and S. Hodgett, "Unusual cause of itching in a pregnancy (cholangiocarcinoma)," *Journal of Obstetrics & Gynaecology*, vol. 28, no. 2, pp. 230-231, 2008.

[6] K. D. Balderston, K. Tewari, F. Azizi, and J. K. Yu, "Intrahepatic cholangiocarcinoma masquerading as the HELLP syndrome (hemolysis, elevated liver enzymes, and low platelet count) in pregnancy: Case report," *American Journal of Obstetrics & Gynecology*, vol. 179, no. 3 I, pp. 823-824, 1998.

[7] M. L. DeOliveira, S. C. Cunningham, J. L. Cameron et al., "Cholangiocarcinoma: thirty-one-year experience with 564 patients at a single institution," *Annals of Surgery*, vol. 245, no. 5, pp. 755–762, 2007.

[8] S. R. Alberts and A. Grothey, "Gastrointestinal Tract Cancers," in *MC. Manual of Clinical Oncology*, D. A. Casciato and Territo, Eds., p. 279, Lippincott Williams & Wilkins, 7th edition, 2012.

[9] K. M. Brown, A. D. Parmar, and D. A. Geller, "Intrahepatic cholangiocarcinoma," *Surgical Oncology Clinics of North America*, vol. 23, no. 2, pp. 231–246, 2014.

[10] M.-A. Castro, M. J. Fassett, T. B. Reynolds, K. J. Shaw, and T. M. Goodwin, "Reversible peripartum liver failure: A new perspective on the diagnosis, treatment, and cause of acute fatty liver of pregnancy, based on 28 consecutive cases," *American Journal of Obstetrics & Gynecology*, vol. 181, no. 2, pp. 389–395, 1999.

[11] J. T. Maier, E. Schalinski, C. Häberlein, U. Gottschalk, and L. Hellmeyer, "Acute Fatty Liver of Pregnancy and its Differentiation from Other Liver Diseases in Pregnancy," *Geburtshilfe und Frauenheilkunde*, vol. 75, no. 8, pp. 844–847, 2015.

[12] S. J. Bacak and L. L. Thornburg, "Liver Failure in Pregnancy," *Critical Care Clinics*, vol. 32, no. 1, pp. 61–72, 2016.

[13] H.-F. Xiong, J.-Y. Liu, L.-M. Guo, and X.-W. Li, "Acute fatty liver of pregnancy: Over six months follow-up study of twenty-five patients," *World Journal of Gastroenterology*, vol. 21, no. 6, pp. 1927–1931, 2015.

[14] Q. Wei, L. Zhang, and X. Liu, "Clinical diagnosis and treatment of acute fatty liver of pregnancy: A literature review and 11 new cases," *Journal of Obstetrics and Gynaecology Research*, vol. 36, no. 4, pp. 751–756, 2010.

[15] F. C. Cobey and R. R. Salem, "A review of liver masses in pregnancy and a proposed algorithm for their diagnosis and management," *The American Journal of Surgery*, vol. 187, no. 2, pp. 181–191, 2004.

[16] A. M. Athanassiou and S. D. Craigo, "Liver masses in pregnancy," *Seminars in Perinatology*, vol. 22, no. 2, pp. 166–177, 1998.

[17] D. T. Purtilo, J. V. Clark, and R. Williams, "Primary hepatic malignancy in pregnant women," *American Journal of Obstetrics & Gynecology*, vol. 121, no. 1, pp. 41–44, 1975.

[18] PM. Zelissen, J. van Hattum, and J. Zelissen PMvan Hattum, "A young woman with a liver tumor and hypercalcemia. Ned Tijdschr Geneeskd," in *J. Zelissen PMvan HattumA young woman with a liver tumor and hypercalcemia. Ned Tijdschr Geneeskd*, pp. 130–1705, 130, 1705-1707, 1986.

[19] S. K. Nakamoto and E. VanSonnenberg, "Cholangiocarcinoma in pregnancy: The contributions of ultrasound-guided interventional techniques," *Journal of Ultrasound in Medicine*, vol. 4, no. 10, pp. 557–559, 1985.

[20] J. P. Marasinghe, S. A. Karunananda, and P. Angulo, "Cholangiocarcinoma in pregnancy: A case report," *Journal of Obstetrics and Gynaecology Research*, vol. 34, no. 1, pp. 635–637, 2008.

[21] M. Wiesweg, S. Aydin, A. Koeninger et al., "Administration of Gemcitabine for Metastatic Adenocarcinoma during Pregnancy: A Case Report and Review of the Literature," *American Journal of Perinatology Reports*, vol. 4, no. 01, pp. 017–022, 2014.

[22] S. Gerli, A. Favilli, C. Giordano, A. Donini, and G. C. Di Renzo, "Mixed hepatocellular carcinoma and cholangiocarcinoma during pregnancy: A case report," *European Journal of Obstetrics & Gynecology and Reproductive Biology*, vol. 187, pp. 76-77, 2015.

[23] W. Y. Lau, W. T. Leung, S. Ho et al., "Hepatocellular carcinoma during pregnancy and its comparison with other pregnancy-associated malignancies," *Cancer*, vol. 75, no. 11, pp. 2669–2676, 1995.

Anastomotic Biliary Stricture Development after Liver Transplantation in the Setting of Retained Prophylactic Intraductal Pediatric Feeding Tube: Case and Review

Patrick T. Koo,[1] **Valentina Medici ⓘ,**[1] **and James H. Tabibian ⓘ**[1,2]

[1]*Division of Gastroenterology and Hepatology, Department of Internal Medicine, University of California Davis Medical Center, Sacramento, California, USA*
[2]*Division of Gastroenterology, Department of Medicine, Olive View-UCLA Medical Center, Sylmar, California, USA*

Correspondence should be addressed to Valentina Medici; vmedici@ucdavis.edu

Academic Editor: Melanie Deutsch

The biliary anastomosis remains a common site of postoperative complications in liver transplantation (LT). Biliary complications have indeed been termed the "Achilles' heel" of LT, and while their prevention, diagnosis, and treatment have continued to evolve over the last two decades, various challenges and uncertainties persist. Here we present the case of a 33-year-old man who, 10 years after undergoing LT for idiopathic recurrent intrahepatic cholestasis, was noted to have developed pruritus and abnormalities in serum liver biochemistries during routine post-liver transplant follow-up. Abdominal ultrasound revealed a linear, 1.5 mm hyperechoic filling defect in the common bile duct; magnetic resonance cholangiopancreatography demonstrated a curvilinear filling defect at the level of the choledochocholedochostomy, corresponding to the ultrasound finding, as well as an anastomotic biliary stricture (ABS). On endoscopic retrograde cholangiography (ERC), a black tubular stricture with overlying sludge was encountered and extracted from the common bile duct, consistent with a retained 5 Fr pediatric feeding tube originally placed at the time of LT. The patient experienced symptomatic and biochemical relief and successfully underwent serial ERCs with balloon dilatation and maximal biliary stenting for ABS management. With this case, we emphasize the importance of ensuring spontaneous passage or removal of intraductal prostheses placed prophylactically at the time of LT in order to minimize the risk of chronic biliary inflammation and associated sequelae, including cholangitis and ABS formation. We also provide herein a brief review of the use of prophylactic internal transanastomotic prostheses, including biliary tubes and stents, during LT.

1. Introduction

The biliary anastomosis, typically constructed via choledochocholedochostomy, remains the most common anatomical site for postoperative complications in LT. Indeed, biliary complications have been regarded as the "Achilles' heel" of LT and are a source of significant morbidity. We present a case of late anastomotic biliary stricture (ABS) development presenting 10 years after LT for idiopathic recurrent intrahepatic cholestasis in the setting of an intraductally retained 5 Fr pediatric feeding tube placed prophylactically at the time of LT and provide a synopsis of the rationale for, use, and outcomes of prophylactic transanastomotic prostheses, including biliary tubes and stents, during LT.

2. Case Report

The patient is a 33-year-old man with a history of progressive idiopathic recurrent intrahepatic cholestasis diagnosed initially at the age of 15. He was managed with ursodeoxycholic acid, cholestyramine, rifampin and naloxone but eventually failed medical therapy as evidence by the development of cirrhosis complicated by ascites, esophageal variceal hemorrhage, pruritus, and progressively rising Model for End-Stage Liver Disease score.

At the age of 22, the patient underwent deceased-donor LT. At the time of LT, the patient's native bile duct was noted to be 10 mm in diameter, while the donor bile duct was 2.5 mm in diameter. In order to make the two orifices more congruent,

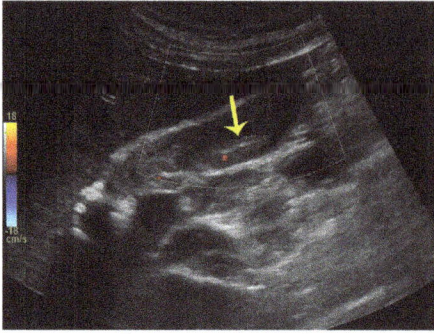

FIGURE 1: Abdominal ultrasound with filling defect in bile duct.

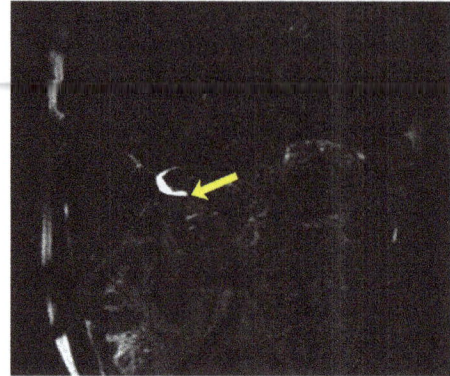

FIGURE 2: MRI/MRCP showing anastomotic biliary stricture, common hepatic ductal dilatation, and subtle curvilinear filling defect within the common hepatic duct.

a ductoplasty was performed with part of the recipient bile duct being oversewn and an end-to-end choledochocholedochostomy being created with running circumferential 5-0 absorbable sutures. The total cold ischemia time was 8 hours, 32 minutes, and the total warm ischemia time was 41 minutes. There were no intraoperative complications, and the patient recovered well following surgery. He was managed on tacrolimus and did well for a decade. Approximately halfway through this period, for geographical and insurance reasons, the patient transferred LT care to our institution. At his 10 year post-LT appointment, the patient endorsed new-onset generalized pruritus and was noted to have developed multiple albeit relatively minor abnormalities in his serum liver test profile, with an alkaline phosphatase of 121 (normal: 35-115 U/L), aspartate aminotransferase of 53 U/L, alanine aminotransferase of 68 U/L, and total bilirubin of 1.2 mg/dL.

Abdominal ultrasound showed no evidence of intrahepatic or extrahepatic biliary ductal dilatation but did note a linear filling defect within the common bile duct (CBD) as seen in Figure 1. MRI/MRCP was thus performed, which was significant for an abrupt change in caliber at the biliary anastomosis consistent with stricture (ABS), dilatation of the common hepatic duct (CHD) to 7 mm, and a curvilinear filling defect at the level of the anastomosis (Figure 2). Given these findings, the patient's original LT operative report was retrieved from the performing institution; this revealed that in addition to the ductoplasty, a 3.5 cm segment of 5 Fr pediatric feeding tube had been placed through the biliary anastomosis to serve as a temporary internal stent.

Given the patient's new-onset pruritus, worsening serum liver tests, and abnormal imaging findings, endoscopic retrograde cholangiography (ERC) was performed. This revealed a small, tortuous native (i.e., recipient) CBD and a short ABS with proximal CHD dilatation. The ABS was first balloon dilated to 6 mm followed by sweeping of the extrahepatic duct was performed with a 9 mm extraction balloon; this first yielded biliary sludge, but with additional sweeps, a 3.5 cm long, black tubular structure with overlying sludge/biofilm was extracted (Figures 3(a) and 3(b)). This was grasped and brought out *per os* using forceps and appeared to be consistent with an oxidized pediatric feeding tube (Figure 4). An 8 mm × 4 cm CRE balloon was then used to further dilate the ABS, and two 10 Fr x 7 cm Cotton-Leung plastic biliary stents were deployed across it. In doing so, the patient's serum laboratory

tests returned to baseline, and his pruritus resolved over the ensuing weeks. The patient now nears completion of serial ERCs at three month intervals as part of a 1-year long maximal stenting protocol in order to achieve durable ABS resolution [1].

3. Discussion

The biliary anastomosis represents the most common anatomical site for postoperative complications in LT and is a cause of significant morbidity. Accordingly, biliary complications have been termed the "Achilles' heel" of LT [2–4]. Biliary strictures are among the most frequent major complications involving the anastomosis and can be classified as either anastomotic (ABS) or nonanastomotic based on location, appearance, and suspected etiology [5]. With respect to the former, a recent meta-analysis of over 14,000 LTs found the incidence of ABS to be approximately 13% [2]. ABSs can develop at any time following LT, but the majority present within one year of LT (mean 5-8 months) [2]. ABSs in the early postoperative period are usually related to surgical technique and/or mismatch of recipient and donor bile ducts, while late-onset ABSs are believed to be secondary to fibrosis from preceding local ischemia or chronic inflammation-related injury [5, 6]. Historically, several surgical techniques have existed for constructing the biliary anastomosis, with additional measures being employed to deal with significant size mismatch between the donor and recipient bile ducts, as in the case of our patient [7, 8]. Early biliary reconstructions included loop choledochojejunostomy, Roux-en-Y choledochojejunostomy (RYCJ), and using the gallbladder as a conduit [7, 8]. In the 1980s, duct-to-duct anastomosis became the most popular technique. Compared to RYCJ and similar surgical techniques, the duct-to-duct anastomosis has the theoretical advantage of no bowel manipulation, less biliary reflux by virtue of an intact sphincter, potentially decreased cholangiocarcinoma risk, and easier endoscopic access (when needed for biliary intervention) [7, 8]. For a number of years, the duct-to-duct anastomosis was constructed over a percutaneous T-tube (irrespective of bile duct size discrepancy) in an effort to bridge the biliary anastomosis

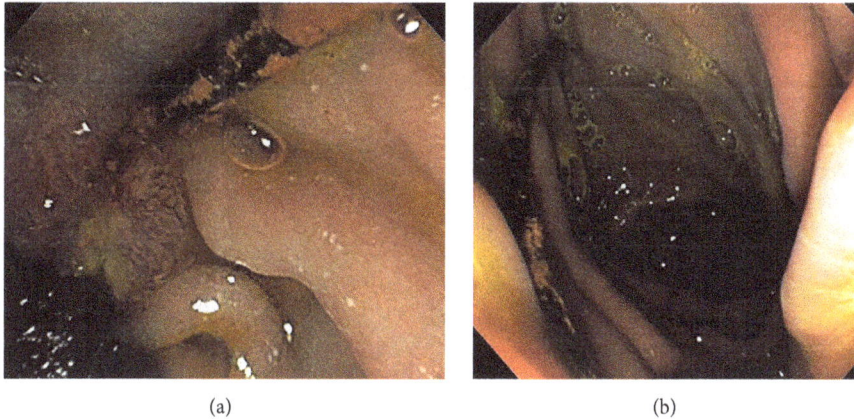

(a)　　　　(b)

FIGURE 3: (a) ERC showing black pediatric feeding tube with overlying biofilm protruding from the papilla. (b) ERC with successful extraction of black pediatric feeding tube from the papilla.

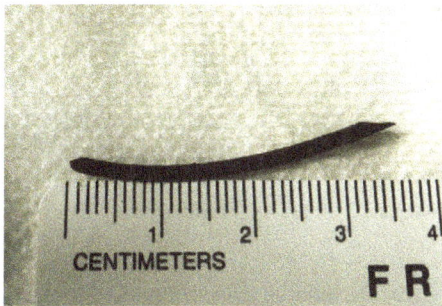

FIGURE 4: Extracted pediatric feeding tube.

and thereby decrease the risk of ABS formation [9]. However, T-tubes have been associated, at least in some studies, with higher rates of biliary complications, especially leakage from the T- tube exit site, and over the last couple decades are thus no longer routinely used in LT at most centers [2, 10]. In cases where there is significant size mismatch between the donor and recipient bile ducts, additional measures which have been employed include: partially closing a patulous recipient CHD or CBD, spatulating the donor duct, everting the recipient CBD, creating a common orifice between the cystic and common ducts, side-to-side ductal anastomosis, or choledochoduodenostomy. These techniques may be performed with or without the use of temporary internal stents.

The use of an internal stent across the biliary anastomosis theoretically eliminates the possible complications associated with T-tubes while preserving the integrity of the biliary anastomosis. Johnson et al. were the first to review the use of prophylactic internal transanastomotic biliary stenting at the time of LT [11]. They placed 6Fr double-J ureteral stents in a transanastomotic, transpapillary fashion and reported a significantly lower biliary complication rate in patients with internal stenting compared to those with T-tubes (18% versus 38%) [11]; there was also a trend towards a lower incidence of ABS development in the internal stent group (7.6% versus 11%) [11].

Multiple studies have since followed with somewhat conflicting findings and thus a lack of convincingly beneficial results. For example, Trachart et al. studied the use of 8 Fr x 2 cm internal stents fabricated from a T-tube and reported a lower rate of ABS compared to the nonstent group (5% versus 15.1%) [12]. Similarly, Jung et al., using 6-8 Fr silastic stents, reported a statistically significant lower ABS rate in the stent group compared to the nonstent group (3.23% versus 11.76%) [13]. In contrast, Mathur et al. found that the use of transanastomotic, transpapillary 5-8Fr silastic pediatric feeding tubes were associated with higher rates of ABS, although the difference was not statistically significant [14]. Mathur et al. concluded that prophylactic internal stenting did not reduce risk of biliary complications and was instead associated with a higher adjusted risk for requiring endoscopic interventions (e.g., ERC) within the first 90 days post-LT [14].

In an effort to minimize the need for endoscopic procedures for stent removal, studies have since been performed using synthetic bioabsorbable stents [15]. Janousek et al. investigated the use of transanastomotic bioabsorbable biliary stents, made from polydioxanone monofilaments. None of the patients in the stent group developed biliary strictures; however, the sample size was small, and long term follow-up was not reported [15]. Most recently, the first randomized control trial assessing the efficacy of prophylactic transanastomotic stenting for duct-to-duct biliary reconstruction in LT was performed [16]. Santosh Kumar et al. randomized LT recipients to either receive a transanastomotic, transpapillary 3-5 Fr ureteric stent or no stent; the authors reported a trend towards higher stricture formation in the stent group compared to the nonstent group (22.6% versus 6.1%), although this was not statistically significant [15]. Given a significantly higher risk of bile leak in the stent group, the trial was terminated early [16].

While the aforementioned studies have varied in the type and size of stents used, the fashion in which they were placed, and the duration for which they were left *in situ*, it is important to note that they all ensured stent passage or removal (or bioabsorption). Johnson et al. reported that 43% of internal stents passed spontaneously, while the remaining

57% required endoscopic removal [11]. Similarly, Tranchart et al. reported that 95% of their patients with internal stents required endoscopic removal, as only 5% of stents were noted to have passed spontaneously [12]. Therefore, it is imperative that sight not be lost of these stents, and that appropriate follow-up (and if needed, removal) be performed, as with other pancreatobiliary stents.

In our patient, while mismatch in donor and recipient bile duct size was a potential risk factor for the development of ABS, it is likely that the prolonged presence of a foreign object in the form of a retained transanastomotic pediatric feeding tube served as a nidus of chronic, low-grade inflammation and ultimately contributed to the development of the patient's late-onset ABS. Therefore, stent removal was recommended, and in doing so, the patient benefitted from symptomatic, biochemical, and cholangiographic improvement.

While we await a more definitive verdict on the efficacy of temporary prophylactic transanastomotic biliary stents in LT, it is clear that if placed, non-bioabsorbable intraductal stents should be removed (if spontaneous passage is not observed) to minimize the risk of developing complications down the road, including cholangitis and/or ABS formation. Our case emphasizes the importance of the routine use of imaging as well as other safeguards following intraductal prosthesis placement to either document spontaneous stent passage or identify patients who may require further evaluation and potentially endoscopic stent removal.

Abbreviations

ABS: Anastomotic biliary stricture
ERC: Endoscopic retrograde cholangiography
LT: Liver transplantation.

References

[1] J. H. Tabibian, E. H. Asham, S. Han et al., "Endoscopic treatment of postorthotopic liver transplantation anastomotic biliary strictures with maximal stent therapy (with video)," *Gastrointestinal Endoscopy*, vol. 71, no. 3, pp. 505–512, 2010.

[2] N. Akamatsu, Y. Sugawara, and D. Hashimoto, "Biliary reconstruction, its complications and management of biliary complications after adult liver transplantation: A systematic review of the incidence, risk factors and outcome," *Transplant International*, vol. 24, no. 4, pp. 379–392, 2011.

[3] R. Y. Calne, "A new technique for biliary drainage in orthotopic liver transplantation utilizing the gall bladder as a pedicle graft conduit between the donor and recipient common bile ducts," *Annals of Surgery*, vol. 184, no. 5, pp. 605–609, 1976.

[4] R. Y. Calne, P. McMaster, B. Portmann, W. J. Wall, and R. Williams, "Observations on preservation, bile drainage and rejection in 64 human orthotopic liver allografts," *Annals of Surgery*, vol. 186, no. 3, pp. 282–290, 1977.

[5] A. Pascher and P. Neuhaus, "Biliary complications after deceased-donor orthotopic liver transplantation," *Journal of Hepato-Biliary-Pancreatic Sciences*, vol. 13, no. 6, pp. 487–496, 2006.

[6] S. K. Satapathy, I. Sheikh, B. Ali et al., "Long-term outcomes of early compared to late onset choledochocholedochal anastomotic strictures after orthotopic liver transplantation," *Clinical Transplantation*, vol. 31, no. 7, 2017.

[7] I. C. Carmody, J. Romano, H. Bohorquez et al., "Novel biliary reconstruction techniques during liver transplantation," *The Ochsner Journal*, vol. 17, no. 1, pp. 42–45, 2017.

[8] P. Leal-Leyte, G. J. McKenna, R. M. Ruiz et al., "Eversion bile duct anastomosis: a safe alternative for bile duct size discrepancy in deceased donor liver transplantation," *Liver Transplantation*, vol. 24, no. 8, pp. 1011–1018, 2018.

[9] A. Shaked, "Use of T tube in liver transplantation," *Liver Transplant Surgery*, vol. 3, pp. S22–S23, 1997.

[10] H. B. Randall, M. E. Wachs, K. A. Somberg et al., "The use of the T tube after orthotopic liver transplantation," *Transplantation*, vol. 61, no. 2, pp. 258–261, 1996.

[11] M. W. Johnson, P. Thompson, A. Meehan et al., "Internal biliary stenting in orthotopic liver transplantation," *Liver Transplantation*, vol. 6, no. 3, pp. 356–361, 2000.

[12] H. Tranchart, S. Zalinski, A. Sepulveda et al., "Removable intraductal stenting in duct-to-duct biliary reconstruction in liver transplantation," *Transplant International*, vol. 25, no. 1, pp. 19–24, 2012.

[13] S. W. Jung, D. S. Kim, Y. D. Yu, and S. O. Suh, "Clinical outcome of internal stent for biliary anastomosis in liver transplantation," *Transplantation Proceedings*, vol. 46, no. 3, pp. 856–860, 2014.

[14] A. K. Mathur, S. N. Nadig, S. Kingman et al., "Internal biliary stenting during orthotopic liver transplantation: Anastomotic complications, post-transplant biliary interventions, and survival," *Clinical Transplantation*, vol. 29, no. 4, pp. 327–335, 2015.

[15] L. Janousek, S. Maly, M. Oliverius, M. Kocik, M. Kucera, and J. Fronek, "Bile duct anastomosis supplied with biodegradable stent in liver transplantation: the initial experience," *Transplantation Proceedings*, vol. 48, no. 10, pp. 3312–3316, 2016.

[16] K. Y. S. Kumar, J. S. Mathew, D. Balakrishnan et al., "Intraductal transanastomotic stenting in duct-to-duct biliary reconstruction after living-donor liver transplantation: a randomized trial," *Journal of the American College of Surgeons*, vol. 225, no. 6, pp. 747–754, 2017.

Permissions

List of Contributors

Carole Massabeau, Virginie Marchand, Sofia Zefkili and Philippe Giraud
Department of Radiation Oncology and Medical Physics, Institut Curie, 75005 Paris, France

Carole Massabeau
Department of Radiation Oncology, Institut Claudius Regaud, 31052 Toulouse, France

Vincent Servois
Department of Radiology, Institut Curie, 75005 Paris, France

Philippe Giraud
Department of Radiation Oncology, European Georges Pompidou Hospital, 75015 Paris, Paris Descartes University, 75005 Paris, France

M. Premkumar, Devraja Rangegowda, Chitranshu Vashishtha, Vikram Bhatia and Badal Kumar
Department of Hepatology, Institute of Liver and Biliary Sciences (ILBS), D-1 Vasant Kunj, New Delhi 110070, India

Jelen Singh Khumuckham
Department of Cardiology, Institute of Liver and Biliary Sciences (ILBS), D-1 Vasant Kunj, New Delhi 110070, India

Erin Gordon and Sameer Kamath
Department of Pediatrics, Division of Critical Care, University of Iowa Children's Hospital, Iowa City, IA 52242, USA

Kamran Qureshi
Section of Gastroenterology and Hepatology, Division of Hepatology, Department ofMedicine, Temple University School ofMedicine, Temple University Health System, 3440 N Broad Street, Kresge BuildingWest No. 209, Philadelphia, PA 19140, USA

Usman Sarwar
Temple University Hospital, 3401 North Broad Street, Philadelphia, PA 19140, USA

Hicham Khallafi
Division of Gastroenterology and Hepatology, Department of Medicine, CaseWestern Reserve University School of Medicine, MetroHealth System, Medical Center, 2500 MetroHealth Drive, Cleveland, OH 44109, USA

Jin Yeon Hwang, Sung Wook Lee, Yang Hyun Baek, Jong Han Kim, Ha Yeon Kim, Suck Hyang Bae and Sang Young Han
Department of Internal Medicine, Dong-A University College of Medicine, Busan 602-715, Republic of Korea

Jin Han Cho and Hee Jin Kwon
Department of Radiology, Dong-A University College of Medicine, Busan, Republic of Korea

Jin Sook Jeong
Department of Pathology, Dong-A University College of Medicine, Busan, Republic of Korea

Young Hoon Roh
Department of Surgery, Dong-A University College of Medicine, Busan, Republic of Korea

Jiten P. Kothadia
Nazih Zuhdi Transplant Institute, INTEGRIS Baptist Medical Center, 3300 NW Expressway, Oklahoma City, OK 73112, USA

Monica Kaminski
Department of Internal Medicine, Coney Island Hospital, 2601 Coney Island Avenue, Brooklyn, NY 11235, USA

Hrishikesh Samant
Division of Gastroenterology and Hepatology, Louisiana State University Health Sciences Center, Shreveport, LA 71103, USA

Marco Olivera-Martinez
Department of Gastroenterology and Hepatology, University of Nebraska Medical Center, 982000 Nebraska Medical Center,Omaha, NE 68198, USA

Lay Lay Win, Hemant Shah, Jordan J. Feld and David K. Wong
Hepatology, TorontoWestern Hospital, University of Toronto, 399 Bathurst Street, 6b-176, Toronto, ON, Canada M5T 2S8

Jeff Powis
Infectious Diseases, Toronto East General Hospital, 825 Coxwell Avenue, East York, ON, Canada M4C 3E7

Stefanie Adolf, Gunda Millonig, Helmut Karl Seitz and Sebastian Mueller
Department of Medicine, Salem Medical Center and Alcohol Research Center, University of Heidelberg, Zeppelinstraße 11-33, 69121 Heidelberg, Germany

Andreas Reiter
Department of Medicine III, Mannheim Hospital, University of Heidelberg, Wiesbadener Straße 7-11, 68305 Mannheim, Germany

Peter Schirmacher and Thomas Longerich
Institute of Pathology, University of Heidelberg, Im Neuenheimer Feld 220/221, 69120 Heidelberg, Germany

Kan K. Zhang, Majid Mayody, Efsevia Vakiani, George I. Getrajdman, Lynn A. Brody and Stephen B. Solomon
Division of Interventional Radiology, Department of Radiology, Memorial Sloan-Kettering Cancer Center (MSKCC), 1275 York Avenue, M276C, New York, NY 10065, USA

Rajesh P. Shah
Stanford Hospital and Clinics, Stanford, CA 94305, USA

Elizabeth Caitlin Brewer and Leigh Hunter
Methodist Hospitals of Dallas, 1441 N Beckley Ave Dallas, TX 75203, USA

Madhumita Prem kumar, Avishek Bagchi, Neha Kapoor, Ankit Gupta, Gaurav Maurya, Shubham Vatsya, Siddharth Kapahtia and Premashish Kar
Department of Medicine, B. L. Taneja Block, Maulana Azad Medical College and Associated Hospitals, Bahadur Shah Zafar Marg, New Delhi 110002, India

Innocent Lule Segamwenge and Miriam Kaunanele Bernard
Department of Internal Medicine, Intermediate Hospital Oshakati, Oshakati, Namibia

Fumio Chikamori
Department of Surgery, Kuniyoshi Hospital, 1-3-4 Kamimachi, Kochi City, Kochi 780-0901, Japan

Nobutoshi Kuniyoshi
Department of Internal Medicine, Kuniyoshi Hospital, 1-3-4 Kamimachi, Kochi City, Kochi 780-0901, Japan

Trinidad Caballero, Mercedes Caba-Molina and Mercedes Gómez-Morales
Pathology Department, San Cecilio University Hospital and School of Medicine, University of Granada, Avenida de Madrid 11, 18012 Granada, Spain

Trinidad Caballero and Javier Salmerón
Networked Biomedical Research Center for Hepatic and Digestive Diseases (CIBERehd), Carlos III Institute of Health, Spain

Anneleen Van Hootegem, Chris Verslype and Werner Van Steenbergen
Liver Unit, Department of Pathophysiology, University Hospital Gasthuisberg, Catholic University of Leuven, 3000 Leuven, Belgium

Amandeep Singh, Nayere Zaeri and Immanuel K. Ho
Crozer Chester Medical Center, One Medical Center Boulevard, Upland, PA 19018, USA

Amandeep Singh
Cleveland Clinic Foundation, 9500 Euclid Avenue, Cleveland, OH 44195, USA

Immanuel K. Ho
Division of Gastroenterology, Pennsylvania Hospital, 230W. Washington Square, 4th Floor, Philadelphia, PA 19106, USA

Masanori Furukawa, Kosuke Kaji, Hiroyuki Masuda, Kuniaki Ozaki, Shohei Asada, Aritoshi Koizumi, Takuya Kubo, Norihisa Nishimura, Yasuhiko Sawada, Kosuke Takeda, Tsuyoshi Mashitani, Akira Mitoro and Hitoshi Yoshiji
Third Department of Internal Medicine, Nara Medical University, Kashihara, Nara, Japan

Masayuki Kubo and Itsuto Amano
Second Department of Internal Medicine, Nara Medical University, Kashihara, Nara, Japan

Tomoyuki Ootani and Chiho Ohbayashi
Department of Diagnostic Pathology, Nara Medical University, Kashihara, Nara, Japan

Koji Murata and Tatsuichi Ann
Division of Gastroenterology, Bell Land GeneralHospital, Sakai, Osaka, Japan

Renato Pascale, Viola Guardigni, Lorenzo Badia, Francesca Volpato, Pierluigi Viale and Gabriella Verucchi
Infectious Diseases Unit, Department of Medical and Surgical Science, S. Orsola-Malpighi Hospital, University of Bologna, Bologna, Italy

Viola Guardigni, Lorenzo Badia and Gabriella Verucchi
Research Centre for the Study of Hepatitis, University of Bologna, Bologna, Italy

Majed M. Almaghrabi
Division of Internal Medicine, University of Toronto, Toronto, ON, Canada

Kyle J. Fortinsky and David Wong
Division of Hepatology, University of Toronto, Toronto, ON, Canada

Ashwinee Natu
Department of InternalMedicine, University Hospitals ClevelandMedical Center, 11100 Euclid Ave., Cleveland, OH 44106, USA

Guiseppe Iuppa
Department of Transplant Surgery, Cleveland Clinic, 9500 Euclid Ave., Cleveland, OH 44195, USA

Clifford D. Packer
Department of Internal Medicine, Louis Stokes VA Medical Center, 10701 East Blvd., Cleveland, OH 44106, USA

Juferdy Kurniawan, Andri Sanityoso Sulaiman and Steven Zulkifly
Division of Hepatobiliary, Department of Internal Medicine, Faculty of Medicine, Universitas Indonesia, Cipto Mangunkusumo National General Hospital, Jakarta, Indonesia

Sahat Basana Romanti Ezer Matondang
Department of Radiology, Faculty of Medicine, Universitas Indonesia, Cipto Mangunkusumo National General Hospital, Jakarta, Indonesia

Toar Jean Maurice Lalisang
Department of Surgery, Faculty of Medicine, Universitas Indonesia, Cipto Mangunkusumo National General Hospital, Jakarta, Indonesia

Ening Krisnuhoni
Department of Pathology Anatomy, Faculty of Medicine, Universitas Indonesia, Cipto Mangunkusumo National General Hospital, Jakarta, Indonesia

G. A. Watson, A. Abu-Shanab, R. L. O'Donohoe and M. Iqbal
St. Vincent'sUniversityHospital, Dublin 4, Ireland

E. Veitsman and Z. Ben Ari
Liver Disease Center, Sheba Medical Center, Ramat Gan, Israel

E. Pras
Institute of Genetics, Sheba Medical Center, Ramat Gan, Israel

E. Pras and Z. Ben Ari
Sackler School of Medicine, Tel Aviv University, Tel Aviv, Israel

O. Pappo
Department of Pathology, Sheba Medical Center, Ramat Gan, Israel

A. Arish and R. Eshkenazi
Hepato-Biliary-Pancreatic Surgery Department, Sheba Medical Center, Ramat Gan, Israel

C. Feray
Department of Hepatology, Henri Mondor Hospital, Créteil, France

C. Feray, J. Calderaro and D. Azoulay
Unite Inserm 955, France

J. Calderaro
Department of Pathology, Henri Mondor Hospital, Créteil, France

D. Azoulay
Department Hepato-Pancreato-Biliary Surgery and Liver Transplantation, Henri Mondor Hospital, Créteil, France

Gregory W. Charville and Richard K. Sibley
Department of Pathology, Stanford University School of Medicine, Stanford, CA 94305, USA

Sukhmani K. Padda
Department of Medicine, Division of Oncology, Stanford University School of Medicine, Stanford, CA 94305, USA

Ajithkumar Puthillath
Stockton Hematology Oncology Medical Group, Stockton, CA 95204, USA

Paul Y. Kwo
Department of Medicine, Division of Gastroenterology and Hepatology, Stanford University School of Medicine, Stanford, CA 94305, USA

Kazuhiro Nishida and Tomohiro Funabiki
Department of Emergent and Critical Care Medicine, Saiseikai Yokohamashi Tobu Hospital, 3-6-1, Shimosueyoshi, Tsurumi, Yokohama-city, Kanagawa 230-8765, Japan

Alan Kawarai Lefor
Department of Surgery, Jichi Medical University, 3311-1 Yakushiji, Shimotsuke, Tochigi 329-0498, Japan

Gary A. Abrams and Robert Chapman
Gastroenterology & Liver Center, Greenville Health System, University of South Carolina School of Medicine Greenville, Greenville, SC, USA

Samuel R. W. Horton
Department of Pathology, Greenville Health System, University of South Carolina School ofMedicine Greenville, Greenville, SC, USA

Felipe Nasser, Joaquim Maurício Motta Leal Filho, Breno Boueri Affonso, Francisco Leonardo Galastri, Rafael Noronha Cavalcante and Diego Lima Nava Martins
Interventional Radiology Unit, Hospital Israelita Albert Einstein, Av. Albert Einstein 627/701, Morumbi, 05652-900 São Paulo, SP, Brazil

Vanderlei Segatelli,
Pathology Department, Hospital Israelita Albert Einstein, Av. Albert Einstein 627/701, Morumbi, 05652-900 São Paulo, SP, Brazil

Lilian Yuri Itaya Yamaga
Nuclear Medicine Unit, Hospital Israelita Albert Einstein, Av. Albert Einstein 627/701, Morumbi, 05652-900 São Paulo, SP, Brazil

Rene Claudio Gansl
Oncology Department, Hospital Israelita Albert Einstein, Av. Albert Einstein 627/701, Morumbi, 05652-900 São Paulo, SP, Brazil

Bernardino Tranchesi Junior
Cardiology Department, Hospital Israelita Albert Einstein, Av. Albert Einstein 627/701, Morumbi, 05652-900 São Paulo, SP, Brazil

Antônio Luiz de Vasconcellos Macedo
General and Oncological Surgery, Hospital Israelita Albert Einstein, Av. Albert Einstein 627/701, Morumbi, 05652-900 São Paulo, SP, Brazil

Atsushi Ono, C. Nelson Hayes, Sakura Akamatsu, Michio Imamura, Hiroshi Aikata and Kazuaki Chayama
Department of Gastroenterology and Metabolism, Applied Life Sciences, Institute of Biomedical & Health Science, Hiroshima University, Hiroshima, Japan

Atsushi Ono, C. Nelson Hayes, Sakura Akamatsu, Michio Imamura, Hiroshi Aikata and Kazuaki Chayama
Liver Research Project Center, Hiroshima University, Hiroshima, Japan

Kazuaki Chayama
Laboratory for Digestive Diseases, SNP Research Center, The Institute of Physical and Chemical Research (RIKEN), Hiroshima, Japan

Jerome Okudo
School of PublicHealth, University of Texas, 1200 Pressler Street, Houston, TX 77030, USA

Nwabundo Anusim
Department of Medicine, Saint Joseph Regional Medical Center, 5215 Holy Cross Parkway, Mishawaka, IN 46545, USA

Gary Golds
Department of Medicine, University of Saskatchewan, 103 Hospital Drive, Saskatoon, SK, Canada S7N 0W8

Lawrence Worobetz
Division of Gastroenterology, Department of Medicine, University of Saskatchewan, 103 Hospital Drive, Saskatoon, SK, Canada S7N 0W8

Yunseok Namn, Yecheskel Schneider and Arun Jesudian
Department of Gastroenterology and Hepatology, Weill Cornell Medical College, New York Presbyterian Hospital, New York, NY, USA

Isabelle H. Cui
Department of Pathology, Weill Cornell Medical College, New York Presbyterian Hospital, New York, NY, USA

Masahiro Takeuchi and Keiji Hirata
Department of Surgery 1, School of Medicine, University of Occupational and Environmental Health, 1-1 Iseigaoka, Yahatanishi-ku, Kitakyushu-shi, Fukuoka 807-0804, Japan

Yoshitaka Sakamoto
Department of Surgery, Moji Medical Center, 3-1 Higashiminatomachi, Moji-ku, Kitakyushu-shi, Fukuoka 801-8502, Japan

Hirotsugu Noguchi
Department of Pathology, School of Medicine, University of Occupational and Environmental Health, 1-1 Iseigaoka, Yahatanishi-ku, Kitakyushu-shi, Fukuoka 807-0804, Japan

Sohsuke Yamada
Department of Pathology and Laboratory Medicine, Kanazawa MedicalUniversity, 1-1Uchinada, Ishikawa 920-0293, Japan

Walid Abboud and Saif Abdulla
Department of Internal Medicine, Zayed Military Hospital, Abu Dhabi, UAE

Mohammed Al Zaabi
Department of Gastroenterology, Zayed Military Hospital, Abu Dhabi, UAE

Ramzi Moufarrej
Department of Critical Care, Zayed Military Hospital, Abu Dhabi, UAE

Malkhaz Mizandari, Tamta Azrumelashvili and Natela Paksashvili
Department of Interventional Radiology, Tbilisi State Medical University, High Technology University Clinic, 0144 Tbilisi, Georgia

Nino Kikodze, Ia Pantsulaia, Nona Janikashvili and Tinatin Chikovani
Department of Immunology, Tbilisi State Medical University, 0177 Tbilisi, Georgia

Ayman Qasrawi and Omar Abughanimeh
Internal Medicine Department, University of Missouri-Kansas City School of Medicine, Kansas City, MO, USA

Mouhanna Abu Ghanimeh
Internal Medicine Department, Division of Gastroenterology, Henry Ford Hospital, Detroit, MI, USA

Simran Arora-Elder
Division of Hematology/Oncology, University of Maryland Medical Center, Baltimore, MD, USA

Osama Yousef and Tarek Tamimi
Division of Gastroenterology, University of Missouri-Kansas City School of Medicine, Kansas City, MO, USA

Thein Swe and Akari Thein Naing
Department of Internal Medicine, Interfaith Medical Center, Brooklyn, NY, USA

Aama Baqui
Department of Pathology, Interfaith Medical Center, Brooklyn, NY, USA

Ratesh Khillan
Division of Oncology, Interfaith Medical Center, Brooklyn, NY, USA

Karen Jiang
Division of Hospital Medicine, Department of Medicine, Brigham andWomen's Hospital, Boston, MA, USA

Ahmad Najdat Bazarbashi and Natalia Khalaf
Division of Gastroenterology, Hepatology and Endoscopy, Brigham andWomen's Hospital, Boston, MA, USA

Sami Dahdal
Department of Internal Medicine, St. John's Riverside Hospital, Yonkers, NY, USA

Adina Voiculescu
Division of Renal Medicine, Department of Medicine, Brigham andWomen's Hospital, Boston, MA, USA

Yonghua Liu, Jinhong Jiang, Qinli Wu, Qiaolei Zhang, Yehui Xu, Zhigang Qu, Guangli Ma, Xiaoqiu Wang, Xiaoli Wang, Weimei Jin and Bingmu Fang
Department of Hematology, Sixth Affiliated Hospital of Wenzhou Medical University, Lishui City, Zhejiang 323000, China

Hiroyuki Sugo, Yuki Sekine, ShozoMiyano, Ikuo Watanobe, Michio Machida and Kuniaki Kojima
Department of General Surgery, Juntendo University Nerima Hospital, Japan

Hironao Okubo
Department of Gastroenterology, Juntendo University Nerima Hospital, Japan

Ayako Ura, Kanako Ogura and Toshiharu Matsumoto
Department of Diagnostic Pathology, Juntendo University Nerima Hospital, Japan

Fahri Yetişir, Omer Parlak, Basar Basaran and Omer Yazıcıoğlu
Atatürk Research and Training Hospital, General Surgery Department, Ankara, Turkey

Akgün Ebru Şarer
Atatürk Research and Training Hospital, Anesthesiology and Reanimation Department, Ankara, Turkey

Hasan Zafer Acar
Natomed Private Hospital, General Surgery Department, Ankara, Turkey

Hesam Keshmiri, Anuj Behal, Shawn Shroff and Charles Berkelhammer
Department of Medicine, Advocate Christ Medical Center, University of Illinois, Oak Lawn, IL 60453, USA

Patrick T. Koo, Valentina Medici and James H. Tabibian
Division of Gastroenterology and Hepatology, Department of Internal Medicine, University of California Davis Medical Center, Sacramento, California, USA

James H. Tabibian
Division of Gastroenterology, Department of Medicine, Olive View-UCLA Medical Center, Sylmar, California, USA

Index

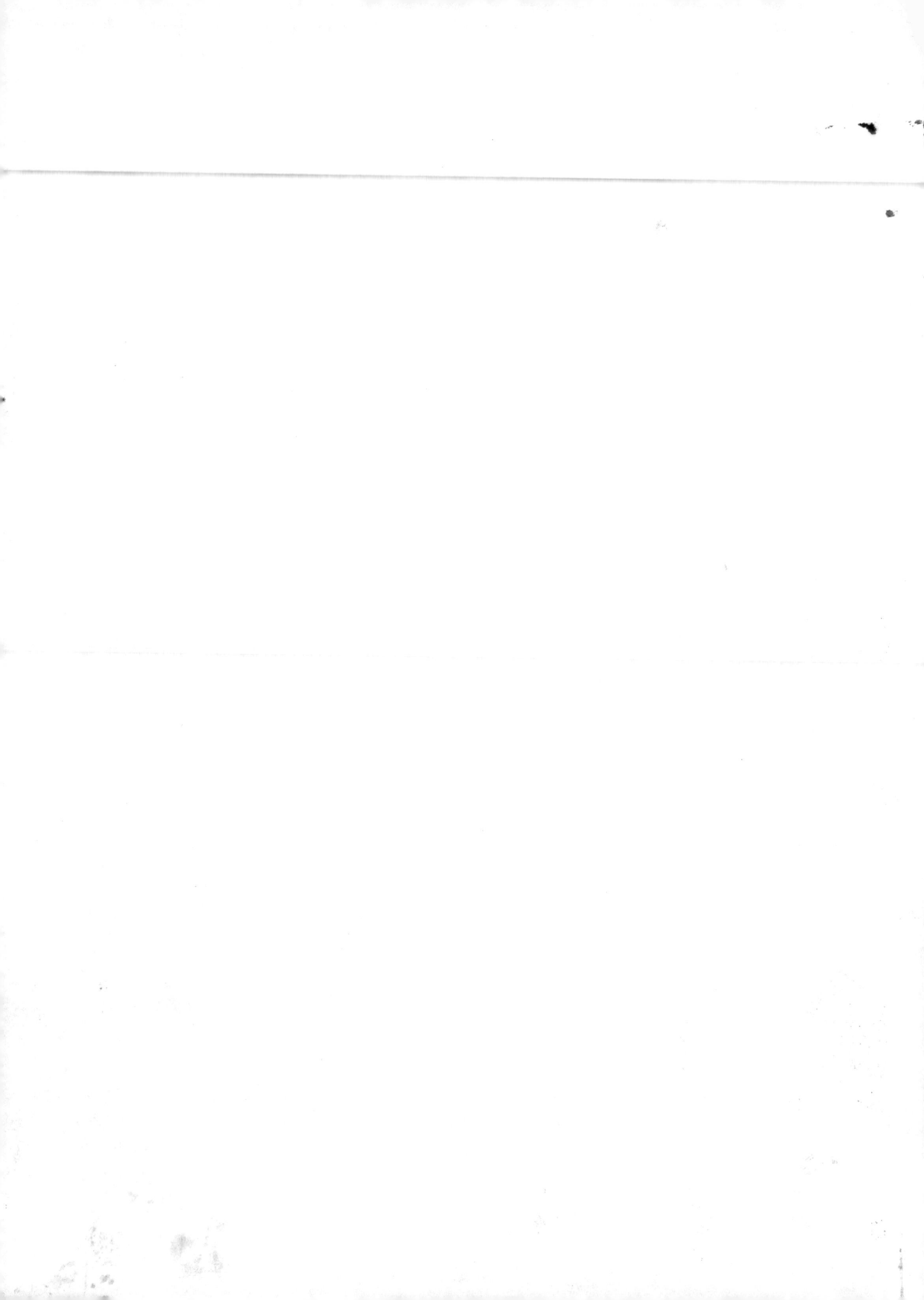